PRINCIPLES OF
EVALUATION
AND RESEARCH
for Health Care Programs

Karen (Kay) M. Perrin, PhD, MPH

Associate Professor, Assistant Dean of Undergraduate Studies

College of Public Health

University of South Florida

Tampa, Florida

JONES & BARTLETT
LEARNING

World Headquarters
Jones & Bartlett Learning
5 Wall Street
Burlington, MA 01803
978-443-5000
info@jblearning.com
www.jblearning.com

Jones & Bartlett Learning books and products are available through most bookstores and online booksellers. To contact Jones & Bartlett Learning directly, call 800-832-0034, fax 978-443-8000, or visit our website, www.jblearning.com.

Substantial discounts on bulk quantities of Jones & Bartlett Learning publications are available to corporations, professional associations, and other qualified organizations. For details and specific discount information, contact the special sales department at Jones & Bartlett Learning via the above contact information or send an email to specialsales@jblearning.com.

Production Credits

Executive Publisher: William Brottmiller
Publisher: Michael Brown
Associate Editor: Chloe Falivene
Editorial Assistant: Nicholas Alakel
Production Manager: Carolyn Rogers Pershouse
Senior Marketing Manager: Sophie Fleck Teague
Manufacturing and Inventory Control
  Supervisor: Amy Bacus

Composition: Cenveo Publisher Services
Photo Research and Permissions Coordinator: Joseph Veiga
Cover Design: Theresa Day
Cover and Title Page Image: © Max Krasnov/ShutterStock, Inc.
Printing and Binding: Edwards Brothers Malloy
Cover Printing: Edwards Brothers Malloy

To order this product, use ISBN: 978-1-284-03896-5

Library of Congress Cataloging-in-Publication Data
Perrin, Kay, author.
  Princples of evaluation and research for health care programs / Kay Perrin.
    p. ; cm.
  Includes bibliographical references and index.
  ISBN-13: 978-1-4496-7436-6 (pbk.)
  ISBN-10: 1-4496-7436-4 (pbk.)
  I. Title.
  [DNLM: 1. Health Services Research—methods. 2. Data Collection—methods. 3. Program Evaluation. 4. Research Design. W 84.3]
  RA440.85
  362.1072—dc23
              2013035793
6048

Printed in the United States of America
18 17 16 15 14   10 9 8 7 6 5 4 3 2 1

To Kevin
My husband

Contents

Preface

This text was written for undergraduate students enrolled in an introductory course related to research or evaluation. The chapters are in a sequential order that forms the foundation for the knowledge needed to understand basic evaluation or research projects. This text is not intended to achieve complete understanding or proficiency in the complex subjects of health science evaluation and research. However, the chapters provide an overview of topics needed to review published literature, collect primary data, analyze data using basic statistics, and present results in written or verbal formats for their intended audiences.

The first three chapters set the stage for evaluation and research. Chapter 1 explains the differences and similarities between evaluation and research, along with how to review literature and develop research questions or goals and objectives that will be addressed in various studies. Chapter 2 introduces ethics, which is a core element in evaluation and research and needs consideration during the development phase. Chapter 3 explores determinants of health, such as health disparities and access to health care. Without regard to social determinants, evaluators and researchers miss key elements in the lives of their target audience that influence health outcomes outside of health care.

The next several chapters define terms and concepts that should be understood prior to planning an evaluation and research study. Chapter 4 introduces various types of theories and models along with examples from current literature on how the theories and models have been used as the framework for project development. The list of theories and models is not intended to be comprehensive, but rather an introduction to examples that are commonly used. Once the research questions or evaluation goals and objectives and an appropriate theory are selected, it is time to explore types of data. Chapter 5 defines the concepts of reliability and validity as well as random and systematic errors. The chapter ends with a detailed description of how to conduct a pilot test and why they are essential. Chapter 6 provides a detailed discussion of qualitative data including types qualitative designs, potential ethical issues, and analyses utilized in qualitative data. Chapter 7 presents some basic elements of research including the difference between basic and applied research, variables, group assignment, constructs, and operational definitions. After these concepts are understood, the three basic types of research design (true experimental, quasi-experimental, and nonexperimental) are defined and examples are provided to enhance understanding. Chapter 8 focuses on survey design, including types of surveys and how to select them. Various tests, inventories, and scales are introduced along with examples and reasons for selecting one survey type over another. A discussion of how culture and diversity influences data collection is included near the end of the chapter.

Chapters 9, 10, and 11 focus on basic skills related to data. Chapter 9 introduces how data are classified as categorical or continuous and then organized using frequency distributions. Building on this knowledge, the concepts of measures of central tendency, the normal curve, standard deviation, and variance are explained in detail with plenty of examples. This chapter serves as the foundation for understanding the next two chapters. Chapter 10 describes terms related to population and samples. There are three main topics covered: sample size considerations, probability and nonprobability samples, and sampling bias. Each topic deserves important consideration when determining the sample size needed for any evaluation or research project. Chapter 11 introduces inferential statistics and defines the terms *scientific hypothesis, research questions, null hypothesis*, and *alternative hypothesis*. The next section presents basic statistical tests (e.g., chi-square, *t*-tests, and correlation coefficients). The chapter ends with a discussion of type I and type II errors.

The last chapters provide skills related to budgets, reports, and presentations, and the text culminates with a case study. Chapter 12 is divided into two sections. The first section describes various types of budgets with examples to practice basic skills. Budget justifications are also presented. The second section defines the types of cost analyses and how each type is used. Chapter 13 illustrates several ways to present results including abstracts, executive summaries, reports, manuscripts, posters, and verbal presentations. Chapter 14 is a lengthy case study reinforcing all aspects presented in this book.

Acknowledgments

During process of writing this book, I received assistance and support from numerous family members, friends, and colleagues.

Kevin, my husband, supported me through the many weekends that were consumed with writing. He allowed me the opportunity to fulfill my dream.

Laura Merrell edited each chapter with great attention to detail. Her superb skills greatly contributed to the quality of this text.

Dr. Richard Riegelman provided guidance and mentoring as I embarked on writing my first textbook. His constructive comments improved the overall quality of this text.

Dr. R. Clifford Blair offered valuable advice throughout the process. As a biostatistician and author, he offered humor and encouragement whenever I got tired of writing.

Over decades of teaching, hundreds of students taught me the skills and expertise needed to write this text.

The University of South Florida College of Public Health granted me time to complete this text.

Most educators say that the best way to learn a subject is to teach it. After writing this text, I have revised this advice to say:

"The best way to learn a subject is not to teach it, but rather to write a book about it."

CHAPTER 1

Purpose

CHAPTER OBJECTIVES

By the end of this chapter, students will be able to:

- Discuss the steps in evaluation
- Prepare a review of the literature for a specific topic
- Develop specific questions for research and evaluations
- Evaluate goal statements and objectives
- Produce a logic model
- Evaluate the positive and adverse influence of stakeholders
- Differentiate the various types of evaluations

KEY TERMS

Goals and objectives

Research questions

Needs assessment

Literature review

Logic model

Stakeholders

Types of evaluations

Introduction

This chapter begins with a discussion about the differences and similarities between evaluation and research. Because this text covers both topics, it is important to learn the definitions of both concepts. The next discussion presents an overview of how to develop research questions and the purpose of conducting a needs assessment. Program planning involves identification of the type and design of program needed; achieving consensus from individuals providing or participating in the program; securing essential financial, personnel, and location resources; and sustained program implementation by staying true to the original design, also called program fidelity. Program evaluation is used for determining the day-to-day program management, short-term results, and long-term program impact. Program evaluations involve data collection and analysis to influence changes to improve program effectiveness.[1] As the first step, researchers read the published literature to determine research questions, whereas evaluators read the published literature to learn about the best practices related to their proposed goals for the planned program. Whether an individual is evaluating a program or conducting research, after reading the published literature, the investigation begins to take shape.

If you are wondering why you need to know about research and evaluation, let's explore the practical side of these skills. Suppose that you are interested in purchasing a new computer. You will plan, research, and evaluate your options prior to making a purchase. The same basic steps are used in research and evaluation.

1. How did you determine that you need a new computer? (Needs assessment)
2. What consumer rating reports will you read to gain information? (Literature review)
3. What questions need to be answered prior to your decision? (Research questions)
4. How will you map out your strategy for making this decision? (Logic model)
5. When visiting stores, what questions will you ask a salesperson? (Qualitative data)
6. What type of numerical data will you obtain online? (Quantitative data)
7. What questions do you ask your friends about their computers? (Qualitative data)
8. Are there budget constraints or stakeholders influencing your decision? (Budget and stakeholders)
9. What type of evaluation is most appropriate? (Evaluation)

10. How will you merge the data and make your final decision? (Data analysis)
11. Purchase a computer, install software, and read the manual. (Final report)

Once you realize the usefulness that research and evaluation skills play in daily life, this text becomes more practical and beneficial. You will learn skills and methods to assist with a wide range of program planning, research, and evaluation methods in your personal and professional lives.

Difference Between Research and Evaluation

Let's begin with some simple definitions followed by more details about the similarities and differences between research and evaluation. Research creates new knowledge[2] with the intention of generalizing results from a sample to the population.[3] Evaluations are conducted to improve an internal situation with no intent to generalize to another population.[2] Now let's compare a few more specific similarities and differences between research and evaluation. Because this text introduces the concepts of both research and evaluation, it is not expected that the reader already understands all of the information provided in **Table 1-1**. Understanding and proficiency will increase as you move through each chapter.

Table 1-1   A Comparison of Research and Evaluation

Research	Evaluation
Creates new knowledge	Improves program effectiveness
Reviews the literature to determine questions that remain unanswered on the topic	Reviews the literature to determine best practices of similar programs
Tests hypotheses	Utilizes facts
Uses a theory for framework and research design	Uses a logic model
Answers specific questions	Answers general questions
Seeks to be value-free[4]	Assigns value to a program[4]
Generalizes results from sample to a population	Recommends improvement for an existing program with a target audience
Uses primary and/or secondary data	Uses primary and/or secondary data
Utilizes statistical test for data analysis	Utilizes statistical test for data analysis
Draws conclusions	Provides useful feedback
Determines what might be significant	Determines what is important
Researcher publishes results	Evaluator writes report for stakeholders

Data from Doherty, T. Research and Evaluation? It's Complicated! Population Health. Department of Health and Human Services of Australia. Available at: www.menzies.utas.edu.au/pdf/Nov%202011%20MRI_final.pdf6. Accessed January 9, 2012.

Because this text covers both evaluation and research topics, the terms related to evaluation and research are presented throughout each discussion. As noted in Table 1-1, many of the same skills, such as development goals or research questions, data collection, data analyses, and report writing, are used in both evaluation and research.[5]

Purpose of Evaluation

Over the past 20 years, because of advances in evaluation, we know that "one size fits all" programs are not effective, and therefore, program planners currently design tailor-made programs to address the unique needs of individuals in a defined community. Keep in mind that the word *community* ranges from students in one specific department, to the employees at a corporation, to the population of an entire city. According to Rossi and Freeman,[6] any tailor-made design requires the evaluator to explore how the proposed program affects individuals and communities. It is also useful to investigate the possible political ramifications and sustainability of the program within the defined community. For example, in 1982, one of first school antidrug programs was initiated by First Lady Nancy Reagan when she developed the "Just Say No" campaign.[7] By 1989, researchers realized that this program was too simplistic to meet the needs of students in diverse cultural, geographic, economic, and social settings. Therefore, it became important to design targeted programs for each population.

Although it seems logical to start any program with the planning phase and end with the evaluation, this logic is not correct. It is essential to design the plan and its implementation in parallel with the evaluation. For example, it is not possible to implement a program that has not been fully planned, nor it is possible to create an evaluation after the implementation phase is complete. Because each phase is intertwined with the other program components, it is important to begin thinking about the following questions related to cost during the planning phase of the program:

- What type of data collection is needed to answer the question?
- Is the target population easily assessable?
- What is the geographical area of the program? Is extensive travel involved?
- Will a control group be used?
- How many staff members will be required to complete the designed program?
- Will incentives be given to recruit participants?
- Are the participants going to be followed over time?

As evaluators begin planning and evaluating a program, there are numerous decisions to make during the initial phase. Before moving into the remainder of this chapter, let's review what types of projects are not either evaluation or research.

As previously stated, research focuses on answering research questions and gaining new knowledge, whereas evaluations concentrate on identifying unmet needs and services, planning effective program implementation, investigating how to improve program services, and assisting staff with program decisions based on cost-effectiveness. Theories are developed, established, and emphasized in research. Although evaluations benefit from using theories, theories are not developed as an evaluation product. So now that research and evaluation have been compared, let's add one more category, called *audit*, that utilizes basic statistics, but is not research or evaluation. Audits are linked to compliance, accreditation, laws, and regulations. For example, the Government Accountability Office utilizes agency and institution data to determine level of culpability in an agency receiving federal funding. Another example is The Joint Commission (TJC, formerly known as the Joint Commission on Accreditation of Healthcare Organizations [JCAHO]). This organization conducts performance and standard measures, health services research, and accountability measures for healthcare institutions across the United States.[8]

The rest of this chapter introduces how to review the literature, conduct a needs assessment, develop questions, identify the type of evaluation, and determine the role of stakeholders in planning programs and evaluations.

Needs Assessment

The purpose of a needs assessment is to identify the strengths, weaknesses, opportunities, and threats (SWOT) in the organization or community. The needs assessment is conducted in collaboration with the stakeholders, such as staff members, community leaders, neighborhood organization members, and political leaders. The goal is to obtain a broad range of opinions about the benefits and worries, because a concern for one group may be an asset for another group.

The first step of the needs assessment is to form a partnership with individuals involved in the organization or community. It is advisable to include at least one member with expertise in conducting a needs assessment to offer an outside perspective to the process. At the introductory meeting, it is important that every member is treated equally and with respect. The neighborhood housing member's opinion and contribution are given the same weight as the city council member's. After getting to know each other, they should coalesce around a few common goals for the needs assessment. It is advisable to focus on two or three goals, so the effort is not too ambitious. After establishing the goals, team members need to address the following questions:

- Who is the target audience for the needs assessment?
- Are there sufficient personnel to staff the needs assessment?
- What funds are available to finance the needs assessment?
- What are the roles, responsibilities, and expectations of each team member?
- Are there data available to ascertain what has been accomplished on this topic previously?
- What is the optimal timeline of the needs assessment?

Once the team answers these questions, it is time to move to the next step. Data collection begins with exploring what types of data are necessary to complete the needs assessment. Generally, data are divided into two categories: qualitative (words) and quantitative (numbers). Qualitative data include but are not limited to focus groups, interviews, town hall meetings, and public forums. The conversations at these events are recorded, transcribed, and analyzed for themes. On the other hand, with quantitative data, the survey responses are converted into numerical data for analysis. For example, the survey question "How would you rate your health today?" provides four scaled choices: excellent (4), good (3), fair (2), and poor (1). The responses are added together and divided by the number of individuals responding, to obtain a mean score or average. In addition, demographic data can be converted to numbers. When asking the respondents how long they have lived in the community, the choices would be: 10+ years (4); 5–9 years (3); 1–4 years (2); less than 1 year (1). As you can see, any type of data may be converted into numbers for quantitative analysis. Besides surveys, quantitative data may come from secondary data sources. When data is collected by another researcher or organization, it is called secondary data. Anyone using secondary data develops her own research objectives and questions. Examples of secondary data include census data, county property tax data, birth and death records, motor vehicle records, acute and chronic disease rates, professional organization licensure data, and so on. These data are public records and are available on city, county, state, federal, organizational, and institutional Internet sites (see **Table 1-2**).

Once the qualitative and quantitative data are collected and analyzed, the team reconvenes to examine the data for direction on how best to proceed with the planning process. Data results also guide refinement of the goals.

Table 1-2   Useful Data Resources

American Cancer Society	www.cancer.org
American Heart Association	www.heart.org
American Medical Association	www.ama-assn.org
American Nurses Association	www.nursingworld.org
American Physical Therapy Association	www.apta.org
Annie E. Casey Foundation: Kids Count	www.kidscount.org
Association of Schools and Programs of Public Health	www.aspph.org
Centers for Disease Control and Prevention	www.cdc.gov
Department of Health and Human Services	www.hhs.gov
Department of Labor	www.dol.gov
Environmental Protection Agency	www.epa.gov
Food and Drug Administration	www.fda.gov
March of Dimes	www.marchofdimes.com
National Institute for Occupational Safety and Health (NIOSH)	www.cdc.gov/NIOSH
National Institutes of Health	www.nih.gov
National Library of Medicine	www.nlm.nih.gov
Physicians for Social Responsibility	www.psr.org
U.S. Census Bureau	www.census.gov

Literature Review

The next step is to review the current published literature. Both researchers and evaluators need to know what other information is published on their topics of interest. Researchers search for what is already known about their topics and what questions remain unanswered. For example, researchers may discover that antidepression Drug A has never been studied on a group of adolescents, even though it has been proven to be effective for adults. This would then suggest a new area of research on antidepression Drug A to see if it would also be effective in adolescents. On the other hand, evaluators review the published literature to discover the best practices on their topics. Best practices are methods or techniques that have consistently been shown to be more effective than others and may be considered benchmarks in a field. For example, evaluators may discover a publication that describes a best practice initiative that reduced back injuries among employees working with elderly patients in assisted-living facilities. At this point, it may be tempting to simply enter your topic into an Internet search engine. Although this technique yields hundreds of websites related to the topic, it does not produce material suitable for a review of the literature. Keep in mind that the constant expansion of information available on the Internet does not mean that it is reliable, because anyone can post information, and it may serve as an infomercial to sell a product, service, or even one individual's opinion on a topic. Generally, a quick way to discern if a website offers valuable information is to glance at the ending of the website address. If the web address ends with .gov, .edu, or .org, chances are the site presents reliable information. However, if the web address ends in .com or .net, you need to proceed with caution when incorporating the information into your literature review.

Rather than entering the topic into a search engine, it is important to read reliable publications that professionals and researchers have written on the topic of interest. This process yields a peer-reviewed literature review. When academic or scholarly colleagues write a manuscript about their research or best practices and submit the manuscript to a professional journal, the journal editor reviews the manuscript and sends it to several other professionals with expertise on the topic. The peer experts examine the manuscript, review the content, inspect for wrong or erroneous information, edit, and decide if the manuscript is suitable to the specific journal. They write comments back to the editor. The editor shares the reviewer comments with the manuscript's authors. If the manuscript is accepted with revisions, the suggested changes are made and the manuscript is resubmitted, reviewed again, and published. This process allows scholarly peers to review the research of their colleagues prior to publication; thus, academic journals are called *refereed* or *peer-reviewed journals*. In contrast, documents posted on Internet sites are not reviewed through a peer-reviewed process and therefore often lack academic rigor, consistency, and attention to detail.

A compelling literature review involves delving into a variety of credible professional reference materials. This process is best accomplished by visiting a university campus library and gaining access to the professional sources through online databases as well as assessing printed materials at the library. If you are not familiar with using databases that house peer-reviewed journals, it is recommended that you review the available tutorial modules or ask a librarian for assistance. As previously discussed, when conducting a peer-reviewed literature review, it is not acceptable to enter the topic into an Internet search engine and use whatever information appears on the screen. This technique yields unreliable information.

To begin a literature review, you need to become familiar with the databases used in health, including but not limited to MEDLINE, CINAHL, FirstSearch, Ovid, and PsychLit. After you access the appropriate database, you may use the "keyword" option to begin your search. This type of search may be limited further by choosing from the following search forms: "any of the words," "at least one of the words," or "must contain all of these words." For example, if you are interested in knowing what has been written about the global efforts to eradicate malaria over the last 10 years, you may wish to use the "must contain all of these words" option. If you do not know much about your selected topic, use the "any of the words" option and cast a wide net related to the topic. Let's say you are interested in childhood obesity. The "any of the words" search results will be voluminous and will not provide the exact information you need, but this search option allows you to explore a wide variety of publications. By reading through a wide variety of publications, you gain knowledge about what research has been done on the topic previously.[9]

In addition to searching by keyword, you can limit your database search by years, language, subjects, or reviews. For example, you can search publications between 2002 and the present, written in English, and limited to human subject research. In addition, you have the choice of selecting review publications. The review publications are useful when starting your search because they provide an overview of the literature written on a specific topic. When you find a few specific and recently published peer-reviewed publications, you learn how other researchers investigated the same issue, including the methods used for the investigation, limitations and challenges, results, conclusions, and suggestions for further research. Although the literature review process is time consuming initially, it saves time later by helping you avoid the mistakes made by other researchers. If you find a peer-reviewed publication of particular interest, you may contact the author to discuss the publication in greater detail. Generally, authors are pleased to discuss their research findings.

To further limit the scope of your search to the most recent publications, it is useful to conduct a Boolean search. This time-saving technique allows you to limit your search efficiently by using three logical operations: OR, AND, and NOT. Keep in mind that some database search engines offer simpler methods, but not identical forms of search statements. It is useful to try a few different search statements until you become accustomed to the database you are using. If you get confused, refer to the help pages provided by the search engines.[10]

Boolean search:

Example 1
Topic: malaria rates
Boolean logic: AND
Search: global AND international malaria rates

Example 2
Topic: air quality
Boolean logic: NOT
Search: indoor NOT outdoor air quality

Example 3
Topic:	sports medicine
Boolean logic:	OR
Search:	adolescent OR teen sports medicine

In addition to using peer-reviewed journal databases, it is also helpful to use other library resources for your review of the literature. The following discussion provides the advantages and disadvantages of printed materials.

Books

Books provide a good starting point for a review of the literature because they offer a valuable general overview on specific subjects. Even though the information is less up-to-date because of publishing time, books should be included in any thorough literature review.

Government Documents

Depending on your field of study, many government documents are posted online through specific agency websites. These documents are extremely useful for a wide variety of topics. For example, if the investigation involves a historical view of HIV/AIDS, it is useful to research political documents to track the success and failure of legislative bills over the years. If you are not familiar with various government databases related to your topic, the reference librarian will offer valuable assistance.

Non-Governmental Organization (NGO) Documents

These organizations post valuable trend data and information related to specific topics. For example, the March of Dimes webpage[11] offers valuable maternal and infant health indicators. If you are not familiar with NGOs, it is best to seek the advice of a reference librarian.

Newspapers

Although newspapers are written for a general audience, the information provides the public a perspective on current events and summaries of recent trend data, such as political polls. It is useful to contrast newspaper articles with other sources for a comparative review of the literature.

Magazines

Like newspapers, magazines are intended for a general audience with the sole purpose of selling advertisements. Unless the topic involves investigating how a specific topic is portrayed in magazines, generally this information is not useful for scholarly literature reviews.

Theses and Dissertations

Because these documents are not published, they are usually only available from the library or through interlibrary loan. Keep in mind that this type of research was conducted by students, so the findings need to be viewed with caution.

Once you have completed your literature research, it is time to compile the information into an organized document. One common mistake made by new researchers is confusing the terms *annotated bibliography* and *review of the literature*. An annotated bibliography contains a brief summary of each citation followed by a short evaluation. The document includes the strengths or weaknesses of the material presented in the citations. For an annotated bibliography, the source citations are presented in alphabetical order, and each citation is presented as a new paragraph. Because citations are provided with each summary, there is no need for a reference page at the end of the document. A review of the literature is a compilation of multiple resources presented in narrative format. The literature review presents all sides of an argument to avoid bias, and areas of dispute are emphasized for the reader. Literature reviews are usually organized around topics rather than presented in chronological order by year of publication. The citations are presented at the end of the paper.

Development of Research Questions or Goal Statements

Once the review of the literature is complete, the next step involves development of research questions or goal statements. Keep in mind that researchers ask questions with the primary goal of generating new knowledge. Evaluators write goal statements and objectives with the purpose of improving an existing program. It is common for new investigators to propose research questions or goal statements that are broad and implausible. After narrowing the topic, it is useful to stop and critically evaluate the proposed project. To assist with this process, refer to **Table 1-3** and read the descriptions for A, B, C, and D. For your topic, circle the letter that best defines your study.

If B, C, or D is circled, the proposed research or program needs reconsideration and modification. With limited resources and time, programs need to concentrate on important and changeable issues. Regardless of which letter is circled, it is useful to reconvene the needs assessment committee to confirm, change, or refute the goals prior to moving forward with the program planning.

Table 1-3   Decision Box

	Important	Not Important
Changeable	A	B
Not Changeable	C	D

A = Important and changeable (Strong)
B = Not important, but changeable (Weak)
C = Important, but not changeable (Weak)
D = Not important and not changeable (Very weak)

It is not unusual for team members to refine the evaluation or research several times prior to finalizing.

Another way to assess program planning is to use the results of the needs assessment and the literature review to answer the following questions:

- What is the perception of the proposed program?
- Do people think the problem is more severe than it might actually be?
- Has a needs assessment confirmed the extent of the problem?
- Are there reliable data available to show the severity of the problem?
- Given limited resources, should this program have high priority?
- Are there other problems that need immediate resources more than this problem?
- Does the long-term or longitudinal data show an increasing trend of this problem?
- What percentage of the population is affected by this problem?
- Will this program solve a portion of the problem?

Finally, by refining the goal and answering the questions in **Box 1-1**, the questions become focused for researchers or evaluators.

BOX 1-1

Research- and Evaluation-Focused Questions

Who?   Identify the target population.

What?   Describe the main purpose of the research or evaluation.

When?   Ascertain the time frame or length of the research or evaluation.

Where?   Describe the specific location.

Let's look at a few examples of focused research questions.

What is the preferred method of health education for newly diagnosed diabetic patients living in a rural area?

Who: Diabetic patients
What: Preferred method of health education:
          Group class, one-on-one education, self-paced workbook, Internet education modules
When: Newly diagnosed
Where: Rural area

Does participation in six weeks of in-house physical therapy prior to a total hip replacement decrease recovery time for elderly patients at their retirement community wellness center?

Who: Elderly patients
What: Physical therapy
When: Six weeks prior to a total hip replacement
Where: Retirement community wellness center

When comparing the use of Brand A surgical bandages with Brand B surgical bandages, which bandage is shown to have lower wound infection rates in the first five days following abdominal surgery?

Who: Brand A and Brand B surgical bandages
What: Lower wound infection rates
When: First five days postoperative
Where: Abdominal surgery sites

The process of writing excellent research questions involves numerous drafts and discussion with team members. Because team members may not have time to physically meet to write the research questions, it is advisable to send drafts via email to receive comments during the process. Once everyone agrees on the wording, it is valuable to schedule a meeting to revisit the results of the literature review and finalize the research questions.

Evaluation: Goals and Objectives

Once the best practices are identified in the literature review, it is time to refine the goal statements and write measureable objectives. For your program, there may be one or more goal statements describing the final impact or outcome of the program. The purpose of each goal statement is to describe an activity using

BOX 1-2

Test Your Skills

Write two goal statements for a program related to decreasing the number of patients who experience falls in a residential nursing home. For each goal statement, write two objectives.

measurable words such as *increase, improve, decrease, establish, deliver, provide,* and *produce.*

Examples of goal statements:[12]

Poor: The course will teach patients about diabetes.

Better: The course will increase the patients' knowledge about diabetes.

Best: The six-week course will increase the diabetic disease management knowledge and blood glucose monitoring for adults recently diagnosed with diabetes.

Once the goal statements are written, objectives are added to describe each of the steps required to accomplish the goals (see **Box 1-2**). Objectives are stated in terms of outcomes rather than processes. Each objective is measurable, identifies the target audience, and specifies the result of the activity with time restrictions.

Examples of objectives:

Poor: Patients attending the diabetic class should understand how to monitor their blood glucose levels.

Better: Patients attending the six-week diabetic course should be able to demonstrate how to monitor their blood glucose levels.

Best: By Week 2, 90% of patients attending the six-week diabetic course should be able to explain the signs and symptoms of low blood sugar and provide a return demonstration of how to monitor their blood glucose levels using their personal monitors.

Now that the evaluation team members have conducted the needs assessment, identified the best practices in the literature, and finalized the goal statements and objectives, it is time to explore the role of stakeholders.

Evaluation: Role of Stakeholders

Because stakeholders such as staff members, community leaders, neighborhood organization members, and political leaders shape how a program is planned, implemented, and evaluated, team members consider the level of influence and power held by stakeholders.[13] Stakeholders have specific roles. When stakeholders learn these roles, each phase of the program design meets diverse needs. Traditionally, stakeholders were viewed as policymakers, program sponsors, program management, evaluation staff, or program staff. Even though target participants were often included in the list of stakeholders, they were not necessarily viewed as equal partners. Over time, the target audience has gained status and equal partnership. Now these stakeholders are viewed as being empowered to sustain community development projects by embracing disenfranchised groups.[14] As shown in **Table 1-4**, stakeholders with low power and high legitimacy represent service recipients or frontline staff. When the high power and low legitimacy stakeholders omit the less empowered individuals from the program design, there is less utilization and sustainability.[15]

Over the past few decades, evaluators have recognized the importance of stakeholder involvement. When stakeholders participate from the first program planning meeting through the evaluation, they are more likely to anticipate problems, provide legitimacy to community partners, share data resources, and assist with final decisions.[14] Stakeholder participation may pose some challenges in addition to these advantages. For example, program funding sponsor (high power) stakeholder opinions may differ from clinic staff (high legitimacy) stakeholder opinions. According to Guba and Lincoln,[15] the team should not avoid such conflict, but rather welcome dissimilar opinions and encourage open dialogue for greater understanding of perspectives. Here are some questions to consider when determining the role of stakeholders:

- How will the low power/high legitimacy stakeholders be assured of equal power throughout the planning and evaluation process?
- How and when will stakeholders be invited to participate in the planning phase?

Table 1-4 Stakeholders and Power

Low Power/High Legitimacy	High Power/Low Legitimacy
Recipients	Policymakers
Frontline staff	Funding agencies
Disenfranchised individuals	Evaluation staff
Target population	Program sponsors
Program staff	Program competitors

Data from Mark MM, Shotland RL. Stakeholder-based evaluation and value judgments. *Evaluation Rev.* 1985;9:605–626.

- Are meetings held at convenient times and locations for low power/high legitimacy stakeholders who have less flexible work schedules?
- Is the program methodology flexible and open to change based on stakeholder opinion?

Stakeholders with various roles and power are critical to the success and sustainability of programs whether in an organization, neighborhood, or community. However, different perspectives and vested interests cause clashing viewpoints for most programs. To overcome this potential conflict, it is essential to find some agreement on common ground among all members. Until all stakeholders agree on the goal statements, there is no purpose in moving forward. Once agreement is achieved on the goal statements, the specific objectives are modified to include diverse views on how to reach the goals. For example, community-based teen pregnancy prevention programs are a common controversial topic at school board and parent-teacher meetings. When the discussion centers around which specific curriculum should or should not be taught, no agreement is reached. However, once the stakeholders agree that a rising teen birthrate is unacceptable in their community, the planning process begins to explore ways to enhance self-esteem and redirect teen activity toward community service projects and part-time opportunities.

Now that the planning process is starting to take shape, it is necessary to introduce the basic components of the evaluation process. As stated at the beginning of the chapter, the evaluation is designed in the context of the program plan. The evaluation should never be an afterthought once the program has been completed. Without incorporating the evaluation in the first step of planning, serious and unresolvable problems will result in the end.

Evaluation: Implementation

After the planning phase is complete, it is time to begin the implementation process. Implementation is defined as the execution of the plan, or simply doing what was planned. The implementation entails a detailed step-by-step process. Think of the implementation with the same level of detail needed for a computer program. Each line of computer code must be correctly executed before the next line of code is read by the computer. The same process is true for implementing a program plan. Although this section focuses on implementation of an evaluation, it is important to note that researchers use the same steps when starting a research study. Research, like evaluation, must follow a detailed plan, so that the research study is completed in a timely and organized manner without omitting any critical details.

To ensure that each step of the plan is considered and implemented, it is useful to develop a timeline. Timelines are developed as a team process, so everyone shares their thoughts, ideas, and concerns. It is essential that team members take responsibility for action items; otherwise, the implementation is delayed. Once the timeline is finalized, it is posted as a visual cue. However, after a timeline is finalized, it is typically expanded and modified throughout the entire implementation process. Some teams use a whiteboard to post the timeline, so it can be easily changed as needed. Depending on the implementation size, timelines are displayed by month, week, day, or even hour, if necessary. In addition, teams may develop a timeline for each phase of the implementation. **Table 1-5** illustrates an example of a timeline for staff training.

Table 1-5   Staff Training Timeline

Month / Week		Action Item	Details	Person Responsible
July	7/3	Team meeting	Finalize implementation timeline	Team leader: JL
	7/10	Curriculum	Order adequate number of copies	Clerk: SA
	7/17	Staff training	Meet with 8 department supervisors to discuss staff training sessions	Team member: FC
	7/24	Staff training	Finalize 16 staff training sessions (2 per department); determine team members who will conduct the staff training	Team member: DE
	7/31	Design observation checklist	Three team members meet to design observation checklist for use during observations	Team members: BR, CD, LR
August	8/7	Practice staff training	Two team members schedule practice training sessions with other team members to finalize timing and quality; receive feedback	Team members: BR, CD
	8/14	Staff training	Two team members complete 16 staff training sessions; ensure fidelity in training by following protocol	Team members: BR, CD
		Track data	Log how many staff members in each department; log how many staff members attended each session	Team members: BR, CD
		Staff members not trained	Schedule additional training dates; contact staff members who did not receive training via in-house email; provide additional training dates and times	Clerk: SA
	8/21	Observations	Using the checklist, assign 4 team members to each randomly observe 2 trained staff members teaching patients	Team members: LR, DE
		Additional staff training sessions	Conduct make-up staff training for those unable to attend previously scheduled training sessions	Team members: BR, CD
	8/28	Fidelity	Team members review results of observation checklists for fidelity	Team members: BR, CD

As shown in Table 1-5, the implementation timeline includes every possible detail, so team members know the expectations for each week. Once one phase has been completed, it is necessary to develop a new timeline for the next phase. Even for large, multiyear programs, it is advisable to develop a timeline for the entire project and then break each segment into workable components for managing daily and weekly activities.

Besides a timeline, the implementation phase entails a method to ensure program fidelity. This method involves the development of all written policies and procedures. For example, as mentioned in Table 1-5, checklist observation documents program implementation. Other written policies include but are not limited to procedures for obtaining informed consent documents, specific instructions, or any procedure that requires adherence to a step-by-step implementation for program fidelity. Once the policies and procedures are in place, the implementation process continues throughout the duration of the program. Parallel to the implementation data collection process, evaluation data are collected at each step of the program. The following discussion introduces the types of evaluation used to assess each phase of programs.

Types of Evaluations

The main purpose of any evaluation is to improve program effectiveness. The complexity of the program and the evaluation determine the type and quality of the decisions. Whether the evaluation is simple or complex, each one requires rigorous and detailed design for success.[16] Although there are numerous types of evaluations, this chapter focuses on the most common types of evaluations: formative, summative, process, outcome, and impact.

Formative Evaluation

Formative evaluation is also called exploratory evaluation. It focuses on the elements of the program and is conducted during the planning and implementation phase. Think of a formative evaluation as ensuring that the program is "formed" correctly. The issues of concern are related to the appropriateness and feasibility of the program materials, messages, and methods used to conduct the program for the target audience. Formative evaluation includes qualitative or quantitative data or a mixture of the two. At each point through the planning, implementation, and evaluation phases, data are collected from the target audience (see **Box 1-3**). For example, during the needs assessment and planning phases, surveys are pilot tested, revised, and completed by a small sample of participants. Such preliminary data determine what changes are needed to improve the readability and understanding of the final survey. Later, during the implementation phase, interviews or focus groups are conducted to confirm the usefulness of the messages and materials. Throughout the program, formative data are collected and portions of the program are modified as needed to address identified concerns.[17]

Summative Evaluation

Summative evaluation determines if the program met any combination of measurement about impact, outcome, or benefits. This type of evaluation is frequently conducted by external evaluators. Generally, quantitative data are used for summative evaluations, because standardized surveys are best suited for

BOX 1-3 Formative Evaluation Questions

Questions for administrators where the program will be implemented:
   What do you know about this program?
   What are the benefits to your facility for agreeing to implement this program?
What problems do you foresee with the implementation of this program in this facility?
What will your staff need to implement this program?
What are the costs associated with the implementation?
Questions for staff in the facility:
   What do you know about this program?
   What have you heard about this program?
   What are the benefits of this program to the staff?
   What are the program barriers experienced by the staff?
   What are the benefits of this program to the participants?
Questions for potential participants:
   What made you decide to attend this program?
   What is most appealing about this program?
   What do you think you will gain by participating in this program?
   Why did you decide to come to this facility for the program?

Summative Evaluation Questions

What type of statistical test was used to analyze the data?
Were statistically significant results found? If so, explain.

measuring specific objectives. For example, a hospital institutes a new discharge planning program to ensure that all patients are educated about their discharge medications. Recently discharged patients are mailed the satisfaction survey along with a self-addressed stamped envelope to return the completed survey. The survey is limited to specific questions about the patient's level of satisfaction related to knowledge about their discharge medications. These data provide a summary of the impact, outcome, and benefits of the hospital's new discharge planning program (see **Box 1-4**).

Process Evaluation

Process evaluation examines all aspects of program implementation. In some situations, this evaluation investigates the organizational and administrative aspects of the program. During a process evaluation, the evaluation monitors the feedback of the program by investigating the issues that influence the implementation as well as the environment surrounding the implementation (see **Box 1-5**).[18]

Process Evaluation Questions

Is the program staying true to the original design (in other words, is there *program fidelity*), and is it maintained in the implementation process?
Are the quality and quantity of the services and products maintained at the capacity level expected?
Is the level of satisfaction sustained across participating groups?
Is there any identified reason why one group of participants is no longer participating?

Outcome Evaluation

Outcome evaluation obtains program data to document short-term results. These descriptive data define output activities, such as the number of individuals calling the toll-free number following a local public service advertisement campaign. Also, data access the short-term program results for the target audience, such as percentage of middle school students showing an increase in awareness of healthy cafeteria food choices after a school health intervention. Other information obtained from outcome evaluation includes knowledge, attitude, or behavioral changes or institutional policy changes (see **Box 1-6**). According to Stead, Hastings, and Eadie,[19] health literacy, social influence, and health policy are the types of action needed for health promotion outcome. Health literacy relates to an individual's knowledge and understanding of a health issue or concern. Social influence explores the availability of personal support and community empowerment. Health policy relates to how strategies are incorporated into organizational practice.

Impact Evaluation

Because of excessive costs and lengthy time commitment, impact evaluations are rarely possible. When feasible, impact evaluation is the most inclusive type of evaluation because of its focus on outcome objectives. Because of external influences, the results are not always attributable to directly to the program. Impact evaluation provides results related to long-term data such as recidivism rates, changes in morbidity and mortality data, or long-term maintenance of a behavioral change (see **Box 1-7**).

BOX 1-6

Outcome Evaluation Questions

Were the short-term goals achieved by the program?

What was the stakeholder's level of satisfaction in the program implementation?

Did specific health knowledge and motivation increase participation among the target population?

Did availability of social support positively affect the participant's health outcome?

Impact Evaluation Questions

What external influences affected the results?

What percentage of participants were lost to follow-up over the longitudinal study?

Was the expected behavior change sustained over the expected period of time?

How did the expected cost compare to the actual cost of the impact evaluation?

Evaluation: Logic Models

Now that the team members have completed the previously discussed tasks, it is time to organize the data and information on one spreadsheet. Even though there are numerous types and designs, all logic models are a graphic depiction of a program from the planning phase through evaluation. Logic models link research questions, goal statements, and objectives to interventions and outcomes. Such models are an excellent way to communicate the big picture to others. This type of communication facilitates buy-in from stakeholders, personnel, and the target audience. Keep in mind that there are whole books written about logic models. See **Table 1-6** for a basic overview of a logic model.[20] It is intended to merely introduce the concept of logic models.

Questions: The questions are listed across the top of the logic model. Each column of the logic model influences how the research questions are answered.

Goal Statements: The goal statements and objectives provide the program overview. Each goal statement is listed and followed by the measureable objectives.

Inputs and Resources: The inputs are defined as the resources available for the program. Inputs include human resources and stakeholders, such as funders, community partners, program staff, collaborators, and volunteers. Fiscal resources are funding, donations, and special grants. Physical resources provide office space and equipment, office and storage space, computers and software, and other special tools, such as cameras and recording devices. Knowledge resources are teaching materials, curriculum, learning competencies, and certification requirements. By listing every resource under the inputs category, it is easy to determine what is missing and needs to be obtained for the program to begin.

Table 1-6   Example of a Logic Model

Goal Statements	Inputs/Resources	Activities	Outputs/Process Evaluation	Outcomes/Impact and Outcome Evaluation		
				Short-term Impact	**Intermediate Impact**	**Long-term Impact**
Overview and objectives	Human resources and stakeholders	Needs assessment	Products	Baseline data collection: knowledge, attitudes, behaviors, and beliefs	Track participation	Documentation of improved outcomes
	Fiscal resources	Baseline data	Services provided		Retention and follow-up rates	Decreased costs due to improved conditions
	Physical resources	Recruitment	Themes	Income generated		
	Educational resources	Focus groups	Profits	Knowledge gained	Implementation strategies for future events	Policy changes due to intervention
		Surveys	Number of persons trained	Stakeholder satisfaction		Strategies for institutional changes
		Interviews				
		Number of training sessions				

External influences: social media, environment effects, political impact

Modified from McCawley P. University of Idaho Extension. Logic Models. Available at: http://www.uiweb.uidaho.edu/extension/LogicModel.pdf. Accessed January 12, 2012.

Activities: Activities involve what needs to be accomplished to achieve the objectives. For example, if an objective requires the development of a community coalition, the activity describes a detailed plan for forming a community coalition. If the objective involves teaching a health course, the activity explains how the resources are used to advertise the course, schedule the date and time, recruit and enroll students, collect fees, invite guest speakers, and so on for the course to be a success.

Outputs: Outputs link the goal statements and objectives to the short-term, intermediate, and long-term outcomes. Outputs may also be viewed as the process evaluation. Although outputs include products, goods, and services as well as the people served by the program, process evaluation monitors the overall implementation activities. Products, goods, and services are webpages, fact sheets, publications, software, curriculum handbooks, community events, courses, and demonstrations. The people served are described by their demographics and characteristics; percentage of target population reached; change in knowledge, attitude, beliefs, and behavior achieved; and overall level of satisfaction expressed.

Outcomes: Outcomes are expressed as short term, intermediate, or long term. Each phase communicates the effect of the program thus far. Short-term outcomes reflect awareness of the issue, motivation to change, and knowledge, attitudes, skills, beliefs, and behaviors needed to make the desired change. Intermediate outcomes build on short-term outcomes and track participation and practices of the target audience; changes in policies within institutions, business, and government agencies; and implementation of strategies by individuals and groups. Long-term outcomes or program impacts follow intermediate outcomes by documenting improved economic, health, educational, social, environmental, or political conditions that relate back to the goal statement. Impact determines permanent change beyond the end of the program. It is the lasting effect of change of institutional policies. For example, over time, the smoke-free indoor air quality goal statement produced a permanent nationwide ban of smoking in restaurants, bars, and domestic air flights.

External influences either support or oppose the goals. Because of the levels of institutional, community, and participant opinions of the goal statement, the program planning process changes to better match the baseline opinion of the community. For example, if the community supports building a free walk-in clinic for the homeless population, the inputs, activities, outputs, and outcomes will differ than if the community opposes a free clinic. If the community has the opinion that a free homeless clinic will increase the number of homeless people, then the program starts at a completely different place. Another type of external influence includes similar and competing programs or services, socioeconomic conditions, governmental policies, and so on.

Summary

This chapter provided an overview of similarities and differences between research and evaluation, starting with the development of questions. The basic difference is that research generates new knowledge, whereas evaluation seeks to improve existing programs. Following a discussion about needs assessments and how to review existing published literature, the remainder of the chapter focused on the identification of program type and design, consensus building among individuals participating in the program, and resources needed such as funding, personnel, and location resources. Program evaluation was defined as day-to-day program management, short-term results, and long-term program impact. Program evaluations include data collection and analysis.

Case Study: Healthy Food/Healthy People

The administrator of a large urban hospital wanted to offer healthier food options in the cafeteria but was not sure what changes needed to occur in the cafeteria. She decided to conduct a needs assessment. Volunteers were recruited from the clinical, financial, administrative, and environmental service staff to serve on the committee. After writing a few broad goal statements, the committee conducted several focus groups with employees from each shift, because night shift food choices may be different from day shift choices. The focus group results showed some general themes, so the committee developed a short survey. The survey was printed on postcards and was made available on the cafeteria tables, at the condiment station, and near the checkout cashier registers. Drop boxes were available at each exit to collect the postcard surveys. This method also allowed both the employees and hospital visitors to participate. The survey was also made available online and on the employee website.

continues

CASE STUDY *continued*

While the survey data were collected over a three-week period, the committee worked with the cafeteria manager. The committee requested secondary data about the most popular and least popular food choices, sodium and sugar content of popular items, and availability of fresh fruit and vegetables. They ranked the current purchased food choices by popularity, cost, and health factors. This grid was compared to the focus group and survey results. After analyzing the needs assessment data, the committee wrote a goal statement and three measureable objectives.

Goal Statement

The hospital administration will change three aspects of the available food and drink choices to encourage healthy eating.

Objectives

1. By the end of May, the hospital cafeteria will offer 50% more fresh fruit and vegetables compared to the baseline data.
2. By the end of June, the hospital cafeteria will replace foods and drinks with excess sodium and sugar with low-sodium and low-sugar foods.
3. By the end of July, the hospital cafeteria will modify its soft drink company contract to exchange the purchase of high-sugar drinks to lower sugar or sugar-free flavored water drinks or pure water.

The committee collected data from the cafeteria manager throughout the first three-month pilot study phase of the cafeteria changes. The baseline data were compared to the pilot study data. The final report was presented to the hospital administrator as the first step in modifying the cafeteria food choices. The results showed that the employees and visitors were spending the same amount of money in the cafeteria, but were purchasing the healthier food choices offered. The committee members agreed that the needs assessment provided valuable baseline data rather than merely making decisions based on a best guess of potential food changes in the cafeteria. Lastly, they expressed high satisfaction from the opportunity to serve on the committee; because it was a representative group of all employees, they got to know people from

continues

CASE STUDY *continued*

other departments, and the process was employee-driven rather than a top-down approach.

Case Study Discussion Questions

1. Discuss other options that might have been used for the data collection.
2. What other types of data could be collected to address the objectives?
3. Now that the baseline data has been collected, what might be the next steps for the committee?

Student Activities

Cubing is an activity that involves exploring one issue from six different directions.[21] For this exercise, divide the class into equal groups of six students per group. Allow each group to select a health science topic of their choice. For this example, the topic is "Bachelor of Science in Health Science (BSHS) degree." Each student is assigned one of the following six questions:

1. *Describe:* What is the Bachelor of Science in Health Science degree?
2. *Compare:* How does the BSHS compare to other undergraduate degrees?
3. *Associate:* What does the BSHS degree make you think of?
4. *Analyze:* What should we look for in the ideal BSHS degree?
5. *Apply:* Apply what we know about undergraduate college degrees to the BSHS degree.
6. *Argue for and against it:* Identify arguments for and against the BSHS degree.

References

1. The Centers for Disease Control and Prevention. IPOM: Immunization Program Operations Manual. Available at: http://www.cdc.gov/vaccines/vac-gen/policies /ipom/. Updated August 6, 2012. Accessed August 21, 2013.
2. Stufflebeam DL. The CIPP Model for program evaluation. In Madaus GF, Scriven M, Stufflebeam DL, eds. *Evaluation Models: Viewpoints on Educational and Human Services Evaluation.* Boston, MA: Kluwer Nijhof; 1983.

3. Priest S. A program evaluation primer. *J Experiential Educ.* 2001;24(1):34–40.

4. Coffman J. Ask the expert: Michael Scriven on the differences between evaluation and social science research. *The Evaluation Exchange.* 2003/2004;9(4). Available at: http://www.hfrp.org/evaluation/the-evaluation-exchange/issue-archive/reflecting-on-the-past-and-future-of-evaluation/michael-scriven-on-the-differences-between-evaluation-and-social-science-research. Accessed on January 8, 2012.

5. Doherty T. Research and Evaluation? It's Complicated! Department of Health and Human Services of Australia. Available at: www.menzies.utas.edu.au/pdf/Nov%20 2011%20MRI_final.pdf. Accessed January 9, 2012.

6. Rossi PH, Freeman HE. *Evaluation: A Systematic Approach.* Newbury Park, CA: Sage; 1993.

7. The Ronald Reagan Presidential Foundation and Library. Just Say No, 1982–1989. Available at: http://www.reaganfoundation.org/details_t.aspx?p=RR1005NRL&h1= 0&h2=0&sw=&lm=reagan&args_a=cms&args_b=10&argsb=N&tx=1203. Accessed January 12, 2012.

8. The Joint Commission. Available at: http://www.jointcommission.org. Accessed June 3, 2012.

9. Shuttleworth M. What Is a Literature Review? Available at: http://www.experiment-resources.com/what-is-a-literature-review.html. Published September 16, 2009. Accessed January 12, 2012.

10. Barker J. Basic Search Tips and Advanced Boolean Explained. Teaching Library University of California, Berkeley. Available at: http://www.lib.berkeley.edu /TeachingLib/Guides/Internet/Boolean.pdf. Accessed January 12, 2012.

11. March of Dimes. Peristats. Available at: http://www.marchofdimes.com/peristats/. Accessed January 12, 2012.

12. University of Connecticut Assessment. How to Write Program Objectives/Outcomes. Available at: http://assessment.uconn.edu/docs/HowToWriteObjectivesOutcomes .pdf. Accessed January 12, 2012.

13. Azzam T. Evaluators responsiveness to stakeholders. *Am J Eval.* 2010;3(1):45–65.

14. Mark MM, Shotland RL. Stakeholder-based evaluation and value judgments. *Evaluation Rev.* 1985;9:605–626.

15. Guba EG, Lincoln YS. *Fourth Generation Evaluation.* Newbury Park, CA: Sage; 1989.

16. Campbell B, Mark MM. Toward more effective stakeholder dialogue: Applying theories of negotiation to policy and program evaluation. *J Appl Soc Psychol.* 2006;36:2834–2863.

17. Posavac EJ, Carey RG. *Program Evaluation: Methods and Case Studies.* Upper Saddle River, NJ: Pearson; 2007.

18. Habicht JP, Victora CG, Vaughan JP. Evaluation designs for adequacy, plausibility and probability of public health programme performance and impact. *Int J Epidemiol.* 1999;28:10–18.

19. Stead M, Hastings G, Eadie D. The challenge of evaluating complex interventions: A framework for evaluating media advocacy. *Health Educ Res.* 2002;17(3):351–364.

20. McCawley P. The Logic Model for Program Planning and Evaluation. University of Idaho Extension. Available at: http://www.uiweb.uidaho.edu/extension/LogicModel .pdf. Accessed January 12, 2012.

21. Orr SK. Exploring stakeholder values and interests in evaluation. *Am J Eval.* 2010;31(4):557–569.

Ethics

Introduction

This chapter provides an overview of ethics. After a description of the role of the federal government in research, two historical landmark cases are presented, followed by definitions of the basic principles of medical ethics. This is followed by a discussion of how these principles are applied to the role of the institutional review board (IRB), development of informed consent documents, and consideration of special populations.

Historical Background

In 1949, following the Nazi Nuremberg trial in Germany, the U.S. National Institutes of Health, Office of Human Subjects Research was founded on the principles of the Nuremberg Code, which contains directives for human experimentation. The following summarizes the Nuremberg Code:[1]

- Voluntary consent is required.
- Research must be of societal value.
- Previous studies justify the need for the research or evaluation.
- Research and evaluation must avoid physical and mental suffering and injury.
- No research may be conducted if prior knowledge suggests the occurrence of death or disability.
- Risks must not exceed humanitarian benefits.
- Program planning and research must protect subjects from injury, disability, or death.
- Research and evaluations may only be conducted by qualified researchers.
- Individuals participating in research or evaluation may withdraw at any time.
- Researchers or evaluators must end their studies if there is cause for concern of subjects regarding their safety.

Later, the U.S. Department of Health and Human Services Office for Human Research Protections (OHRP) was created for the protection of the rights of individuals involved in research and to provide clarification, guidance, and advice; distribute educational information; and maintain regulatory oversight.[2] In 1979, the U.S. National Commission for the Protection of Human Subjects of Biomedical and Behavioral Research wrote the Belmont Report to describe the ethical principles that apply to human subject research. In 1981, the U.S. Department of Health and Human Services and the Food and Drug Administration revised the Belmont Report to be compatible with current statutes.[3]

It is important to review U.S. historical landmark cases that involved unethical practices in medical research. The two cases discussed here are the U.S. Public Health Service Syphilis Study in Tuskegee and the case of Henrietta Lacks.

U.S. Public Health Service Syphilis Study in Tuskegee

Syphilis is a sexually transmitted infection of great importance to public health because it may not present symptoms for years, increasing chances of it being spread among people before being treated. Syphilis causes many health problems including painful lesions and sores and, if left untreated, dementia in later life. Syphilis may also be passed from an infected mother to her newborn child. In 1932, the U.S. Public Health Service started a research study about the progression of syphilis in Macon County, Alabama, near Tuskegee. Of the 600 impoverished African American males in the study, 399 had syphilis and 201 did not have syphilis. The men were never told that they were involved in a research study, and they did not receive proper medical care to treat syphilis. For study participation, the men received free medical exams, meals, and burial insurance; however, they were never allowed to quit participating in the study. In 1936, the study's first clinical report was published. In 1947, penicillin was available to effectively treat syphilis, yet the men never received treatment. During World War II, 250 men in the study registered for military service, were diagnosed with syphilis, and obtained treatment for syphilis. After 40 years, in 1972, the assistant secretary for Health and Scientific Affairs announced the end of the Tuskegee Study, and an advisory panel declared the study was unethical. By the time the study ended, 74 men were alive. Of the original 399 men, 28 had died of syphilis, 100 had died of related complications, 40 wives had been infected, and 19 children had been born with congenital syphilis. In 1973, a class-action lawsuit was filed on behalf of the men and their families. In 1974, an out-of-court settlement was reached for $10 million, plus lifetime medical benefits and burial services to all living participants. In 1975, the benefits were extended to wives, widows, and children. The last study participant died in January 2004, and in 2009 the last widow receiving benefits died. As of this writing, there are 15 remaining children receiving medical and health benefits. The Tuskegee Study left a legacy of mistrust among the African American community toward the medical establishment and many public health efforts.[4] On May 16, 1997, after 65 years, President Clinton apologized for government's syphilis study in Tuskegee, Alabama.[5]

Henrietta Lacks

Henrietta Lacks was an African American who lived in Virginia and worked as a tobacco farmer. In 1951, at age 30, she was diagnosed with cervical cancer. A physician from Johns Hopkins Hospital in Baltimore used a piece of her cervical tumor to grow a cell line to be used for medical research. Neither Ms. Lacks nor her family had any knowledge that her cells were used for research. They never signed an informed consent document. The immortal cell line was named HeLa from the first two letters of her first and last names. This cell line was the first human cells to ever grow in a culture medium. Henrietta's cells were used to develop the polio vaccine, cloning, gene mapping, and in vitro fertilization, among other scientific advancements. Her cells were used for 25 years after her death.[6] It remains unclear why her cells never died. The story was uncovered when writer Rebecca Skloot researched the history of HeLa cells. Ms. Skloot revealed that the Lacks family was unaware that researchers sold vials of their mother's cells, never receiving any money. Ms. Skloot wrote a book, titled *The Immortal Life of Henrietta Lacks*, about what she found. The Henrietta Lacks Foundation was started to provide financial assistance to needy individuals who have made important contributions to scientific research without their knowledge or consent.[7]

Basic Principles of Medical Ethics

Medical ethics are a system of moral principles and values applied to medical, health, and biological science judgments and decision making. To understand ethics, it is important to learn basic terminology. The basic ethical principles are respect for persons, beneficence, and justice. After learning the definitions, it becomes apparent that each principle is understandable on its own. However, when several ethical principles are considered jointly, the overlap can lead to contradiction.

Respect for persons or autonomy is divided into two sections. First, each individual is treated with respect and is given adequate information to make an informed decision, including having no treatment or alternative treatments. Informed decisions should be made without excessive influence of others. Second, individuals with diminished decision-making capacity require extra protection, depending on the risk of harm and the likelihood of benefit. Throughout research involvement, autonomy should be reassessed to ensure that participating individuals maintain their self-determination and understand risks and benefits. All participants are shown respect, and no reasonable information is withheld. For example, when enrolling prisoners in a research study, they have a right to volunteer for research, but the prison living conditions should not lead to coercion or undue influence over the protocol.[3] Questions of respect for persons or autonomy include the following:

- Does each potential subject have the personal capacity to willfully choose to participate in the research or evaluation?
- Is anyone feeling internal or external pressure to participate?
- Are the subjects free to withdraw from the research?

Beneficence is aligned with the Hippocratic Oath principle of "do no harm," protecting individuals from harm by maximizing possible benefits and minimizing possible risks. In medical research, experimental medical treatments are ethical when the chance of possible benefit outweighs the risk of possible harm. However, in medical research, because it is not known if the experimental treatment will benefit or harm the participant, it is necessary to recognize that benefits and risks may result while gaining knowledge. Beneficence assumes that risks are minimized as individuals and society benefit from participation in research. Beneficence is often ambiguous, especially when the research involves more than minimal risk with no definitive and measurable benefits. At this point, the participant's choice must be free of coercion, and he or she must be given all possible choices to make a completely informed decision. The researcher is required to stop the research at any time when it becomes clear that the participants are harmed.[8] Questions of beneficences include the following:

- Is the research providing benefits to the subjects?
- Is the research needed to move science forward?
- Is it possible that the researchers stand to gain more from the research than the subjects do, such as data collection for academic publications and future grant applications to promote their personal careers?
- Are the subjects protected from possible risks of harm, or are they being used as data points with limited regard for their well-being?

Justice requires a fair distribution of burden and benefits, so that every person with the same condition has an equal chance of being exposed and an equal chance of benefitting from the treatment.[8] There are two levels of justice: individual and social. Individual justice occurs when specific volunteers are recruited because they would potentially benefit from the research and other volunteers are specifically not recruited due to undesirable traits or medical conditions. Social justice requires the equal distribution of research benefit or burden across the target population rather than a select portion of the population.[3] When a researcher recruits volunteers, it is essential to justify the selection process. Volunteer research participants cannot be chosen simply because of their availability or their compromised position in society, but rather for reasons directly related to the research question. On the other hand, justice requires that when new medical technology is successfully developed, every individual with the medical condition should have equal access to the benefits of the new technology, regardless of ability to pay. Questions of justice include the following:

- Is there a fair distribution of burden and benefits?
- Does every person in the target audience have the same chance of being selected for the research?

- Are the patients with the same illness seeking care at the local county health department being recruited at the same rate as patients seeking care at a private physician's office?
- Because of lack of random assignment, is one group of patients serving as the nontreatment group while another group of similar patients is benefitting from the treatment?

Although respect for persons, beneficence, and justice are the main ethical principles, there are additional ethical principles—nonmaleficence, paternalism, and utilitarianism—often noted in medical research.[3]

Nonmaleficence is defined as refraining from causing harm or acting with malice toward a person. Questions of nonmaleficence include the following:

- Even if the research or evaluation is not causing harm, is it possible that it is not refraining from malice?
- What does a subject gain by being asked to disclose his sexual or criminal activity for the purpose of research or evaluation?
- Even if the subject signed the informed consent paperwork, does answering personal questions cause the subject to experience anxiety?
- If a person is involved in a longitudinal study for several years, do the constant reminders to remain involved feel like an invasion of privacy over time regardless of the research topic?

Paternalism involves a relationship of uneven power between a healthcare provider and a patient. For example, it is paternalistic for a healthcare provider to insist on a treatment without informing and educating the patient about all available options. In this case, without the patient's consent, the healthcare provider takes the role of a parent and places the adult patient in the role of a child. Questions of paternalism include the following:

- Did the healthcare provider treat the adult patient as a child?
- Was medical information withheld from the adult patient because the healthcare provider did not think the person should be told about the medical diagnosis?
- Was the adult patient given information about alternative medical treatments, or was the patient only given information on the treatment the healthcare provider thought was best?

Utilitarianism is the decision, behavior, or action that achieves the greatest good for the greatest number of people.[8] For example, some healthcare providers might think it is ok to recruit cancer patients to determine the dosage of a new medication. The research is not designed to help these current cancer patients, but rather to determine the correct dosage for future patients. This type of research design involves questionable ethics. Questions of utilitarianism include the following:

- Is the research design aimed at current or future patients?
- Is only one specific group, such as Medicaid patients, recruited for a research study, but all patients with the same medical condition will benefit from the research?

Ethical Links Between Research and Evaluation

Building on the historical background and basic ethical principles already discussed, let's explore the ethical links between research and evaluations. Keep in mind that the purpose of research is to create new knowledge, whereas the purpose of evaluation is to improve programs. Any type of research that involves collecting any type of data (interviews, tissue samples, survey completion, etc.) from human subjects must involve an ethical review to ensure the physical, psychological, and social safety of the human subjects. Now let's discuss evaluations. Even though evaluations are not creating new knowledge like research, most evaluations do involve collecting data from human subjects. Although there are differences between the purpose of research and purpose of evaluation, the need to protect human subjects remains the same. That being said, there can sometimes be some blurring between research and evaluation on certain projects. It is possible for one project to involve both research and evaluation. For example, a funded project conducts research to develop an innovative teen pregnancy prevention curriculum for after-school programs, and the same team implements the innovative curriculum and conducts the evaluation to determine if teen pregnancy rates have dropped over the five-year longitudinal evaluation. Because the team involved is conducting both the research and the evaluation (often at the same time), it would be wise to hold both activities to the same research standards.

Confidentiality of Medical Information and Research Data

Confidentiality of medical information and research data is an essential component of health care as well and research and evaluation studies. After obtaining informed consent from an individual, healthcare providers and investigators are responsible for protecting every aspect of their personal information including contact information, survey responses, medical data, test results, and interview responses. They are responsible for maintaining this protection for the duration of the research and until seven years after the completion of the research. It cannot be emphasized enough that all data must be stored in locked cabinets or in password-protected databases. More elaborate procedures are necessary when the collected data involves sensitive information such as criminal activities or sexual behaviors. When studies involve assigning codes for identifiers, the investigators must separate the actual names from the assigned codes to maintain confidentiality. Investigators are responsible for ensuring that their staff receives the required training on federal guidelines related to data confidentiality. For example, hospital administrators must ensure confidentiality of patient medical records just as investigators must protect data collected from study participants.

The most common training for patient and data confidentiality is related to the Health Insurance Portability and Accountability Act (HIPAA), which passed in 1996 under President Bill Clinton. Title I of HIPAA protects health insurance coverage for workers and their families if they change or lose their jobs. Title II of HIPAA is known as *administrative simplification* and establishes the national standards for electronic healthcare transactions and national identifiers for providers, health insurance plans, and employers.[9] For the consumer, HIPAA provides individuals the right to determine who may read or receive a copy of their medical records, add corrections to their medical records, give permission for sharing health information, and file a complaint with the healthcare provider, health insurer, or the federal government. If anyone feels that their medical records have been handled inappropriately, they may file a complaint at the U.S. Department of Health and Human Services website, www.hhs.gov/ocr/hipaa/. The type of medical information that is protected includes information added to the individual's medical record, conversations shared between healthcare providers about an individual's care, personal medical information in computer system databases, and billing information.[10]

Whether in health care or research, hospital administrators, principal investigators, and head researchers are responsible for ensuring that each person providing health care or working on research is familiar with the details of HIPAA and knows how to protect the privacy of patient data, records, conversations, surveys, and any other information that is collected. There are several websites that offer training for HIPAA and research certification, including the following:

http://www.unc.edu/hipaa/training.htm
http://privacy.health.ufl.edu/training/visitors/instructions.shtml
http://www.hhs.gov/ocr/privacy/hipaa/understanding/training/index.html

Table 2-1   Professional Codes of Ethics

Health Education	http://www.nchec.org/credentialing/ethics/
Nursing	http://www.nursingworld.org/codeofethics
Medicine	http://www.ama-assn.org/ama/pub/physician-resources/medical-ethics/code-medical-ethics.page
Pharmacy	http://www.pharmacist.com/code-ethics
Physical Therapy	http://www.apta.org/EthicsProfessionalism/
Public Health	http://www.apha.org/NR/rdonlyres/1CED3CEA-287E-4185-9CBD-BD405FC60856/0/ethicsbrochure.pdf
Public Health Leadership Society	http://www.phls.org/home/section/3-26/
American Evaluation Association	http://comm.eval.org/codeofconduct/

Healthcare Providers: Medical Care Versus Medical Research

Medical research poses ethical concerns because healthcare providers have the ethical obligation to "do no harm" and protect individuals by maximizing possible benefits and minimizing possible risks. However, the role of healthcare providers changes when they conduct medical research. In research, healthcare providers are conducting experiments to gain new knowledge and answer research questions, rather than to treat an individual's illness. To answer research questions, individuals are recruited to voluntarily participate in medical research. In the research planning phase, it is the researcher's responsibility to review basic ethical principles and confirm that any possible violations are minimized as much as possible. For example, during the informed consent process, it is not possible for a healthcare provider to be certain that the research will protect individuals from harm. The research may involve comparing Drug A and Drug B against the currently available standard of care, Drug C. Medical research never intends to harm volunteers, but individuals may experience a negative reaction to the experimental drug. On the other hand, research may show that Drug A is superior over Drug B and Drug C, so the researcher needs to switch all participating volunteers to Drug A to maximize benefits and reduce risks. Let's revisit the ethical principles by examining the following questions:

- Does the proposed research involve a special population, such as pregnant women, individuals with mental or physical disabilities, elderly individuals, or prisoners?
- What training does the research staff need prior to recruiting subjects?

- If the subjects are involved in the research for several years, how often are the subjects reeducated on the research and asked to sign a new informed consent form?
- If the subjects benefit from participation, is there a fair distribution of the anticipated benefits?
- If the research involves observing subjects in public locations, would a reasonable person be offended by the invasion of their privacy?
- How has the researcher planned for maintaining the confidentiality of the data?

Before moving on, let's apply the ethical principles to a few case studies.

Physical Therapy Example

A 76-year-old patient had heart surgery. After surgery, he moved into the hospital-owned inpatient rehabilitation center for eight weeks of physical therapy. He started to improve during the first few weeks, but lately he has been skipping appointments and stays in his room. The patient told the physical therapist that he wants to go home. His physician thinks the gentleman needs to stay for the full eight weeks. The patient needs his physician's signature to check out of the clinic. From notes in the patient's chart, his physician knows the gentleman wants to go home. The physician is intentionally not responding to the patient's telephone calls, because he knows that the gentleman is not strong enough to go home and care for himself. Is the physician making an ethical decision for this patient?

Nursing Example

It is common for nurses to work in various medical specialties within a hospital. One day the nurse may be asked to move from a medical floor to a postsurgical floor because of a shortage of nurses. For this type of move, the nurse is using approximately the same skills for both types of patients. When a nurse is asked to cover a nursing shortage in a pediatric critical care unit, the nurse is presented with an ethical dilemma. Because the nursing code of ethics focuses on patient safety, should the nurse oblige her employer and work her shift in the unfamiliar critical care unit or adhere to patient safety and refuse to work in the critical care unit?

Medical Example

A second-year resident is asked by her attending physician to obtain patient consent for a surgical procedure to reduce the patient's shoulder pain following a sports injury. After reviewing the patient's chart, the resident realizes that the scheduled procedure is not required to eliminate the shoulder pain. At a recent conference, the resident learned that a simple injection of cortical steroid has been proven to be just as effective for this type of shoulder pain. The resident is not comfortable obtaining the patient's signature on the surgical consent form, because she knows that the procedure is not necessary, is expensive, and requires several hospital days for postoperative recovery. What ethical principles are being violated in this situation?

Hospital Administration Example

Healthcare providers in a hospital setting observe situations where they cannot help but think about the cost associated with caring for a terminally ill patient who would be better served in the hospital hospice unit. Caring for terminally ill patients on a medical floor involves spending valuable healthcare dollars that some would argue might better serve other patients with a higher chance of survival. What ethic principle includes this type of argument?

Hospital Ethics Committee Example

A 36-year-old quadriplegic patient of sound mind requests to be removed from life-support systems during his current hospitalization. He has been a quadriplegic for 18 years and does not wish to continue to live in this medical condition. He obtained a do-not-resuscitate (DNR) order a few years ago. His healthcare practitioners refuse to remove his life-support devices. The patient and the healthcare practitioners refer the case to the hospital ethics committee for resolution. What ethical principles does the committee need to discuss?

Evaluation Example

An evaluation team from the state university was hired by the state health office to provide a recommendation on whether the clinic should remain open. The university and the state senator were both from the city where the clinic was located. The evaluation team was aware of these political challenges, but they decided they would accept the project. During the first month, the clinic administrator arranges personal interviews with a few select clinic board members as a way to assist the evaluation team with making connections. A few weeks later, the clinic financial officer offered to supply billing data. During the second month, the evaluation team was told by several employees that the number of patients seen at the clinic was lower than what was recorded in the electronic medical records and that the submission of fraudulent insurance claims was a common practice. However, these staff members also stated their fear of being unemployed if the clinic closed. The evaluation project was getting complex and teeming with a variety of ethical issues. Although it is not the job of evaluators to become investigative detectives, they do need to be aware of underlying legal and politics issues. What ethical principles apply to this situation? How should the evaluation team proceed?

Institutional Review Board

An institutional review board (IRB) is a committee that serves to formally approve, monitor, and review every type of biomedical and behavioral research that involves human subjects. The purpose of the IRB is to protect the rights and welfare of the research subjects. At the national level, the U.S. Food and Drug Administration (FDA) and the U.S. Department of Health and Human Services (DHHS) oversee the IRB regulations including approval, required modifications of research, and disapproval of research.[11] Keep in mind that each agency or division under the FDA and DHHS has its own rules and regulations for biomedical and behavioral research and evaluation. At the local level, institutions have their own IRB committees, such as universities, hospitals, clinics, health departments, and school districts. Every IRB committee performs oversight functions of all research conducted on human subjects within their institutions. In some situations, researchers must obtain IRB approval from more than one committee. For example, if a university researcher receives state funding to conduct an evaluation at a local health department clinic, the investigator must receive IRB approval from the university IRB as well as the local health department IRB committee.[3]

To accomplish the purpose of the IRB, the committee members review research protocols, informed consent documents, recruitment brochures, surveys, interview and focus group question guides, and all other materials related to the research. The IRB also reviews procedures involving previously collected patient data or secondary data, such as patient charts, lab and medical test results, prescription drug data, satisfaction surveys, financial information, and any other type of outcome data. The protocol is to assess the research ethics and methods, and to ensure that participation is informed and voluntary and that all subjects are capable of making personal decisions. The IRB committee approves research and evaluations that provide informed consent for subjects, shows that the risks to the subjects are balanced with potential societal benefits, and proves that subject selection is fair with equal distribution of risks and benefits to eligible participants.[12] Each IRB committee requires a written application with the following required components:[3]

- Research protocols and amendments
- Written informed consent forms
- Participant recruitment procedures and advertisements
- Written information provided to participants
- Research or evaluation plan
- Information about availability of compensation and schedule of payments
- Safety information to accommodate any adverse conditions resulting from the research, including name and contact information of lead researcher, evidence of the researcher's qualifications, and names of all personnel involved with any aspect of research

Depending on the type of research, IRB committees request additional information and multiple document revisions prior to making a final approval decision. Applications of the general principles to the conduct of research leads to consideration of the following requirements: informed consent, risk/benefit assessment, and selection of individuals for research.

Informed Consent

Informed consent is the hallmark of human subject research because it reflects the individual's right to respect and autonomy. Informed consent is not a one-time encounter to obtain an individual's signature, but rather an ongoing process to ensure that human subjects continue to understand that their involvement is voluntary. According to the DHHS,[12] informed consent must include the following components: full disclosure, comprehension, adequate compensation, and voluntary choice.

Full disclosure: Full disclosure involves revealing the purpose and expected duration of the subject's participation, procedures involved, description of potential risks and benefits, appropriate alternative procedures or treatments, confidentiality of records, and a statement affirming that participation is voluntary and that refusal or withdrawal will not result in a penalty or loss of entitled benefits. All informed consents must be written using laypeople's words with simple sentence structure and presented in the preferred language of each potential human subject for maximum comprehension. Here are a few examples of how to simplify medical terminology: bruise instead of hematoma, arms instead of upper extremities, pills instead of medications. In addition, informed consent documents include information on the researcher's name and how to contact them to answer questions, as well as information about the ability to withdraw at any time from the research without penalty. It is important that participants know that their participation is not required for their care and understand the range of risks and benefits involved. The written informed consent document is given to the person and orally discussed by the researcher each time, and in some situations there must be a third party present to witness the process as well as the person's and researcher's signatures.[12]

Informed consent problems arise when certain aspects of the research are likely to change a patient's response or behavior; for example, if the research involves healthcare provider interactions with patients. If healthcare providers are told that their patient interactions will be videotaped, it is likely that the healthcare provider will act differently. In this case, it is sufficient to invite healthcare providers to participate in a quality improvement study and inform them that the exact purpose will be revealed when the research is concluded. Whenever research involves incomplete disclosure, it is required that incomplete disclosure is essential to complete the research, undisclosed risks are no more than minimal, and debriefing sessions are planned along with dissemination of results. Full disclosure may never be withheld to increase recruitment or cooperation.[3]

Comprehension: When researchers or evaluators are explaining the informed consent document, it is important that participants understand every aspect of the research. This understanding means that the document must be written in the preferred language of the individual and at an appropriate written and verbal literacy level. The time and location of obtaining consent are considered. Consents are obtained during normal business hours in a quiet location. Individuals may wish to have family members present to hear the explanation and ask questions, although the participating individual makes the final decision. For example, if research is explained quickly in a noisy hospital waiting room, chances are that the individual will not be allowed sufficient time to make an informed choice. Obtaining the informed consent is viewed as an educational process. It is the researcher's responsibility to ensure that individuals understand and comprehend the information. As potential risks increase, so does the obligation of complete understanding prior to giving consent. Sometimes an added safeguard is used, such as asking the individual to repeat the explanation of the research. IRB committees need to make every effort to enhance the subject's comprehension. Even with the best intentions, a researcher may communicate every aspect of the informed consent document, but the subject fails to fully understand his participation in the study. The reasons for lack of understanding may be, for example, mental capability being diminished by age or physical or mental disabilities;

being under the influence of medications, alcohol, or other substances; fear of reduced healthcare services; need for monetary compensation; or real or imaginary feelings of coercion. When research involves a specific medical condition, such as dementia, an individual's legal guardian is asked to sign the informed consent, make surrogate decisions, and protect him or her from harm.[12]

Adequate compensation: Adequate compensation for participation in research is not specifically stated in the federal regulations. The IRB committee determines the risk of possible coercion as well as reasonable compensation for each situation. Incentives must not be so attractive that potential participants are blinded to the risks or conceal accurate information for admission into the lucrative research. Compensation does not need to be a cash payment. Other types of compensation include bus tokens, travel reimbursement, babysitting services, movie tickets, or gift cards.[12]

Voluntary choice: Voluntary choice involves an agreement to participate in research after individuals understand every aspect of the study. In addition, they must be free of coercion and undue influence. Coercion occurs when a person in power threatens harm if individuals do not agree to participate in the research and sign the consent form. For example, a prisoner would experience coercion if the warden announces that all prisoners must participate in the study or else special privileges will be evoked. Undue influence happens when an excessive incentive is offered for participation; for example, if a pharmaceutical company expedites patient recruitment by offering $1,000 to every Medicaid patient with hypertension to take eight doses of a new experimental hypertension drug. Because Medicaid patients likely need $1,000, they could sign consent forms without asking questions in order to receive the excessive cash payment. Undue influence also occurs when a family member is persuaded to convince the patient to participate in the study, thus removing the patient's choice. Threatening to revoke healthcare services is also a threat of undue influence.[3]

Other considerations of informed consent involve observational research, active and passive consents, secondary data, and cultural and diversity concerns.

Observational research: When human behavior is observed, researchers request an informed consent waiver because subjects may act differently when observed. For example, researchers may wish to observe human behavior, so they stage a biker hitting a pedestrian at a crowded intersection. For this type of research, IRB committees apply common sense and consider the degree of risk for the subjects involved without their consent.

Active consent and passive consent: These terms are commonly used in a school setting when research involves noninvasive study with students under age

18 years. When a passive consent form is used, the researcher gives the students a document to take home to their parents or guardians. With passive consent, the parent or guardian may read about the noninvasive research. If the document is not returned to school, the student will participate in the research. If the parent or guardian does not wish the student to participate, the signed form must be returned to school. Because it is common that students do not give such forms to their parents, some parents are never made aware of the research. In this case, regardless of the reason the parent never responds, the student is allowed to participate in the research. To clarify, passive consent means the student participates by passive parental consent. For active consent, the researcher sends the document home with the students. In this case, however, the student is unable to participate unless the document is signed by the parent and returned by the student. Parents need to be "active" for their child to participate. In this case, the researchers offer incentives for students to return the signed form in a short period of time. For example, the class with the greatest number of returned signed forms by Friday receives a pizza party, or each student who returns a signed form receives a school t-shirt.

Secondary data: Common examples of secondary data include patient medical charts, birth and death certificates, traffic violations, motor vehicle records, medical billing records, school attendance records, and insurance company vehicular claims data. Most secondary data are obtained in the form of aggregate data, which is defined as records that do not contain any personal or identifying information that could be linked back to a specific individual. For example, hospital administrators use secondary data to determine if the rate of patient readmissions due to nosocomial or hospital-acquired infections has increased or decreased during a specified period of time. Secondary aggregate data provide specific information about patients who were readmitted to the hospital within 30 days of discharge. Data are deidentified and do not include patient names, addresses, or contact information. By linking the initial diagnosis with the readmission diagnosis, hospital administrators are able to pinpoint the possible cause of the infection by specific location within the hospital, type of procedure or treatment, type of infection, medical specialty, and so on. Biased data would result if patients are readmitted to another hospital with an infection.

Cultural and diversity issues: IRB committees verify that the research staff has appropriate cultural and diversity sensitivity training so that participating individuals are treated with respect. If participating individuals feel comfortable, they are more likely to respond honestly to personal questions. For example, even though the researcher from one culture views the interview question as routine, the responding person from another culture may view the identical question as intrusive. Topics that may be considered sensitive in various cultures include diverse marriage and parenting attitudes, sexual behaviors, employment loyalty, loyalty to healthcare practitioners, religious beliefs and practices, use of traditional medical treatments, and so on. Researchers and evaluators need to be comfortable with not only the topic but also the potential ethical issues that may arise when recruiting individuals from various cultural backgrounds.[12]

Risk/Benefit Assessment

The risks and benefits of research are carefully weighed by the IRB committee, researcher, and participating individual. Based on known data, risk is defined as the chance that harm may occur. Risk is usually viewed as high, moderate, or low. Risks may include psychological, physical, legal, social, or economic harm. A benefit is viewed as a positive health or welfare value. The risk–benefit ratio assessment is considered as the probability and extent of possible harm versus anticipated benefits. In the IRB application, it is essential to clearly state known risks according to the medical literature as well as available alternative choices. When risk–benefit ratios are unknown, the researcher is unable to disclose the information in the informed consent. This situation is called *equipoise* and is defined as the uncertainty of the therapeutic treatment effectiveness. This issue requires that the informed consent document state that the effectiveness of the experimental treatment is unknown.[13] Risk–benefit ratios are also a concern when the research participant is pregnant or becomes pregnant in the future. Again, the informed consent document must include a statement about the possibility of unforeseeable risks, including risks to the current or future embryo or fetus, the ability to become pregnant, and for males the ability to impregnate a partner in the future. Lastly, for researchers, the risk–benefit ratio must be fully disclosed in the informed consent document as well as in the research design. For the IRB committee, any potential risks must be justified and offset by benefits when feasible. Participating individuals must understand the risk–benefit ratio, have the opportunity to ask questions throughout the research, and know that they can withdraw from the study at any time.

Selection of Individuals and Special Populations

When IRB committees review an application, particular attention is paid to special populations that may be recruited for participation in the research or evaluations. Each category of special populations poses unique considerations related to informed consent. Depending on the degree of risk and therapeutic component, some groups of individuals are more suitable for recruitment than others, unless the research is related to a specific medical condition, such as depression among institutionalized individuals. Also, individuals who are dependent on public healthcare services should not bear the burden of research when advantaged individuals are also recipients of benefits. Other special populations receive specific IRB regard. For example, children or individuals with mental health disabilities may not be able to understand the scope of the research. As for prisoners or institutionalized individuals, it is questionable if their consent is truly voluntary or perceived as mandatory. Hospitalized and very sick patients may have diminished comprehension because of medications, emergency treatment, or pain management. These patients may concede their rights to gain additional or faster medical benefits or enroll in research to please their healthcare practitioners. Such individuals need protection against research recruitment for reasons like convenience, medical diagnosis, or socioeconomic status.[12] In research studies or evaluation projects, recruiting pregnant women is an ethical slippery slope. On one hand, if the research involves enhancement of prenatal care, pregnant women need to be enrolled in research to move prenatal science forward, but on the other hand, there is a fundamental obligation to the health and well-being of the woman and the fetus. Lastly, the elderly constitute a special population, and their issues incorporate many of the previously stated concerns for all special populations. Overall, the investigators and the IRB committee must be aware of the unique ethical concerns when recruiting individuals from special populations. IRB committees must not overprotect special populations to the detriment of research, and one group of subjects should not bear more risks for the benefits of another group. Adequate representation of special populations is important, especially in research that may disproportionately affect that same population.[3]

Summary

This chapter provides a historical overview of medical ethics, including two landmark cases that violated federal laws and doctrine. This discussion was followed by a discussion of the basic principles of medical ethics with examples. The next section described the purpose of the institutional review board and how to design comprehensive informed consent documents, including the consideration of special populations.

Case Study: *Diaz vs. Hillsbourgh County Hospital Authority*

In 1987, Karen Perrin reported to the high-risk perinatal outpatient clinic at Tampa General Hospital with affiliation to the University of South Florida in Tampa. She was looking forward to a busy day and the change of pace. Karen had worked at Tampa General since January 1986. Her normal assignment was labor and delivery, but as a part-time nurse, it was not unusual for her to fill in elsewhere. For the next two weeks, Karen worked at the outpatient high-risk pregnancy clinic while Sue, the clinic's head nurse, took time off for her wedding. In total, Karen was assigned to work in the clinic for a total of four weeks. She worked in the clinic for two weeks, returned to her regular position for two weeks, and then was again temporarily assigned to the clinic for two additional weeks because Sue's daughter became ill.

Among other clinic tasks, Karen cared for high-risk pregnant women who came to the clinic for amniocenteses. Amniocentesis is a procedure in which a needle is inserted through a women's abdomen to extract amniotic fluid for testing.[14] Karen entered each patient's name, hospital number, and Medicaid or insurance number into the "amnio" record log at the desk. She took the patient's weight and blood pressure, measured her belly, and checked her urine. She set up the tray of amniocentesis needles and test tubes and labels for the tubes. She explained the procedure to the patients, offered reassurance, and asked if they had any questions.[15]

During her clinic assignment, Karen noticed something unusual. The pregnant women did not ask questions about the procedure. "I kept seeing all these women having amnios. Over and over and over. I'd see them one week, I'd say, "Why are you back again?" I'm looking in their chart and I'm seeing that this is amnio #5, amnio #6. . . ."[15] When she talked with the pregnant women, it was clear that they did not understand why they were having so many amniocenteses. Their response was always the same: "The doctor told me, if I don't do them, my baby will die."[16]

continues

CASE STUDY *continued*

An Inquiry

In late 1987, Karen consulted her supervisor. A meeting was schedule with the vice president of nursing and director of the perinatal unit. They told her that the pregnant women were part of a medical study that had been approved by university and hospital institutional review boards. Therefore, they considered the matter closed. Her supervisor told her to drop the issue and not pursue additional investigation into the matter. Karen did not stop because she suspected that the women were unaware of a medical study. She continued to press for further investigation. In February 1988, a final meeting was held and the vice president of nursing made it clear that she had not taken any action and that she did not intend to investigate the matter further.

The Next Step

Karen shared her concerns with a friend who was a civil rights attorney, Stephen Hanlon. At the advice of Mr. Hanlon and the American Nursing Association, Karen was instructed to gather the evidence. She went to the high-risk clinic, took the amnio record log, made a copy, and returned the log to the clinic drawer. She returned a few days later to copy the last few pages, only to discover that "someone had taken a razor blade and cut all the pages out of the book. The pages were gone, and they were never found again. This was our only evidence."[15] She provided the copied amnio record log to Stephen Hanlon. She also found the contact information for 10 women in the log who had multiple amnioceteses. She contacted them by mail and stated that their rights may have been violated and invited them to contact her. Only one woman, Flora Diaz, age 16, responded.

The Lawsuit

In January 1990, Stephen Hanlon filed a federal class action lawsuit accusing the university, the hospital, and two physician researchers of ignoring DHHS regulations on informed consent. Although the lawsuit

continues

CASE STUDY *continued*

was initially filed in response to a fetal lung study[17] involving approximately 280 women, investigation revealed some 30 studies at Tampa General involving 5,000 pregnant women between November 1986 and January 1990. Because none of the women or their babies were harmed, this case is not about malpractice but rather a matter of dignity. The women were used as research subjects without their informed consent.

Doctors' Perspective

Walter Morales, MD, one of two physician researchers in the lawsuit, denied any wrongdoing. "I can assure you I would never do anything to a research subject that I wouldn't do to my own wife."[18] Furthermore, he noted that he wished the case had gone to trial instead of being settled because he did not believe that the facts would show the patients were coerced into signing the forms.[16] The results of the study were published in the *Journal of Obstetrics and Gynecology*, and as a result, the combined use of corticosteroids and thyrotropin-releasing hormone is now common practice in many hospitals.[19]

The Settlement

After almost 10 years of litigation, the case was settled out of court. Under the agreement, the university and the state of Florida paid $2.7 million and Tampa General Hospital paid $1.14 million.[20] In addition to the cash payment, the hospital and university agreed to revise record keeping so that information on study participants was easily accessible in a database. Tampa General Hospital and the University of South Florida also agreed to apply a standard readability test to their consent forms before submitting future projects to the IRB.

A Postscript

Karen Perrin, whistle-blower in this case, was removed from patient care and was laid off from the hospital in September 1990.[21] The hospital made attempts to revoke her nursing license, but she successfully

continues

CASE STUDY *continued*

defended her actions with the assistance of the American Nursing Association.[22] Karen completed her master's in public health in 1990 and her PhD in 1996 from the College of Public Health at the University of South Florida. Currently, she is an associate professor at the University of South Florida and lectures on medical ethics.[15] Dr. Perrin is the author of this text.

Case Study Discussion Questions

1. What other actions could the nurse have taken?
2. What is the role of the medical residents in this case?
3. What is the role of the nurse supervisor?

Student Activity

1. Write a 200-word case study describing a violation of an ethical principle related to an area of healthcare interest.
2. Obtain two examples of IRB applications from a local hospital, health clinic, school district, or university. Compare and contrast the information required on each document.
3. Obtain an advanced directive or living will from three different states. Compare and contrast the information required on each document.

References

1. National Institutes of Health Office of Human Subjects Research. Regulations and guidelines, directives for human experimentation, Nuremburg code. Reprinted from *Trials of War Criminals Before the Nuremberg Military Tribunals Under Control Council Law* No. 10, Vol. 2, pp. 181–182. Washington, DC: U.S. Government Printing Office; 1949. Available at: http://www.recerca.uab.es/ceeah/docs/Nuremberg%20 code.pdf. Accessed January 12, 2012.
2. United States Department of Health and Human Services Office for Human Research Protections. HHS Announces Proposal to Improve Rules Protecting Human Research Subjects. Available at: http://www.hhs.gov/ohrp/index.html. Accessed January 12, 2012.

3. United States Department of Health and Human Services. The Belmont Report. Available at: http://www.hhs.gov/ohrp/humansubjects/guidance/belmont.html. Accessed January 12, 2012.

4. Centers for Disease Control and Prevention. The U.S. Public Health Service Syphilis Study at Tuskegee: The Tuskegee Timeline. Available at: http://www.cdc.gov/tuskegee/timeline.htm. Accessed January 12, 2012.

5. Centers for Disease Control and Prevention. The U.S. Public Health Service Syphilis Study at Tuskegee: A Presidential Apology. Available at: http://www.cdc.gov/tuskegee/clintonp.htm. Accessed January 12, 2012.

6. Zielinksi S. Henrietta Lacks' "immortal" cells. *The Smithsonian*. January 22, 2010. Available at: http://www.smithsonianmag.com/science-nature/Henrietta-Lacks-Immortal-Cells.html. Accessed January 12, 2012.

7. Rebecca Skloot. About *The Immortal Life of Henrietta Lacks*. Available at: http://rebeccaskloot.com/the-immortal-life. Accessed January 12, 2012.

8. The Joint Commission. *Hospital Accreditation Standards*. Oakbrook Terrace, IL: JCAHO; 2009.

9. Centers for Medicare and Medicaid Services. HIPAA: General Overview. Available at: https://www.cms.gov/hipaageninfo/. Accessed January 12, 2012.

10. National Hospice and Palliative Care Organization. Summary of the HIPAA Privacy Rule. Available at: http://www.caringinfo.org/files/public/ad/HIPPA_Privacy_Rule.pdf. Accessed January 12, 2012.

11. U.S. Department of Health and Human Services. Regulations. Available at: http://www.hhs.gov/ohrp/humansubjects/index.html. Accessed January 12, 2012.

12. U.S. Department of Health and Human Services Office for Human Research Protections. IRB Guidebook. Available at: www.hhs.gov/ohrp/archive/irb/irb_guidebook.htm. Accessed January 12, 2012.

13. Petrini C. Ethical issues in translational research. *Perspect Biol Med.* 2010;53(4): 517–533.

14. O'Connor TL. *A Patient Guide to Amniocentesis.* Tampa, FL: Tampa General Hospital; 1987.

15. Werner D. Personal communication with Dr. Karen Perrin in preparation for forthcoming book. Donna Werner, PhD, Philosophy Chairperson, Humanities Department, St. Louis Community College, St. Louis, MO.

16. Aronson P. A medical indignity. *National Law Journal.* 2000:A1.

17. Morales WJ, O'Brien WF, Angel JL, Knuppel RA, Sawai S. Fetal lung maturation: The combined use of corticosteroids and thyrotropin-releasing hormone. *Obstet Gyneco.* 1998;73:111–116.

18. Hanlon S. Clinical Research Trials and Tribulations. Presentation, American Bar Association, November 10, 2000.

19. Kaighin A. Physician defends research on fetuses. *Tampa Tribune.* February 3, 1990.

20. Ricks D. Court case mars legacy of helping doctor: Research was based in compassion. *Orlando Sentinel.* March 26, 1990.

21. *Diaz v. Florida Board of Regents*, 8:90-cv-00120-HLA (2000).

22. Washington W. Hospital, USF settle 'dignity' suit. *St. Petersburg Times.* March 11, 2000.

3

Determinants of Health

CHAPTER OBJECTIVES

By the end of this chapter, students will be able to:

- Describe three historical health changes that have taken place over the last century
- Define the concept of health disparities
- Examine how *Healthy People 2020* relates to the social determinants of health
- Rate which social determinants of health are most essential for optimal health outcomes
- Create a MAP-IT project for a local community health issue

KEY TERMS

Health disparities   Social determinants of health
Healthy People 2020

Introduction

This chapter introduces how researchers and evaluators look beyond disease and disability when studying health programs. Before jumping to the chapter, let's begin with laying a foundation by presenting a brief overview of historical achievements in health. It is difficult to plan and evaluate future health programs without knowing some of the past success stories. The historical background is followed by an introduction to a discussion of health disparities and social determinants as viewed by the U.S. Department of Health and Human Services *Healthy People 2020*. At the end of the chapter, an evaluation tool called MAP-IT (Mobilize, Assess, Plan, Implement, Track) describes a method to achieve the *Healthy People 2020* objectives in program planning, research, and evaluation.

Historical View of Achievement in Health

In the last century, individuals in the United States enjoyed improved health and life expectancy thanks to many public health achievements (see **Table 3-1** and **Table 3-2**).[1-4] For example, fewer people died from infectious diseases such as

Table 3-1 Ten Great Public Health Achievements in the United States, 1900–1999

Cardiovascular disease[5]	Fewer deaths from stroke and coronary heart disease thanks to smoking cessation, blood pressure control, and early detection and treatment
Contraceptive and family planning options	Altered social and economic roles of women such as smaller family size, longer intervals between pregnancies, fewer maternal and infant deaths
Fluoridation of drinking water[6]	Reduction of childhood tooth decay and tooth loss in adults
Food safety	Less microbial contamination and increase in nutritional content
Healthier mothers and babies	Improved hygiene and nutrition, antibiotics, greater access to health care, and maternal and neonatal medical advances
Highway safety[7]	Safer motor vehicles, improved vehicles and highway engineering, and increased use of seatbelts, child safety seats, and motorcycle helmets
Infectious disease control	Clean water and improved sanitation, antimicrobial therapy for tuberculosis and sexually transmitted diseases
Occupational safety[8]	Fewer injuries in the workplace environment thanks to safer protective equipment, improved ventilation, fewer toxic exposures, and shorter work hours
Tobacco control	Recognition of tobacco use as a health hazard, successful antismoking campaigns that changed social norms to reduce initiation of tobacco use, increase cessation, and reduce environmental tobacco smoke exposure
Vaccinations[9]	Reduced number of childhood diseases: measles, mumps, rubella, chicken pox; latest HPV vaccine to reduce cervical cancer

Adapted from Centers for Disease Control and Prevention. Ten great public health achievements—United States, 1900–1999. *MMWR*. 1999;48(12):241–243. Available at: http://www.cdc.gov/mmwr/preview/mmwrhtml/00056796.htm. Accessed January 12, 2012.

Table 3-2 Top Ten Causes of Death from 1900 to 2007 in the United States

Rank	1900*	1920	1950	2007**
	Life expectancy: 49.2 years	Life expectancy: 54.1 years	Life expectancy: 68.2 years	Life expectancy: 77.8 years
1	Influenza/pneumonia	Influenza/pneumonia	Heart disease	Heart disease
2	Tuberculosis	Heart disease	Cancer	Cancer
3	Diarrhea/enteritis	Tuberculosis	Stroke	Stroke
4	Heart disease	Stroke	Accidents	Chronic lower respiratory disease
5	Stroke	Kidney disease	Infant death	Accidents
6	Kidney disease	Cancer	Influenza/pneumonia	Diabetes
7	Accidents	Accidents	Tuberculosis	Alzheimer's disease
8	Cancer	Diarrhea/enteritis	Arteriosclerosis	Influenza/pneumonia
9	Senility	Premature birth	Kidney disease	Kidney disease
10	Diphtheria	Childbirth conditions	Diabetes	Septicemia

Adapted from Centers for Disease Control and Prevention. Leading Causes of Death. Available at: http://www.cdc.gov/nchs/fastats/lcod.htm. Accessed January 12, 2012; Centers for Disease Control and Prevention. Leading Causes of Death, 1900–1998. Available at: http://www.cdc.gov/nchs/data/dvs/lead1900_98.pdf. Accessed January 12, 2012; National Center of Health Statistics. *National Vital Statistics Report: Fast Facts A to Z*. Atlanta, GA: Centers for Disease Control and Prevention; 2006.

tuberculosis and dysentery after people understood the importance of clean water and sanitation. Deaths caused by motor vehicles decreased after the production of safer vehicles, the introduction of seatbelt laws, and the advocacy of Mothers Against Drunk Driving (MADD). As a result of these and other changes, life expectancy has increased by more than 30 years over the last century. Not only are people living longer, but *how* people are dying has also changed over the same time period.

Before moving on, take a closer look at Table 3-2 by answering the following questions:

1. What happened between 1920 and 1950 that caused influenza to drop from first to sixth place?
2. Why did cancer move from eighth in 1900 to sixth in 1920 to second in 1950 and 2007?
3. What made chronic lower respiratory disease appear on the list in 2007?
4. What changed to move diabetes from tenth in 1950 to sixth in 2007?

5. Why has kidney disease remained ninth since 1950?

6. What other changes are puzzling across time?

(Answers appear at the end of the chapter.)

Over the years, the leading causes of death changed from infectious disease to chronic disease influenced by behavioral choices, such as tobacco usage, poor diet, lack of physical activity, and alcohol consumption.[10] Building on the shift to chronic disease, in 1979, the U.S. Department of Health and Human Services published the Surgeon General's report *Healthy People: The Surgeon General's Report on Health Promotion and Disease Prevention.* This document described the current health of the U.S. population and set goals for the future. Every decade since that time, the document is updated with a new health focus.[11]

As researchers study and evaluators plan health programs, *Healthy People 2020* serves as a valuable resource for the national goals and objectives. For example, if researchers wish to study the relationship between diabetes and hypertension, it is beneficial to search *Healthy People 2020* to determine the national goals and objectives in comparison to their study population (see **Table 3-3**).[12]

Before moving forward, let's step back and put the pieces together. So far, we have discussed the historical background in which the leading causes of death moved from infectious to chronic diseases and how this change initiated the creation of *Healthy People* over the decades. Using these two discussions as the foundation, next we define the concepts of health disparities and social determinants of health. As previously stated, researchers refer to *Healthy People 2020* to

Table 3-3   Example of a Goal and Objectives from *Healthy People 2020*

Topic	Diabetes
Goal D-7	Increase the proportion of the population with diagnosed diabetes whose blood pressure is under control.
Baseline	51.8% of adults aged 18 years and older with diagnosed diabetes had their blood pressure under control in 2005–2008.
Target	57.0%
Target setting	10% improvement
Data source	National Health and Nutrition Examination Survey (NHANES), Centers for Disease Control and Prevention (CDC), National Center for Health Statistics (NCHS)

Adapted from Healthy People 2020. 2020 Topics and Objectives. Available at: http://www .healthypeople.gov/2020/topicsobjectives2020/objectiveslist.aspx?topicId=8. Accessed May 3, 2013.

establish the national baseline goals and objectives for numerous health topics. However, it is important not to merely plan programs and evaluations around goals and objectives. It is critical to look at other factors, for example, health disparities and social determinants of health that influence the health outcome of individuals.

Health Disparities

Let's begin with the definition of health disparities. *Healthy People 2020* provides the following definition of a health disparity:

> A particular type of health difference that is closely linked with social, economic, and/or environmental disadvantage. Health disparities adversely affect groups of people who have systematically experienced greater obstacles to health based on their racial or ethnic group; religion; socioeconomic status; gender; age; mental health; cognitive, sensory, or physical disability; sexual orientation or gender identity; geographic location; inequities in income, education, and access to health care and other characteristics historically linked to discrimination or exclusion.[13]

In addition, health disparities lead to an individual's inability to achieve and maintain optimal health, for example, in the cases of higher infant mortality and low birth weight rates, shorter life expectancy, and higher rates of chronic disease, stroke, and substance abuse.[14] Health researchers acknowledge that health disparities are interconnected with biological, environmental, and lifestyle behaviors that negatively affect health outcomes. For example, an elderly African American woman living with a disability in a rural area has multiple health disparities. Through no fault of negative lifestyle choices, she is likely to experience poor health outcomes.

As researchers study health programs, they need to take into account the participants' level of health disparities. For example, if a pharmaceutical drug company wishes to study the effectiveness of a newly developed gestational diabetes drug at a local health department clinic, researchers need to be aware that pregnant women may not comply with the required weekly clinic visits in the research protocol. The pregnant women may wish to participate and receive the cash incentive, but because of their inflexible work hours, lack of transportation, or limited healthcare choices, they are unable to comply with the research protocol of attending nonessential weekly clinic visits. Without applying knowledge related to health disparities, the pharmaceutical researchers may falsely conclude that the pregnant women were noncompliant.

Social Determinants of Health

As we move from health disparities to the social determinants of health, let's remember that good health does not always equal the mere absence of disease. Social determinants of health are the complex relationship of factors that influence an individual's or population's health, such as safe and affordable housing, access to education, public safety, availability of healthy foods, local emergency/health services, and environments free of life-threatening toxins[15] (see **Figure 3-1**). In *Healthy People 2020*, social determinants of health explore ways to improve an individual's social and physical environments to improve health (see **Table 3-4**).[16]

Even though it is important, sometimes evaluators find it difficult to step back and view the whole individual who is participating in a specific study. When an evaluation has a narrow and specific focus, it is necessary for evaluators to recall the health disparities and social determinants that each participant may be experiencing on a daily basis. **Table 3-5** provides a scenario about the reasons individuals are not taking their medications.

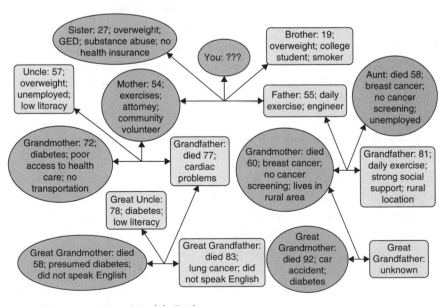

FIGURE 3-1 Your Health Risks

Table 3-4   Examples of Social Determinants of Health

Resources	Available safe resources for daily living, such as safe food and housing
Safety	Exposure to crime, violence, and social disorder within specific communities; residential segregation
Education	Access to quality education, language, and literacy
Employment	Job opportunities and job training
Stress	Socioeconomic conditions, concentrated poverty, and stressful living conditions
Social support	Social support, social norms, and attitudes (e.g., discrimination, racism, and distrust of government)
Health care	Access to healthcare services
Activity	Availability of community-based resources in support of community living and opportunities for recreational, cultural, and leisure-time activities; physical activity
Transportation	Transportation options and public safety
Technology	Access to technology, such as cell phones and the Internet

Referring back to the list in Table 3-4, the following discussion provides a detailed description of a few social determinants of health, including physical activity, education, access to health care, and the resources of safe food, safe housing, and employment. Keep in mind that when evaluators plan and evaluate health programs, it is important to take into account how social determinants of health have an effect on program planning as well as the evaluation and results. For example, healthcare clinic staff may wish to determine how many adults in the community have hypertension. They may decide to conduct a neighborhood health fair that includes free blood pressure screening. Although the health fair sounds like a good idea, it is important to consider the consequences on how to advise individuals identified as at-risk for hypertension. Looking at the previous discussion on health disparities and social determinants of health, the healthcare staff would need to ask the following questions: (1) Do the at-risk individuals have access to health care at the local clinic, or is the clinic at capacity and only taking a few new patients per month? (2) Is there adequate public transportation for the at-risk individuals to get to clinic? (3) Are systems in place at the clinic to accommodate more patients in need of translation services or low literacy health education classes? Are the health education classes already filled? and (4) Does the neighborhood have safe public spaces for walking and other physical activities to lower the rates of obesity in the community? These and other questions need to be considered when researchers ask even a simple question such as "How can we determine the number of people in this community who are at-risk for hypertension?"

Table 3-5   Linking Health Care, Health Disparities, and Social Determinants of Health

---

A team of healthcare providers determines that there is a need to hire an evaluation team to increase hypertensive medication compliance among patients in the internal medicine clinic. The evaluation team, along with the healthcare providers (nurses, pharmacists, social workers, and physicians), plans an evaluation to study what health disparities and social determinants of health create barriers to medication compliance.

Healthcare Provider Concerns	Health Disparities and Social Determinants of Health	Ways to Reduce Barriers
Patients may not understand the importance of taking the medicine each day for long-term benefits.	Education	Provide low literacy health education classes.
Patients may not purchase their medications because their employers do not offer access to health insurance benefits.	Employment and healthcare access	Provide community resources to obtain medications.
Some patients do not speak English, so they may not understand the instructions.	Language barrier	Use translation services.
Patients may not purchase their medicine because they lack transportation to the pharmacy.	Lack of transportation	Offer clinic pharmacy services.
Patients may not take their medication because of undesirable side effects. Their daily lives may be too complex to comply with multiple clinic appointments.	Stress	Allow flexible appointments and phone counseling for minor medication adjustments.
Patient may lack social support and suffer from depression; no willingness to improve health.	Social support	Explore interest in health education classes.
Patient's obesity may contribute to hypertension.	Physical activity	Introduce free community physical activity classes.
Patient's neighborhood violence and stress may contribute to hypertension.	Safety	Investigate other living opportunities to lower stress.

Patients have numerous reasons for medication noncompliance. As healthcare providers learn more about health disparities and social determinants of health, they begin to understand why their patients are not taking their medications rather than simply labeling the patient as noncompliant.

Physical Activity

As previously stated, *Healthy People 2020* is an excellent starting point for developing research questions or for determining how specific topics of social determinants are related to research questions. For example, if the research questions are related to obesity, it is useful to refer to the physical activity section of *Healthy People 2020* in **Table 3-6**. It is well documented that lack of physical activity and excessive sedentary behaviors contribute to increased health disparities in

---

Table 3-6   Physical Activity Objectives

Healthy People 2020

Goal PA-1	Reduce the proportion of adults who engage in no leisure-time physical activity.
Goal PA-2	Increase the proportion of adults who meet current federal physical activity guidelines for aerobic physical activity and for muscle-strengthening activity.

Sub-Goal PA-2.1	Increase the proportion of adults who engage in aerobic physical activity of at least moderate intensity for at least 150 minutes/week, or 75 minutes/week of vigorous intensity, or an equivalent combination.
Sub-Goal PA-2.2	Increase the proportion of adults who engage in aerobic physical activity of at least moderate intensity for more than 300 minutes/week, or more than 150 minutes/week of vigorous intensity, or an equivalent combination.
Sub-Goal PA-2.3	Increase the proportion of adults who perform muscle-strengthening activities on 2 or more days of the week.
Sub-Goal PA-2.4	Increase the proportion of adults who meet the objectives for aerobic physical activity and for muscle-strengthening activity.

Adapted from Healthy People 2020. 2020 Topics and Objectives. Available at: http://www .healthypeople.gov/2020/topicsobjectives2020/objectiveslist.aspx?topicId=8. Accessed May 3, 2013.

diabetes, hypertension, cardiovascular disease, and some types of cancer among non-white racial/ethnic minority groups.[17-19]

When health researchers study diseases related to obesity, it is important to consider the possible reasons individuals lack physical activity. As with the other intertwined social determinants of health, lack of physical activity does not occur as a single item. For example, an obese adult with type 2 diabetes did not become obese in a few months, but rather over a long period of time. When researchers study obesity, they investigate the physical, psychological, and social aspects that determine the individual's health, not merely the medical condition related to obesity. As shown in **Box 3-1**, when analyzing obesity data, researchers learn that obesity is a multilevel condition with no easy, one-step solutions.

Education

When researchers and evaluators investigate health programs, they assess the literacy level of the target population prior to the study development. When written documents or verbal instructions are above the literacy level of the recipient, the result is a lack of comprehension. It is up to the investigators to verify that the written and verbal information conveyed in a study is at the proper health literacy level. According to the U.S. Department of Health and Human Services, health literacy is defined as the extent that individuals have "the capacity to

BOX 3-1

Facts About Obesity in the United States

- Adult obesity is increasing for all income and education levels.
- Men: Education achievement and obesity are not related for men.
- Women: Women with college degrees are less obese than women with less education.
- More than one-third of adults and almost 17% of youth were obese in 2009–2010.[20]
- There was no change in the prevalence of obesity among adults or children from the previous year.[20]
- Obesity prevalence did not differ between men and women.[20]
- Adults aged 60 and over were more likely to be obese than younger adults.[20]
- No state has met the nation's *Healthy People 2010* goal to lower obesity prevalence to 15%. The number of states with an obesity prevalence of 30% or more has increased to 12 states in 2010.[21]
- In 2009, nine states had obesity rates of 30% or more. In 2000, no state had an obesity prevalence of 30% or more.[21]
- In 2008, medical costs associated with obesity were estimated at $147 billion; the medical costs paid by third-party payers for people who are obese were $1,429 higher than those for people of normal weight.[21]

obtain, process, and understand basic health information and services needed to make appropriate health decisions."[22] It is estimated that 12% of adults lack the health literacy skills required to manage their health needs.[23] Adults with health disparities often also have low health literacy and are more likely to report their health as poor and lack health insurance.[24] Essentially, the same individuals dealing with health disparities are also the populations most likely to experience low health literacy (e.g., elderly, racial and ethnic minorities, people with less than a high school degree or GED certificate, people with low income levels, nonnative speakers of English, and people with compromised health status). Low health literacy is also linked to poor health outcomes, less utilization of preventive services, and higher healthcare costs.[25]

When investigators recruit individuals for any type of health study, it is common to ask for personal health information. If the recruited individuals have low literacy skills, they may become overwhelmed with stress because of the unfamiliar situation. When the informed consent documents are not written and explained verbally in a low literacy format, individuals are unable to give true informed consent to participate in the study. Whether or not the health information is connected to a research protocol, individuals with low literacy skills need basic health education to understand and retain the medical information needed for self-care, medication regimes, follow-up treatment, or the initial cause of their illness and prevention of a future recurrence.

Researchers and evaluators also need to realize that health literacy skills involve not only words but also numbers. Some basic math is needed when tracking blood glucose levels, measuring liquid medications, and understanding prescription labels. Both healthcare providers and investigators benefit by communicating in plain language for maximum comprehension and understanding. Documents written in plain language use the following techniques:

- Placing the most important information first
- Grouping information together to increase understanding
- Writing in active voice
- Using simple one- to two-syllable words rather than standard medical terminology
- Providing a phonetic pronunciation of medical terms

The readability score of plain language documents should not exceed a fifth-grade reading level. Most word processing software packages include readability level tools.

From an investigator's standpoint, when writing health documents, it is important to know the intended audience and to test materials several times during the development process. After achieving a fifth-grade readability score, the next step is to consider the spoken word. When explaining health information, it is essential to avoid using medical terminology, abbreviations, and medical jargon. Plain language applies to written and spoken health information.[26] See **Box 3-2** for an example of plain language.

Lastly, researchers and evaluators should be aware that participating individuals may have excellent literary skills in one language, but limited language proficiency in another language. Many global citizens experience this situation during international travel, especially when faced with unfamiliar alphabets. Even with a limited working knowledge of another language, individuals struggle to explain their health history and immediate need for treatment. It is important for investigators and healthcare providers to determine an individual's level of literacy in

BOX 3-2

Sample of Plain Language

High Health Literacy

Good morning, Mrs. Smith. Have you voided enough for the UA sample? Your doctor ordered a CBC, CMP, and INR for this morning. You will be NPO tonight. After the heart cath in the a.m., you will be moved to CCU for a 24-hour observation.

Low Health Literacy

Good morning, Mrs. Smith. How are you feeling this morning? Have you been able pee into the white plastic hat that I put in the toilet to collect your urine? After you finish your breakfast, a person from the lab will be back to stick your arm again for a few more blood tests that your doctor ordered. I will remind you again, but after midnight tonight, you will not be able to eat or drink anything. In the morning, your doctor is planning to repeat the procedure on your heart that you had last week. After the procedure, you will be moved to another room. I will tell your husband about this room change when he comes in later today. Your doctor wants to have you in the intensive care unit for heart patients. In case you have any heart problems, the specially trained nurses will be able to care for you immediately. Do you have any questions? If not, I'll be back in with your medicine in a few minutes. If you think of any questions, I will try to answer them when I return. Enjoy your breakfast.

their native language before assuming a lack of health knowledge. For example, if an English-speaking patient became ill while traveling to China, or if a Chinese patient became ill while traveling to the United States, a translator is required for understanding (see **Table 3-7**).

Table 3-7   Example of English to Chinese Translation

English	Chinese
I speak only a bit of English.	我只能说一点英语。
I have no fever or pain.	我没有发烧或疼痛。
I have been vomiting for three days.	我已经呕吐三天了。
I feel weak. Please help me.	我感到虚弱。请帮助我。

Access to Health Care

When researchers and evaluators investigate why some individuals do not come to the clinic until their illness or medical condition is severe enough to require hospitalization, it is important to consider if the individual was blocked from accessing medical care because they lacked insurance. As with other social determinants of health, access to health care does not solely predict health outcomes but, when linked to other health disparities, leads to poor health outcomes. Investigators are challenged to keep one eye on the big picture of reaching optimal health outcomes, while studying ways to improve a few factors related to health disparities or social determinants of health. Lastly, it is important to understand that increased healthcare spending does not equal improved health and longer life expectancy (see **Box 3-3**).[27]

Resources: Safe Food, Safe Housing, and Employment

This section presents the closely linked cycle within social determinants of health: food security, safe housing, and employment. When investigators find ways to recruit and retain individuals struggling to secure food, housing, and employment for themselves and their families into studies or evaluations, both investigators and individuals benefit from the effort. Investigators gain valuable insight and data from an often marginalized sample of the population, and the participating individuals are empowered by the opportunity to have their voices heard and their health data included in studies.

Safe Food

According to *Healthy People 2020*, food security is defined as the availability of nutritious, adequate, and safe food, and the ability to acquire acceptable foods without stealing or using emergency food supplies. On the other hand, food insecurity is a household economic condition of uncertainty about availability to

BOX 3-3

Access to Health Care in the United States

As of 2009, 50.7 million people in the United States did not have health insurance.[28] The Institute of Medicine estimates that uninsured individuals between 25 and 64 years of age have a mortality (death) rate 25% higher than insured individuals in the same age group.[29] Uninsured adults with chronic diseases often delay or skip medical appointments and refilling of prescriptions. When chronic diseases are not managed, the condition escalates into a serious medical emergency. Because of a lack of preventive screening, uninsured individuals are diagnosed with late-stage cancers rather than having early-stage cancers detected by screening or clinical examination. When care is inaccessible, uninsured individuals die of trauma and serious acute conditions, such as strokes and heart attacks, because they avoid seeking emergency medical care.[30] There are also situations in which individuals have health insurance but lack the ability to pay for healthcare services not covered by health insurance, such as copayments, tests not covered by health insurance, and prescription drugs.

regularly obtain nutritious, adequate, and safe foods, whereas hunger is an individual's condition resulting from food insecurity (see **Table 3-8**).[12]

Safe Housing

Affordable housing is defined as a family paying less than 30% of its annual income on housing.[31] When the costs for housing exceed 30% of their income, families have difficulty paying for food, clothing, transportation, and medical care.[31] In the United States, it is estimated that 12 million renter and homeowner households now pay more than 50% of their annual incomes for housing.[31] A family with one full-time worker earning the minimum wage cannot afford the local fair-market rent for a two-bedroom apartment anywhere in the United States. The lack of affordable housing is a significant hardship for low-income households, preventing them from meeting their other basic needs, such as nutrition and healthcare, or saving for their and their families' futures.[32,33] In 2009, an individual had to earn $14.97 per hour to afford a one-bedroom apartment.[34] The lack of affordable housing led to increased rent and overcrowding in affordable and substandard housing. After reviewing **Table 3-9**, take a minute to calculate what percentage of your income is spent on housing.

Table 3-8   Food Insecurity

Healthy People 2020

Topic	Nutrition and weight status
Goal NWS-12	Eliminate very low food security among children.
Goal NWS-13	Reduce household food insecurity and, in doing so, reduce hunger.
Baseline	14.6% of households were food insecure in 2008.
Target	6.0%
Target method	Retain 2010 target.
Data source	Food Security Supplement to the Current Population Survey, U.S. Department of Commerce, Census Bureau

Adapted from Healthy People 2020. 2020 Topics and Objectives. Available at: http://www .healthypeople.gov/2020/topicsobjectives2020/objectiveslist.aspx?topicId=8. Accessed May 3, 2013.

Employment

Without adequate and stable employment, individuals are forced to make difficult choices regarding their ability to pay for housing, food, child care, health care, and education. When housing consumes more than 50% of the household

Table 3-9   Salary and Cost of Housing

Year of Minimum Wage Increase	U.S. Federal Minimum Wage (Hourly Rate and Annual Salary)	Average National Cost of Rent (Imputed) Monthly	Percentage of Salary for Housing Alone
1968	$1.15 = $2,392	$92	46%
1970	$1.30 = $2,704	$105	47%
1972	$1.60 = $3,328	$120	43%
1976	$2.30 = $4,784	$166	42%
1979	$2.90 = $6,032	$226	45%
1980	$3.10 = $6,448	$252	47%
1981	$3.35 = $6,968	$277	49%
1990	$3.80 = $7,904	$464	70%
1991	$4.25 = $8,840	$489	66%
1996	$4.75 = $9,880	$565	68%
1997	$5.15 = $10,712	$588	66%
2007	$5.85 = $12,168	$835	82%
2008	$6.55 = $13,624	$865	76%
2009	$7.25 = $15,080	$874	69%

Data from Lincoln Institute of Land Policy. Rent-Price Ratio. Available at: http://www.lincolninst .edu/subcenters/land-values/rent-price-ratio.asp; Accessed January 12, 2012.

income, families are at risk of becoming homeless. When individuals are living on the edge of poverty, only one illness, accident, or missed paycheck pushes them into homelessness. In the cycle of food insecurity, unsafe housing, and unemployment, there are other factors that force individuals into homelessness. As with all social determinants of health, these factors may be the reasons for homelessness or may amplify other existing factors, such as new or long-term disability,[35] domestic violence,[36] mental illness,[37] and addiction disorders.

Using *Healthy People 2020* to Study Health Disparities and Social Determinants of Health

Now that you have learned how the concepts of health disparities and social determinants of health fit into research and evaluation, in this section we explore how to use a tool called MAP-IT (**M**obilize, **A**ssess, **P**lan, **I**mplement, **T**rack). As stated earlier in this chapter, *Healthy People 2020* reflects the nation's high-priority health issues and the need to decrease health disparities and improve social determinants of health for enhanced health outcomes. To accomplish these goals, it is suggested that investigators use *Healthy People 2020* and MAP-IT to study ways to achieve optimal health for individuals, communities (e.g., organizations, institutions, corporations, universities), and the nation.[38] **Table 3-10** presents how to use MAP-IT with the example of reducing falls among elderly patients at a local hospital.

Table 3-10   MAP-IT: Research Related to Reducing Falls Among Admitted Elderly Patients in the Hospital

MAP-IT	Objectives	Questions to Ask	Reducing Patient Falls
Mobilize	Gather a broad representation of key individuals and organize a partnership/coalition.	What are the vision and mission of the coalition?	The vision and mission of the hospital is to improve health and wellness.
	Identify roles for partners and organizations.	Who should be represented?	Representative sample of staff (physicians, nurses, certified nursing assistants, physical therapists) and two community members.
	Assign responsibilities to move process forward.		

continues

Table 3-10 MAP-IT: Research Related to Reducing Falls Among Admitted Elderly Patients in the Hospital *continued*

MAP-IT	Objectives	Questions to Ask	Reducing Patient Falls
Assess	Assess both needs and resources in the community. Set priorities: feasibility, effectiveness, and measurability. Collect state and local data to determine local needs. Explore social determinants of health related to the issue: Is the health of the community affected by the physical environment? Does every individual in the community have access to health services? Is the health of the community affected by the social environment (e.g., employment, education level, language, transportation)? Does individual lifestyle behavior affect the health issue being addressed? What will it take to improve the health of the community?	Who is affected and how? What resources do we have, and what resources do we need?	Retrieve hospital data regarding elderly patient falls over the past 12 months: location of fall, type of injury sustained, diagnosis of patients who fell, nursing unit where fall occurred, and so on. Social determinants: Did the physical environment (bed rails, wet floor, bathroom facilities, etc.) increase the likelihood of the elderly patient's fall? Did the elderly patients fall because they misunderstood the instructions given by the staff? Were instructions presented with appropriate literacy level and in the appropriate language of the elderly patient? Did the elderly patient's obesity contribute to his/her fall risk? Was the elderly obese patient placed in an adequate-size hospital bed? After reviewing the data, what will it take to reduce the number of elderly patient falls in the hospital?
Plan	Use *Healthy People 2020* to determine the goals and objectives. Clear objectives are needed in a good plan. Write concrete steps for achieving each objective. Assign responsibilities and activities to each team member. Search for best practices and other tested interventions.	What is the goal? What is needed to reach the goal?	Goal: Improve the health, function, and quality of life of older adults.* Write clear objectives and concrete steps for achieving each objective. Assign responsibilities and activities to each team member. Conduct a review of literature for best practices of fall prevention and precautions among the elderly.

*http://healthypeople.gov/2020/topicsobjectives2020/overview.aspx?topicId=31

continues

Table 3-10 MAP-IT: Research Related to Reducing Falls Among Admitted Elderly Patients in the Hospital *continued*

MAP-IT	Objectives	Questions to Ask	Reducing Patient Falls
Implement	Create a detailed work plan.	Is the plan being followed?	Determine if the plan is being followed.
	Share reasonability by assigning a specific person to each activity.	Is there a way to improve the plan?	Determine if improvements are needed in the plan.
	Celebrate accomplishments.		
Track	Evaluate each segment to track progress over time.	Is the plan evaluated at each step?	Evaluate the fall prevention program at each step.
	Check data collection for standardization, reliability, and validity.	Is the plan being followed?	Are the number of falls among elderly patients decreasing in the hospital?
	Share progress with partners.	Was goal reached?	
	If you see a positive trend in data, issue a press release or announcement.		

Adapted from Healthy People 2020. Implementing Healthy People 2020. Available at: http://www.healthypeople.gov/2020/implementing/default.aspx. Accessed May 3, 2012.

Summary

This chapter presented information about health disparities and social determinants of health. From this discussion, it is apparent that health is "a state of complete physical, mental, and social well-being and not merely the absence of disease or infirmity."[39] Although some individuals reach optimal health, other individuals lack optimal health because of factors outside their control. In other cases, individuals make poor personal health choices, such as use of tobacco products or lack of exercise and proper weight management. In any case, investigators planning health programs, conducting health research, or evaluating health programs need to understand the effect of health disparities and social determinants of health on health outcomes.

Case Study

After reading the following case study, make a list of the health disparities and social determinants of health that shape the health outcome.

continues

CASE STUDY *continued*

Jim and Nancy Hawthorne, ages 58 and 54, respectively, are African American, have been married for 35 years, and teach elementary students in the small rural school district about 90 miles from a metropolitan area. They are both about 20 pounds overweight and have a family history of diabetes and hypertension. Because of their hectic schedules, they do not take time to exercise. Their combined net income is $70,000 annually, or $5,833 per month. They spend 35% of their income on their home mortgage. With a tight budget for household expenses, they pay a portion of living expenses for their two children in college and give a little money to Nancy's parents, who live in their home on a fixed retirement income.

Jim and Nancy's health insurance is available through the school district and costs $260 per month for the family. Because the family does not have any chronic health conditions, they selected the lower monthly cost premium with the higher annual deductible cost of $1,000 per person for an annual cost of $4,000 for the Hawthorne family. For example, after Nancy pays $1,000 of her medical bills, the insurance company begins to pay 80% of medical bills, and then Nancy pays 20% of her medical bills for the remainder of the calendar year. They admit they probably do not know enough about health, nutrition, and exercise, but they feel fine.

In January, Nancy's elderly mother's health declined rapidly. Because her father was unable to be the primary caregiver, Nancy's parents moved into Jim and Nancy's home. Nancy began to experience extreme stress trying to juggle her children, work responsibilities, and having her parents join the household. With the money her parents saved on rent and utilities, Nancy was able to hire a part-time home health aide for a few hours each day. The home health aide was kind, but spoke only a little English, so her parents were not comfortable with the arrangement. Nancy applied for a leave of absence and cared for her mother until she died in March. Nancy's dad continued to live with Jim and Nancy, because he does not drive and would be isolated from any social interaction if he moved back to his home. Her father's health declined, but he was able to stay alone during the day, so Nancy's stress decreased and she returned to work in April.

continues

CASE STUDY *continued*

In May, Jim experienced mild chest pain while walking on the tread-mill at the local gym. After telling Nancy about his chest pain, Jim scheduled an appointment with their family physician in their small town. Dr. Williams referred him to a cardiologist, Dr. Cintron, for further evaluation. Dr. Cintron's office was located in the metropolitan area 90 miles from their home. After admitting Jim to the university hospital, Dr. Cintron conducted a nuclear medicine heart stress test and scheduled a heart catheterization for the following day. During the procedure, Dr. Cintron placed three stents in Jim's blocked arteries with minor complications. While Jim remained in the hospital for two days, Nancy stayed at a nearby hotel. She was worried about leaving her father alone, but a neighbor agreed to check on him each day.

The total $120,000 hospital bill included the doctor's office visits, anesthesiologist, radiologist, nuclear medicine, operating room time, cardiologist, medications, and hospital room charges. Because Jim had not yet paid his $1,000 annual health insurance deductible, he was required to pay the first $1,000 of the medical bill plus 20% of remaining $119,000—a total amount of $24,800. Jim and Nancy did not have enough money in savings, so they established a 36-month payment plan of $688 per month with the hospital. Fortunately, the hospital did not charge any interest. This additional monthly expense put further strain on all aspects of the family budget. Jim's heart condition required another hospitalization in June, and their 20% portion of the bill pushed their monthly hospital payment to more than $800. Because of his declining heart condition, Jim was required to retire early from the school district and they sold their second car. Living on Jim's small retirement check and Nancy's salary, they could no longer afford to pay a portion of their children's tuition, so their children transferred to a local community college and moved home. Within two years, the Hawthorne family declared bankruptcy, foreclosed on their home mortgage, and moved into a small apartment in an undesirable section of their rural community. Fortunately, their children received associate degrees in health fields, so they are employed at the university hospital in the metropolitan area, share an apartment in the city, and take the bus to work.

continues

CASE STUDY *continued*

Case Study Discussion Questions

1. If you were the case manager for this family, when would you begin to intervene?
2. What other options did Jim and Nancy have early in their financial problems?
3. What would you have done in their situation?

Student Activity

For the national data, it is useful to become familiar with the U.S. census data at http://factfinder2.census.gov/faces/nav/jsf/pages/index.xhtml.

Census FactFinder Treasure Hunt
Easy

1. The decennial census does what? This survey collects data every 10 years about households, income, education, home ownership, and more for the United States, Puerto Rico, and the island areas.
2. The American Community Survey does what? This nationwide survey was designed to provide communities a fresh look at how they are changing.
3. Find the 2000 population for Johnston City, Illinois, from a table describing its general demographic characteristics.
4. Quickstart is made up of two boxes. In the text box on the left, type the topic you are looking for, in this case, "Population." In the text box on the right, type the geographic location you are looking for, in this case, "Johnston City, Illinois." Click "Go" to see a list of the search results. Search results are organized by year, starting with the most recent. Find the table labeled "Profile of General Demographic Characteristics: 2000."
5. In 2000, 3,557 people lived in Johnston City, Illinois.
6. What are the different geographic types one may filter data by? Nation, state, county, city or town, congressional district, census tract, metro/ micro area, zip code/ZCTA.

7. According to the U.S. Popclock projection, there is one birth in the United States every _____ seconds. 8

8. Using the address search function, what census tract does 1600 Pennsylvania Ave. NW, Washington, DC 20500 reside in? 62.02 District of Columbia.

Medium

1. What percentage of the population ages 25 years and older have obtained a bachelor's degree?
   a. Total population 25 years and older: 204,288,933
   b. Those with bachelor's degrees: 36,244,474
   c. Percentage: 17.7%

2. What percentage of the U.S. population ages 25 years and older have obtained any level of schooling past high school?
   a. Some college, no degree: 21.3%
   b. Associate's degree: 7.6%
   c. Bachelor's degree: 17.7%
   d. Graduate or professional degree: 10.4%
   e. Total: 57%

3. Using the 2010 American Community Survey one-year estimates table DP03, how many Americans had no healthcare coverage during the year? 47,208,222
   a. What percentage of the total population does this represent? 15.5%

4. Create a map showing state populations by density. (Requires that students view the four-minute "Create a Map" tutorial.)

5. You may filter the tables by population group. How many Native American tribal groups are tracked by the U.S. Census Bureau? 542

6. For the United States in 2010, in the age group 85 to 89, are there more men or women? The number of women in this age group is almost double the number of men: 1,273,867 men versus 2,346,592 women, or 54.3 men for every 100 women.

7. Using the American Community Survey (2005–2009), what percentage of all women aged 15–50 who gave birth in the past 12 months were married? 33.4%, using the fertility table under the American Community Survey (S1301).

Hard

1. Using the 2010 American Community Survey one-year estimates table DP03, what percentage of families makes less than $35,000 annually?
   a. Total number of households: 114,567,419
      i. Less than $10,000 a year: 7.6%
      ii. 10,000–14,999: 5.8%
      iii. 15,000–24,999: 11.5%
      iv. 25,000–34,999: 10.8%
   b. Total percentage: 35.7%, or 40,900,568 families (that is, 40,900,568/114,567,419)

2. Using the same table, what percentage of families makes less than $10,000 a year? 8,707,123 families/114,567,419 = 7.6%

3. In the United States in 2009, how many employees worked for the healthcare and social assistance industry? Under topics, choose "Business and Industry," then choose "Employment, "then "Employees." In 2009, County Business Patterns (CB0900A1 table) you will find a list of industry types. Under health care and social assistance, you will find the answer: 17,531,142

4. On average, how much does a person in the healthcare and social assistance industry make yearly? From the same table, you will find a column that says "Annual Payroll ($1,000)." This is the amount of money, in thousands, that is paid each year in this industry. To find this figure, you must multiply the number found for healthcare and social assistance by $1,000, and then divide by the number of workers in that industry. 735,531,215 X 1,000 = 735,531,215,000; 735,531,215,000/17,531,142 = $41,955/year.

5. According to the most recent data, how many people live in the zip code 28306? This is one zip code for Fayetteville, North Carolina. As of 2010, there were 39,683 people residing in this zip code.
   a. Of those, how many were of American Indian, Alaskan Native, Native Hawaiian, or other Pacific Islander racial descent?
      i. American Indian or Native Alaskan: 1,142
      ii. Native Hawaiian or other Pacific Islander: 106
      iii. Total: 1,248
   b. What percentage of the total population does this represent? 1,248/39,683 = 3.1%

In most situations, it is possible to locate state and local data from the U.S. census data. Specific data requires accessing local databases, and such data may be password protected to protect personal information and therefore are not published on the Internet.

References

1. The Centers for Disease Control and Prevention. Ten great public health achievements—United States, 1900–1999. *MMWR*. 1999;48(12):241–243. Available at: http://www.cdc.gov/mmwr/preview/mmwrhtml/00056796.htm. Accessed January 12, 2012.
2. The Centers for Disease Control and Prevention. Leading Causes of Death. Available at: http://www.cdc.gov/nchs/fastats/lcod.htm. Accessed January 12, 2012.
3. The Centers for Disease Control and Prevention. Leading Causes of Death, 1900–1998. Available at: http://www.cdc.gov/nchs/data/dvs/lead1900_98.pdf. Accessed January 12, 2012.
4. National Center of Health Statistics. *National Vital Statistics Report: Fast Facts A to Z*. Atlanta, GA: Centers for Disease Control and Prevention; 2006.
5. Joint National Committee on Prevention, Detection, Evaluation, and Treatment of High Blood Pressure. *Arch Intern Med*. 1997;157:2413–2446.
6. Burt BA, Eklund SA. *Dentistry, Dental Practice, and the Community*. Philadelphia, PA: WB Saunders Company; 1999:204–220.
7. Bolen JR, Sleet DA, Chorba T, et al. U.S. Department of Health and Human Services, Centers for Disease Control and Prevention. Overview of efforts to prevent motor vehicle-related injury. In: *Prevention of Motor Vehicle–Related Injuries: A Compendium of Articles from the Morbidity and Mortality Weekly Report, 1985–1996*. Atlanta, GA: U.S. Department of Health and Human Services, CDC; 1997.
8. Centers for Disease Control and Prevention. Fatal occupational injuries—United States, 1980–1994. *MMWR*. 1998;47:297–302. Available at: http://www.cdc.gov/mmwr/preview/mmwrhtml/mm5016a4.htm. Accessed January 12, 2012.
9. Bunker JP, Frazier HS, Mosteller F. Improving health: Measuring effects of medical care. *Milbank Q*. 1994;72:225–258.
10. Mokdad AH, Marks JS, Stroup DF, Gerberding JL. Actual causes of death in the United States, 2000. *JAMA*. 2004;291(10):1238–1245.
11. Healthy People 2020. About Healthy People. Available at: http://www.healthypeople.gov/2020/about/default.aspx. Accessed May 3, 2012.
12. Healthy People 2020. 2020 Topics and Objectives. Available at: http://www.healthypeople.gov/2020/topicsobjectives2020/objectiveslist.aspx?topicId=8. Accessed May 3, 2013.
13. U.S. Department of Health and Human Services, The Secretary's Advisory Committee on National Health Promotion and Disease Prevention Objectives for 2020. Phase I Report: Recommendations for the Framework and Format of Healthy People 2020: Section IV, Advisory Committee Findings and Recommendations. Available at: http://www.healthypeople.gov/hp2020/advisory/PhaseI/sec4.htm#_Toc211942917. Accessed January 6, 2010.

14. Healthy People 2020. The History and Development of Healthy People. Available at: http://www.healthypeople.gov/2020/about/history.aspx. Accessed May 3, 2012.

15. Gornick ME. Disparities in Health Care: Methods for Studying the Effects of Race, Ethnicity, and SES on Access, Use, and Quality of Health Care, 2002 [Revised by Swift EK]. Available at: http://www.iom.edu/~/media/Files/Activity%20Files /Quality/NHDRGuidance/DisparitiesGornick.pdf. Revised March 7, 2002. Accessed August 23, 2012.

16. Healthy People 2020. Social Determinants of Health. Available at: http://www .healthypeople.gov/2020/topicsobjectives2020/overview.aspx?topicid=39. Accessed May 3, 2012.

17. U.S. Department of Health and Human Services, Centers for Disease Control and Prevention, National Center for Chronic Disease and Prevention and Health Promotion. *Physical Activity and Health: A Report of the Surgeon General.* Atlanta, GA: DHHS; 1996.

18. Eisenmann JC, Bartee RT, Smith DT, Welk GJ, Fu Q. Combined influence of physical activity and television viewing on the risk of overweight in US youth. *Int J Obes.* 2008;32(4):613–618.

19. Flegal KM, Carroll MD, Ogden CL, Curtin LR. Prevalence and trends in obesity among US adults, 1999–2008. *JAMA.* 2010;303(3):235–241.

20. Centers for Disease Control and Prevention. Signs: State-specific obesity prevalence among adults—United States, 2009. *MMWR.* 2010;59(30);951–955.

21. Finkelstein EA, Trogdon JG, Cohen JW, Dietz W. Annual medical spending attributable to obesity: Payer and service specific estimates. *Health Aff.* 2009;28(5): 5w822–w831.

22. Kirsch IS, Jungeblut A, Jenkins L, Kolstad A. *Adult Literacy in America: A First Look at the Results of the National Adult Literacy Survey (NALS).* Washington, DC: National Center for Education Statistics, U.S. Department of Education; 1993.

23. Centers for Disease Control and Prevention. *Simply Put: A Guide for Creating Easy-to-Understand Materials.* Atlanta, GA: Centers for Disease Control and Prevention; 2010. Available at: http://www.cdc.gov/healthliteracy/pdf/Simply_Put.pdf. Accessed August 23, 2013.

24. National Center for Education Statistics. *The Health Literacy of America's Adults: Results from the 2003 National Assessment of Adult Literacy.* Washington, DC: U.S. Department of Education; 2006.

25. Plain Language Action and Information Network. What Is Plain Language? Available at: http://www.plainlanguage.gov/whatisPL/index.cfm. Accessed January 12, 2012.

26. U.S. Department of Health and Human Services. *National Standards for Culturally and Linguistically Appropriate Services in Health Care.* Washington, DC: Office of Minority Health; 2001.

27. Wardrip KE, Pelletiere D, Crowley S, eds. *Out of Reach: 2009.* Washington, DC: The National Low Income Housing Coalition; 2009.

28. DeNavas-Walt C, Proctor BD, Smith JC. *Income, Poverty, and Health Insurance Coverage in the United States: 2009.* Washington, DC: U.S. Census Bureau; 2010:60–238.

29. Institute of Medicine, Committee on Health Insurance Status, Consequences Board on Health Care Services. *America's Uninsured Crisis: Consequences for Health and Health Care.* Washington, DC: The National Academies Press; 2009.

30. Stanton MW. The high concentration of U.S. health care expenditures. *Research in Action.* June 2006;19. Rockville, MD: Agency for Healthcare Research and Quality;

2006. Available at: http://www.ahrq.gov/research/ria19/expendria.htm. Accessed August 23, 2013.

31. U.S. Department of Housing and Urban Development. Affordable Housing. Available at: http://www.hud.gov/offices/cpd/affordablehousing/. Accessed May 3, 2012.

32. Lincoln Institute of Land Policy. Rent-Price Ratio. Available at: http://www.lincolninst .edu/subcenters/land-values/rent-price-ratio.asp. Accessed January 12, 2012.

33. DeNavas-Walt C, Proctor BD, Lee CH. *Income, Poverty, and Health Insurance Coverage in the United States: 2005.* U.S. Census Bureau, Current Population Reports, P60-231. Washington, DC: US Government Printing Office; 2006.

34. The U.S. Conference for Mayors. A Status Report on Hunger and Homelessness in America's Cities: 2007. Available at: http://usmayors.org/hhsurvey2007/hhsurvey07 .pdf. Accessed January 12, 2012.

35. The U.S. Conference for Mayors. A Status Report on Hunger and Homelessness in America's Cities: 2005. Available at: http://www.usmayors.org/hungersurvey/2005 /HH2005FINAL.pdf. Accessed January 12, 2012.

36. American Civil Liberties Union. Domestic Violence and Homelessness. Available at: http://www.aclu.org/pdfs/dvhomelessness032106.pdf. Accessed January 12, 2012.

37. Alzheimer's Association. Major Milestones in Alzheimer's and Brain Research. Available at: http://alz.org/Research/science/major_milestones_in_alzheimers.asp. Accessed January 12, 2012.

38. Healthy People 2020. Implementing Healthy People 2020. Available at: http://www .healthypeople.gov/2020/implementing/default.aspx. Accessed May 3, 2012.

39. The World Health Organization. Definition of Health. Available at: http://www .who.int/about/definition/en/print.html. Accessed January 12, 2012.

Answers to Questions Pertaining to Table 3-2

1. Antibiotics were developed and widely used.
2. The number of deaths from cancer increase as the number of deaths from infectious diseases decrease. Also poor lifestyle choices, such as smoking, increase the number of cancer deaths.
3. Smoking over a long period of time causes chronic obstructive pulmonary disease (COPD).
4. Increased obesity rates caused an increase in diabetes rates.
5. Kidney dialysis and kidney transplants were developed, but prevention of kidney disease remains stable.
6. How long is your list?

CHAPTER 4

Theories and Models

CHAPTER OBJECTIVES

By the end of this chapter, students will be able to:

- Explain the difference between inductive and deductive reasoning
- Evaluate theories and models to determine the most appropriate application for the proposed research
- Produce action plans and time management charts for projects
- Assess each segment of a SWOT (strengths, weaknesses, opportunities, and threats) analysis for quality improvement

KEY TERMS

Action plans	SWOT analysis
Models	Theories

Introduction

After discussing the role of deductive and inductive reasoning related to theory, this chapter covers the topic of theories and models from two viewpoints. First, we explore various theories and models related to building, planning, and evaluating frameworks. Beginning with broad universal theories, we move through system, community, organization, and individual behavior change theories. Second, theories and models near the end of the chapter focus on strategic planning techniques to achieve goals in the allotted time. It is important to note that some references in this chapter are several decades old. These older references are linked to established theories and models that have been stable, valid, and reliable when used in research and evaluation over an extended period of time. This chapter also introduces some theories and models that are current but have only been used in a few studies.

Let's begin with definitions. Depending on the discipline, theories and models are defined using approximately the same terms. In other disciplines, models are used to develop theories or are used independent of theories. A theory is a set of related concepts that present a systematic view of events, issues, and situations in order to explain them or make predictions, whereas generally, models represent interactions between concepts in order to show patterns.[1] In science, theory is based on tested and observable facts. Once a scientific theory is developed, the facts are interpreted or investigated by other scientists, but the facts remain the same. Theories are based on facts, laws, and principles while leaving room for unanswered questions. Over time, theories are challenged and tested. Scientists confirm or refute theories based on reviews within the scientific community. Theories either stand the test of time or are deemed to be lacking credibility. Theories are used to increase and validate knowledge. Some theories are limited to one discipline, whereas other theories are used across disciplines. For example, behavioral change theories are used across disciplines to modify individual behavior and improve health outcomes. Theories are used to test a hypothesis, investigate a phenomenon, or validate an existing body of knowledge. In some disciplines, such as nursing, theories are used to establish and guide practice. The remainder of this chapter provides examples of universal scientific theories followed by theories and models related to systems, communities, and individual behaviors. The chapter ends with a presentation of theories used for strategic planning.

Deductive and Inductive Reasoning

There are two types of reasoning used in the development of theories: deductive and inductive. First, deductive reasoning is used to gain knowledge. Deductive reasoning moves from theory to observations or findings. The conclusion must be true provided that the previous statements are true:

1. 90% of all children like ice cream.
2. Sally is a child.
3. Therefore, the probability that Sally likes ice cream is 90%.

Deductive reasoning moves from general to specific. The steps include (1) starting with a theory, (2) developing a specific hypothesis to test, (3) collecting observations to confirm or refute the hypothesis, and (4) confirming the theory.[2]

The following example illustrates deductive reasoning. Healthcare providers know from well-established research that obesity increases the risk of cardiac conditions. Each time healthcare providers see an obese patient in a clinic, the providers discuss the relationship of obesity and increased cardiac problems. If the obese patients do not reduce their weight, they are likely to experience detrimental cardiac symptoms in the future.

Second, inductive reasoning works in the opposite direction. The steps include (1) observing specific behaviors and measures, (2) identifying specific patterns among the collected data, (3) formulating a proposed hypothesis, and (4) developing a conclusion, model, or theory.[2] Other researchers repeat the observations to confirm or refute the theory. See **Box 4-1** for an example of inductive reasoning from the literature.

Types of Theories and Models

Universal Theories

Among the most well known of universal theories is gravitational theory. In the late 16th century, Galileo developed the hypothesis that all objects fell at the

---

BOX 4-1

Acquired Immune Deficiency Syndrome (AIDS)

In the early 1980s, healthcare providers began treating men with signs of impaired immunity followed by development of *Pneumocystis carinii* pneumonia.[3] Some men also developed a skin cancer called Kaposi's sarcoma.[3,4] Within less than a year, healthcare providers observed that the men lost weight rapidly and most of the men died. Later, as this same phenomenon became more common, researchers from the U.S. Centers for Disease Control and Prevention (CDC) formed a task force to develop a hypothesis to monitor the outbreak. After observing a pattern of symptoms among the patients, the condition was named *acquired immune deficiency syndrome* (AIDS).[5]

same rate because of air resistance. Newton expanded this hypothesis into the theory of gravity. Newton added that gravity gives weight to objects, thus causing objects to fall to the ground when dropped. In addition, gravity keeps the planets in their orbits around the sun, and the moon in orbit around the earth.[6] In 1915, after many trials and errors, Einstein developed the general theory of relativity by expanding the theory of gravity.[7] Although this text is not about physics, this example shows the powerful effect of scientists building on previous theories to move physics forward over several centuries.

System Theories

System theory involves breaking apart a concept for the purpose of studying each segment independently. After a thorough study, segments are reassembled with greater knowledge of the entire entity within the system. For example, healthcare providers study human anatomy and physiology to understand function and interaction of each part of the whole being. The same is true for hospital administrators, in that the budget, personnel, purpose, and interaction of each department must align in order to achieve a finely tuned, successful healthcare facility.

The following discussion introduces two examples of system theories: the Theory of Goal Attainment and the Ecological Model. Both theories illustrate how to break concepts into parts for a closer examination. Keep in mind that there are numerous examples of system theories across multiple disciplines. The two examples selected for this discussion are related to healthcare systems. The Theory of Goal Attainment was created by a nursing theorist,[8] and the Ecological Model presents the interaction between behavioral patterns and social/environmental factors.

Theory of Goal Attainment

Imogene King's Theory of Goal Attainment is an example of a system theory. This theory focuses on personal system concepts, interpersonal system concepts, and social system concepts.[8] The first level of this theory begins with the individual as a whole or the personal system concepts including perception, self, body image, personal space, time, and coping. The second level explores how the individual perceives his environment or interpersonal system concepts (objects, persons, events, stress, and communication). The third level investigates the social system concepts (authority, power, status, and organizations).[8] Because King's theory is related to nursing practice, the theory focuses on how the nurse interacts with the patient and the environment to achieve maximum well-being. See **Box 4-2** to read a summary of how this theory was used in a recent publication by Alligood.[9] See **Box 4-3** to practice your skills using a case study.

BOX 4-2

Family Health Care with King's Theory of Goal Attainment

In 2010, Alligood used King's Theory of Goal Attainment to organize issues related to health care, including pediatric mental illness, diabetes, asthma, and chronic obstructive pulmonary disease. Across all healthcare issues, the concepts of each system are discussed. By applying the Theory of Goal Attainment, the author emphasizes that when the family unit becomes the patient-and-caregiver dyad, the first level becomes the personal system concepts of the dyad rather than those of an individual patient. For example, concepts of perception, time, and coping are all involved with how the patient/caregiver dyad function in the healthcare system. At the second level, families stress the change in family roles, and long-term stress is also discussed. At the third level, how the dyad functions within the healthcare system is discussed, especially when making healthcare decisions for the patient. Alligood concludes the publication with the assertion that King's Theory of Goal Attainment remains useful and relevant for today's research because of its strong nested framework of personal, interpersonal, and social systems.[9]

BOX 4-3

Case Study: King's Theory of Goal Attainment

Recently, Alice graduated from nursing school, and she is anxious to begin her career at the local hospital. In nursing school, she wrote a paper about King's Theory of Goal Attainment, so she is familiar with the theory. After a few months of working, Alice was asked by her supervisor to join a nursing team to improve patient care on the 24-bed medical and surgical unit. Alice was thrilled and talked about King's theory at the first meeting. The nurses remembered learning this theory and decided to conduct a small study to determine if patient satisfaction would improve if they implemented the principles in King's theory. After patients signed the informed consent form, the nurses distributed surveys to patients during the evening shift the night before their discharge.

continues

BOX 4-3 *continued*

Following King's theory, which defines the environment as objects, persons, and events, the nurse researchers defined "objects" as furniture in the patient's hospital room, "persons" as staff nurses who provided day-to-day care, and "events" as the restricted 8:00 a.m. to 8:00 p.m. visiting hours. Here is a sampling of the survey questions:

Furniture: Was the lounge chair in your hospital room comfortable when you were able to move from the bed? Was the furniture in your hospital room comfortable for your visitors?

Staff nurse: Do you feel that there were an adequate number of nurses per shift to provide excellent care? Did the nurses have time to chat with you?

Visiting hours: Would you like to have 24-hour visiting hours? Would you like to retain the restricted 12-hour visiting hours?

These questions, plus many other questions, allowed the nurse researchers to use King's theory to evaluate how the hospital environment influences patient satisfaction and, ultimately, their recovery process while in the hospital. Once the data were analyzed, the nursing team made recommendations to hospital administration on ways to improve the patient environment.

Ecological Model

In 1979, Bronfenbrenner developed the Ecological Model, also sometimes called the socioecological model or ecological framework, with a focus on the interaction between behavioral patterns and social environmental factors.[10,11] The five main constructs of this model include (see **Figure 4-1**):[12]

Intrapersonal factors: Is an individual willing to change one or more characteristics, such as knowledge, attitudes, skills, or intention, to conform to a social norm? For example, individuals with a desire to stop smoking seek smoking cessation information. They are trying to stop smoking to conform to the social norm.

Interpersonal relationships: Are social networks (family, friends, coworkers, and acquaintances) providing positive or negative influences on a person's health behavior? For example, an individual who drinks excessive amounts of alcohol enjoys partying with other alcoholic friends because negative health behavior is

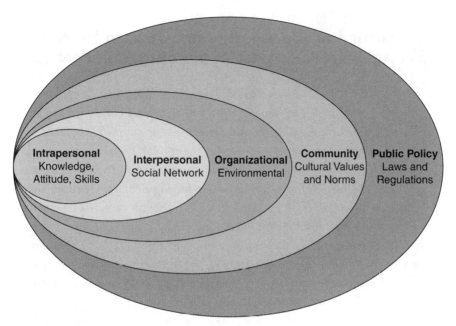

FIGURE 4-1   The Ecological Model
Adapted from American College Health Association. Healthy Campus 2020. Ecological Model. Available at: http://www.acha.org/healthycampus/ecological_model.cfm.

the social norm of the group. When individuals join Alcoholics Anonymous, they establish a new, positive social norm with recovering alcoholic friends.

Organizational factors: Is the organization providing positive or negative influences on the health of the staff? For example, prior to establishing a smoke-free campus, a hospital could offer smoking cessation classes and support groups, nicotine gum and patches at no cost, free gym memberships, and lowered health insurance rates for nonsmoking employees after one year. These positive influences and incentives demonstrate a long-term commitment to the employees' health and wellness.

Community factors: Are the individuals in power at the community level providing positive or negative influences on the overall health of others? (*Community* can be defined as family, church, informal social networks, or geographic area.) Because communities compete for scarce resources, there needs to be a coordinated effort to allocate resources equitably. Too often those individuals with the most serious health problems (e.g., poor, rural, disabled, uneducated, homeless, unemployed, minorities) receive the fewest services. For example, if a city council voted to build well-lit sidewalks around the perimeter of the low-income housing development, the environmental change could have numerous positive

BOX 4-4

Using the Ecological Framework to Explore Aging in Place Research, Policy, and Practice

In 2011, Greenfield used the ecological framework to explore what type of support individuals may need when they choose to remain in their current residences as their need for support increases as they age. After a brief overview of the model, the author explores multiple aspects. For example, there are environment-focused dimensions, such as the need for wide doorframes for wheelchairs. There are also social aspects, such as interpersonal relationships with caregivers. Person-focused dimensions include an elderly individual's willingness to accept assistance with personal care needs and professional help for regaining strength. At the end of the publication, the author summarizes how to apply the ecological framework to aging through a comprehensive list of examples of questions for research, practice, and policy.[13]

health and social benefits, including increased cardiovascular activity and weight loss, enhanced social support networking among neighbors, improved safety, and community pride.

Public policy: Is the purpose of the proposed national, state, or local public policy aimed at improving and protecting the population's health? For example, when the required immunization schedule changes for admission into elementary school, decisions are based on research of specific infectious disease outbreaks and how best to protect children from acquiring and spreading the disease.

See **Box 4-4** for an example of how the ecological framework has been used in a recent publication related to aging.

Community and Organizational Theories and Models

This section includes a discussion of three theories and models related to communities and organizations, including Social Networks and Social Support Theory,[14] Diffusion of Innovations Theory,[15] and the RE-AIM Model.[16]

Social Networks and Social Support Theory

In 1985, Gottlieb developed the Social Networks and Social Support Theory to recognize how behavior change occurs when individuals have social networks and social support in their community.[14] Social networks are groups of family members or friends and include the following characteristics:

Structure: Is there a defined group size with common goals or activities?

Interaction: Does the relationship among members include mutual sharing? Do the members contact each other frequently? Are the relationships long-term?

Functional: Do the relationships offer social support, resource connections, and a sense of social identity?

Social support includes the following characteristics:

Emotional support: Do the individuals listen and show concern toward each other?

Instrumental support: Do the individuals offer actual tangible or physical support, such as financial support or time?

Informational support: Do the individuals give genuine advice, directions, or resource referral information?

Appraisal support: Do the individuals provide positive feedback to each other? Keep in mind that not all social networks offer genuine social support to the individuals involved.

Be cautious in evaluating social support organizations. Some organizations claim to offer social support, but upon further investigation, social support ends when individuals fail to pay mandatory membership fees, question the organizational mission statement, or miss too many meetings. For example, the American Cancer Society offers Reach To Recovery social support groups for women with breast cancer. The groups are free, open to the public, and provide advice and support to those women going through breast cancer treatment and recovery. On the other hand, some organizations welcome individuals who pay required membership dues and may not maintain continuous social support if individuals fall on hard times. For example, a weight loss organization could require weekly dues and offer support, advice, and positive feedback for reaching weight loss goals. However, as soon as the individual stops paying weekly dues, the support, guidance, and praise stop immediately. See **Box 4-5** for an example of social support.

Diffusion of Innovations Theory

Diffusion of Innovations Theory explains how individuals adopt new ideas, products, and social practices across a community or from one community to

BOX 4-5

Social Networks and Social Support

In 2012, Benson published research related to how support networks affected psychological adjustments directly and indirectly. The research data were collected from 106 mothers of children with autism spectrum disorder. The mothers completed surveys and participated in home interviews. The measures included network characteristics, perceived social support, depressed moods, subjective well-being, and parent, child, and family characteristics. The results indicated that network size and proportion of network members who provided emotional support increased perception of social support and well-being, and decreased perception of depressed moods. Also, the results showed that when the mothers perceived increased interpersonal conflict within the mother's network, their perceived depressed moods increased.[17]

another.[15] For the diffusion process to work, it is necessary to describe adopters and rate of adoption. Adopters are individuals who accept change at various rates:

Innovators: Individuals who seek out the latest technology, product, or activity.
Early adopters: Individuals who like innovation but are not the first in line at the store.
Early majority: Individuals who wait until they receive some external motivation before getting involved in the change.
Late majority: Individuals who are not willing to make any change until most people have made the change; they have a wait-and-see attitude toward change.
Laggards: Individuals who are last to buy into the change in spite of constant exposure, or who have limited access to the typical communication networks.

Engaging the innovators is critical for success and involves studying the characteristics of innovation. These characteristics include the following:

Relative advantage: Is this change or innovation perceived as better than the current product or service?
Compatibility: Is the change or innovation perceived as consistent with the past experiences?

Complexity: Is the change or innovation perceived as difficult to understand or use?

Flexibility: Is it possible for the adopter to try out the change or product prior to adopting the change?

Observability: Is it possible for the adopter to observe others use or adapt to the change or innovation?

For example, when "smartphones" were first available, manufacturers emphasized the advantages over current phones on the market. They offered innovator adopters compatibility with retention of current phone numbers and service providers. Some manufacturers offered a 30-day free trial period and discount pricing to first-time buyers. Lastly, innovator adopters increased product exposure by allowing individuals in their social networks to observe the convenience and ease of using a smartphone.

Keep in mind that an individual may be an early adopter for one behavior or product and a late adopter for another innovation. For example, some individuals are innovators for the latest technology product, but they are laggards about fashion trends. For each adoption process, individuals engage in the five-step innovation decision process:

1. *Knowledge:* What does the individual know about the innovation? Does she need or desire additional information?
2. *Persuasion:* Based on sufficient information and understanding, has the individual been persuaded to adopt the innovation?
3. *Decision:* Has the individual determined that this innovation is the correct decision or product for him?
4. *Implementation:* Is the individual satisfied with the product or innovation? Is she seeking modifications in the product?
5. *Confirmation:* Does the individual continue to adopt the innovation and incorporate its use into daily life?

Over time, individuals accept or reject the innovation, or perhaps adopt a later version of the same innovation after further modifications are made to increase consumer satisfaction. For example, when e-book readers were introduced, some people purchased the product but may have become dissatisfied because of the black-and-white screen and inability to read in bright sunlight because of glare on the screen. After the product was modified and offered in a color, nonglare screen, dissatisfied consumers readopted the innovation.

Lastly, without successful communication, the innovation is not successful. There are two basic communication channels: interpersonal and mass media.

Interpersonal or face-to-face communication is considered the most effective method of innovation adoption. Second, mass media channels are a rapid and effective way to create awareness and knowledge about the innovation. Mass media channels include radio, television, newspapers, billboards, magazines, brochures, direct mail marketing, phone solicitation, and social media websites. Although mass media reaches a larger audience, it is less effective in changing individual behaviors. For example, when manufacturers developed a gum to help people stop smoking, they used communication to make the product successful. The company gave free gum samples to clinics so healthcare providers could distribute the gum to patients face-to-face and talk about the health benefits related to smoking cessation. Soon after the clinic distribution, the company focused on mass media by advertising in print media with discount coupons and mail-in rebates, along with radio and television advertising. Many smokers considered the gum as a way to stop smoking, even though limited research was conducted on the effectiveness of the gum in smoking cessation. See **Box 4-6** for an example of Diffusion of Innovations Theory in research.

BOX 4-6

Diffusion of Innovations and Telemedicine with Low-Income Minorities

In 2012, George, Hamilton, and Baker reported the results of their study that determined what patients living in underserved urban areas thought about telemedicine as a way to increase their access to specialty medical care. The researchers conducted 10 focus groups with 43 African Americans and 44 Latinos. The groups were conducted in English and Spanish to meet the needs of the participants. The results showed that the participants perceived the advantages of telemedicine as increased access to specialty medical care and less wait time, but the disadvantages included concerns about confidentiality, privacy, and the lack of physical presence of the healthcare provider. The researchers concluded that prior to the adoption of telemedicine, issues related to patient satisfaction and provider–patient interactions must be addressed in the diffusion of innovation through tailored marketing strategies.[18]

RE-AIM Model

The purpose of RE-AIM is to evaluate program interventions to determine the effect of programs.[16] Programs are assessed at the individual, organization, and community levels using five dimensions: reach, efficacy, adoption, implementation, and maintenance.

Reach: Reach pertains to the individual level and establishes the number or percentage of people who receive the program. To calculate the percentage, it is necessary to know the denominator (total population) and the number of participants. Although it is ideal to collect demographic data on participants and nonparticipants, ethical issues arise because nonparticipants may not have consented to the research. In some cases, if a large community intervention is studied, researchers use census data. At this level, similarities or differences between participants and nonparticipants are verified at the baseline.

Efficacy: Efficacy relates to the individual's assessment of positive and negative program outcomes and the need to include physiologic, behavioral, quality of life, and participant satisfaction outcomes.

Adoption: Adoption refers to the organization or community and establishes the percentage of locations such as worksites, health departments, and schools that adopted the program. Direct observation, interviews, and surveys determine the level of adoption. At the same time, barriers to adoption are investigated.

Implementation: Implementation is the fidelity of the program, or the extent to which the program was provided as intended. At the individual level, participant adherence and follow-through is measured as the outcome. At the organization or community levels, implementation measures staff involvement and implementation fidelity.

Maintenance: Maintenance is the most challenging at the individual, organization, and community levels. Individuals relapse into previous behaviors. Unless polices are changed and enforced at the organization and community levels, health behavior programs are not sustained. See **Box 4-7** for a case study using the RE-AIM Model.

Individual Behavior Theories and Models

Numerous theories attempt to explain, predict, or change human behavior. As with any theory, these theories have been modified for improvement. For this discussion, four theories are presented: the Health Belief Model,[19] the Stages of Change Model (Transtheoretical Model),[20] the Theory of Reasoned Action,[21] and the Social Learning Theory (Social Cognitive Theory).[22]

RE-AIM Case Study

BOX 4-7

As of January 1, the hospital administration enacted a smoke-free policy. This community health facility is the only hospital in this rural county. In June, the hospital used RE-AIM to prepare for the smoke-free policy change.

Reach: It was necessary to determine approximately how many individuals were at the hospital, including employees, healthcare providers, patients, delivery personnel, volunteers, and visitors. Once that number was estimated, the hospital used county statistics to estimate how many individuals in contact with the hospital were smokers and how many were nonsmokers. Surveys and interviews were conducted with representative groups to determine knowledge, attitudes, and beliefs about the upcoming smoke-free policy and how best to implement it.

Efficacy: The hospital initiated a number of smoking cessation classes and provided free nicotine gum in the gift shop and at all patient nursing units. The healthcare providers provided the nicotine patch for appropriate patients and employees without medical contraindications. Data were collected on the positive and negative consequences as well as the participants' satisfaction.

Adoption: On January 1, as planned, the hospital enacted the smoke-free policy. Extra staff were available to answer questions, provide smoking cessation options, and direct individuals wishing to smoke to a designated smoking area near the back of the parking garage. Nicotine gum and patches were available for inpatients wishing to smoke. Surveys were collected and interviews were conducted by graduate students to determine the success of the adoption phase with a special emphasis on the barriers to adopting the smoke-free policy. Data were collected on the number of individuals smoking in non-designated areas who had been given verbal and written reminders about the new smoke-free policy.

Implementation: After one month, prepolicy data, first month of policy data, and end of first month data were analyzed to determine the effectiveness of the implementation. Were there fewer individuals

continues

BOX 4-7 *continued*

> smoking in nondesignated areas? How many individuals were reg-
> istering, attending, and completing the four-session smoking ces-
> sation classes? How many prescriptions for nicotine patches were
> written by healthcare providers? How many nicotine gum packets
> were distributed by the gift shop and nursing units in patient care
> areas? Were the numbers decreasing or increasing?
>
> *Maintenance:* Six months after the smoke-free policy was enacted, data were
> collected again to verify that the policy had been institutionalized
> and the number of individuals smoking in the hospital and in the
> community was decreasing.

Health Belief Model (Rosenstock, 1974)

The Health Belief Model was developed in the 1950s by psychologists who
assumed that individuals fear disease and that the degree of fear determines their
motivation to seek preventive health services. Simply put, actions to reduce fear
motivate individuals to act. The Health Belief Model consists of four constructs
related to perceived threats and net benefits (see **Table 4-1**).[19]

Table 4-1   The Health Belief Model Constructs and Related
Research Questions

Construct	Question	Example
Perceived susceptibility	Does the individual think she is at risk of getting the health condition or disease?	A 60-year-old female does not perceive a personal risk for breast cancer because no one in her family has ever had breast cancer.
Perceived severity	How serious does the individual think the health condition or disease is?	A 20-year-old female does not perceive the need for Pap test because she is not aware of the potentially serious and long-term conditions that may result from an undiagnosed sexually transmitted disease.
Perceived benefits	Does the individual believe the suggested action would decrease the risk of impact of the health condition or disease?	An overweight 48-year-old male with diabetes does not perceive any value or health benefits from losing 10–15 pounds because he has been a diabetic for more than 10 years.
Perceived barriers	What is the individual's opinion on the real or psychological costs of the suggested action?	A female adolescent is afraid to mention a changing mole on her shoulder because she is afraid she might need surgery and will have a scar on her shoulder.

The Health Belief Model incorporates cues to action, which are internal or external events that motivate individuals to act. An internal event is feeling a breast lump and scheduling a mammogram appointment. An external event is having a close relative be diagnosed with a specific disease or health condition, viewing a public service announcement, or reading a healthcare brochure. The external examples activate an individual's readiness to take action. For example, an overweight male who smokes two packs of cigarettes each day reads multiple brochures about weight loss and smoking cessation, but he does not begin to change his behavior until his health insurance premiums increase because of his risk status.

In 1977, Bandura[23] added self-efficacy to the Health Belief Model. Self-efficacy is the individual's confidence that he or she has the ability to perform the suggested action successfully. For example, if a woman does not believe she has the ability to remember how to correctly use the exercise machines at her gym, she is less likely to use the machines for fear of sustaining an injury from misuse (see **Box 4-8**).

Stages of Change Model, or Transtheoretical Model (Prochaska and DiClemente, 1983)

In the early 1980s, Prochaska and DiClemente published the Stages of Change Model, or Transtheoretical Model, which describes the stages of an individual's

---

BOX 4-8

Developing Culturally Appropriate Health Materials Using the Health Belief Model

In 2012, researchers reported results related to using the Health Belief Model to develop culturally appropriate weight management materials for African American women. Seven focus groups ($n = 50$) were conducted. Results revealed that the women reported that the perceived benefits to losing weight were reduced risk of health problems and improved physical appearance. The perceived barriers were lack of social support, motivation, and accurate dieting information. Motivators were reported as a health problem diagnosis, physical appearance, and saving money on clothing purchases. Self-efficacy was shown to be related to the women's frustration with their history of dieting. The conclusion of this research reveals the need for specific messages to the target audience.[24]

Table 4-2   The Stages of Change Model or Transtheoretical Model

Stage	Question	Example
Precontemplation	Is the individual aware that the behavior is a problem?	Patient is not ready to stop smoking.
Contemplation	Has the individual seriously thought about changing the behavior in the near future?	Patient wants to quit smoking in the next few months.
Preparation	Is the individual planning to take action? Is the individual making arrangements prior to changing behavior?	Patient is going to quit smoking on his next birthday and is investigating various methods.
Action	Is the individual implementing a specific action plan to modify behavior and surroundings?	By using nicotine gum, patient stopped smoking on her birthday and threw away all cigarettes.
Maintenance	Is the individual continuing the desirable actions? Is the individual repeating the actions to prevent lapses and relapse?	Patient has been smoke-free for three months without relapse.
Termination	Does the individual have the ability to resist temptation and relapse?	Patient is able to resist smoking when visiting friends who continue to smoke cigarettes.

readiness to change a specific health behavior.[20] The six-stage model is used to predict either adding a positive behavior or dropping a negative behavior (see **Table 4-2**).

The Stages of Change Model is a circular rather than a linear model. Often, individuals revert back to undesired behavior during the action or maintenance stage. It is common for individuals to go through the stages several times prior to achieving the success of extinguishing a negative behavior or engaging in a positive behavior. See **Box 4-9** for a case study involving the Stages of Change Model.

Theory of Reasoned Action (Fishbein and Ajzen, 1975)

In 1975, the Theory of Reasoned Action was developed to predict and understand human behavior; it has four constructs (see **Table 4-3**).[21] For an example of the Theory of Reasoned Action from the literature, see **Box 4-10**.

Social Learning Theory (Bandura, 1977), or Social Cognitive Theory (Rotter, 1954)

Social Learning Theory combines interactive factors to understand human behavior (see **Table 4-4**).[22,23,25]

BOX 4-9

Using Stages of Change for Sunscreen Promotion

In 2012, researchers reported findings of their study related to enhancing sunscreen use at different stages of change. There were 292 participants in the study including three groups: (1) the group with no intention of using sunscreen ($n = 51$), (2) the group with high intention but no regular use of sunscreen ($n = 102$), and (3) the group that uses sunscreen on a regular basis ($n = 139$). The results showed that communication about a plan to use sunscreen was the most effective for the high-intention group. In conclusion, the findings showed the need for interventions to match the stage of each segment of the target audience to be most effective.[26]

Table 4-3   Constructs in the Theory of Reasoned Action

Four Constructs in the Theory of Reasoned Action	Example
One: Individuals believe that if a behavior is performed, a given outcome will occur.	Individuals believe that if they receive an annual flu vaccine, their chances of getting severe flu symptoms are reduced.
Two: Behavior is influenced by motivation to comply with social norms.	If their workplace is offering free flu vaccines in the company lobby from 11:00 a.m. to 1:00 p.m. every Friday in September, workers are likely to follow social norms and be motivated by coworkers to receive the flu vaccine.
Three: Attitude plays a role in behavior. If an individual has a positive attitude, the outcome is likely to be favorable; if an individual has a negative attitude, the outcome is likely to be less favorable.	Individuals who received the flu vaccine previously and *did not* get the flu are more likely to receive the vaccine again. Individuals who received the flu vaccine previously and *did* get the flu are less likely to get the vaccine again. Also, individuals who never received the vaccine and never got the flu are less likely to receive the vaccine.
Four: Subjective norms affect beliefs. If an individual believes his social peer group is in favor of or opposed to a certain behavior, this perception affects the motivation to comply with peers.	If individuals believe (with or without evidence) that their coworkers received the flu vaccine, then they are more likely to also receive the flu vaccine.

BOX 4-10

A Test of the Theory of Reasoned Action: Oral Hygiene

In 2012, research findings were reported on using the Theory of Reasoned Action to influence oral hygiene behavior and gingival outcomes. With a sample size of 113, data were collected from baseline examinations and self-report questionnaires. Results revealed that higher self-efficacy to baseline was linked to higher frequency of oral health behaviors at 3 months. Females were linked to more normative beliefs and greater self-efficacy. Overall, the results showed that greater oral hygiene at 3 months predicted gingival outcomes at 12 months.[27]

Table 4-4 Constructs of Social Learning Theory

Construct	Question	Example
Behavioral capability	Does the individual have the knowledge and skills necessary to perform a specific behavior that affects future actions?	After attending five classes, did individuals with type 2 diabetes obtain the knowledge and skills necessary to give themselves insulin injections?
Expectations	Does the individual expect a specific outcome for performing a behavior?	After attending five classes, did individuals with type 2 diabetes expect that the insulin injections and prescribed food plan would lower their blood glucose?
Self-efficacy	Does the individual have an adequate sense of self to do what it takes to change a behavior?	After attending five classes, did individuals with type 2 diabetes have a personal desire to follow the insulin injection and prescribed food plan to lower their blood glucose?
Environment	How is the individual changing his or her environment and at the same time being changed by the environment?	After attending five classes, did individuals with type 2 diabetes learn how to eliminate unhealthy food choices from their kitchen and replace the items with positive food choices? After this change, did the individuals report that it was easier to follow the food plan because the unhealthy food choices were no longer readily accessible?
Reinforcement	What type of reinforcement is influencing an individual to change a behavior?	After attending five classes, what type of reinforcement did individuals with type 2 diabetes receive for attempting the required behavioral changes? Did the individuals' hemoglobin A1C drop as a positive long-term reinforcement?

In addition, the theory involves three types of reinforcement to influence behavior change: (1) direct reinforcement, where the individual receives a reward for performing the behavior, (2) vicarious reinforcement, where the individual sees someone receive a reward for performing the behavior, and (3) self-management/self-control reinforcement, where the individual gains control by tracking personal behavior and personal rewards reinforce the positive behavior. For example, when individuals join a weight loss group, they learn (behavioral capacity) how to eat healthily and exercise more. They see others in the group record a weight loss each week, so they have an expectation of losing weight. The weekly meetings offer the type of environment to assist individuals seeking a healthy weight loss program. Their behavior is reinforced, because they lose weight each week (direct) and observe others (vicarious) receive applause and certificates each week for achieving weight loss goals. By tracking their prescribed food and exercise plan, they gain control over food and exercise to achieve and maintain their ideal weight.

See **Box 4-11** for an example of the Social Learning Theory. Note that the reference for Box 4-11 is from the proceedings of the 2012 National Conference on Undergraduate Research (NCUR). It illustrates how undergraduate students are involved in research studies.

BOX 4-11 Social Learning Theory: Extended Families in the African American Community

In 2012, Armstrong presented results from collecting qualitative data from document analysis techniques and from conducting interviews with African American families. The operational definition includes two types of families: (1) *extended family* is defined as multiple generations with aunts, uncles, grandparents, and so on, and (2) *nuclear family* consists of primarily a mother and father. From an economic standpoint, results show that extended families collect greater financial resources than the nuclear family and therefore are considered the composition of the ideal family.[28]

Strategic Planning Models

Whether you are planning a new project, evaluating an existing project, or determining procedures to revamp an organization, strategic planning skills are required. The easiest way to define strategic planning is to answer the following questions:

Where is the project currently?

Where does the project hope to be in one year?

What needs to be accomplished to meet the goal, and how can it be done?

There are numerous benefits of strategic planning; it provides a roadmap for how the project is conducted from beginning to completion. A few examples of how a project benefits from strategic planning include (1) establishing realistic and achievable objectives for each goal, (2) developing a sense of ownership among the team members, (3) prioritizing use of key resources, (4) allowing the opportunity to listen to team member opinions prior to initiating the first step of the project, (5) creating and reviewing the time management chart together to avoid time conflicts in the future, and (6) addressing potential internal conflicts among team members. To avoid complaints that strategic plans are developed but never used, it is important to update and refer to it at regular intervals. Think of the strategic plan as a process rather than a final product. For example, it serves no purpose for healthcare providers to spend several weeks revamping the clinic's strategic plan to improve staff retention and patient satisfaction if the recommendations in the plan are never implemented or never revisited a few months after the implementation.

There are two common types of strategic planning models. One is goal based and the other is issue based. Goal-based strategic planning involves starting with a goal or mission statement and then developing the action plan to meet the goals, for example, to improve clinic staff retention. Issue-based strategic planning begins with examining the issues or problems that need to be addressed, then prioritizing the issues and working toward an action plan to solve the problems, for example, the increasing cost of training new clinic staff, the number of clinic staff resignations in the past 12 months, the specific type of clinic staff resigning, results of exit interviews to determine reasons for resignation. For maximum collaboration and participation, engagement of diverse stakeholders is ideal in the development of either type of action plan. Once the action plan is developed and agreed upon, it is necessary to use a time management chart to ensure timely completion of the project.

This section describes several tools to assist with tracking the progress of the action plan over time. There are many ways to manage simple to complex projects including elaborate computer software programs. Gantt charts, action plans, and SWOT analyses are described in this discussion. Regardless of the tracking tool selected, it is important to utilize a management system tool for each project.

Gantt Charts

Gantt charts illustrate schedules, tasks, and activities over a specific period of the project (see **Figure 4-2**). Because Gantt charts are viewed by the entire team, everyone is aware of start and finish dates of each aspect of a project. By using shading for percentage completed, the vertical line stays current to the present. Some Gantt charts provide details of relationships between activities as well as the team members responsible for the completion of each task.

Action Plans

Action plans track each activity related to goals, objectives, activities, and the person responsible (see **Table 4-5**). This type of action plan reduces confusion about who is responsible for ensuring that each activity is completed on time. Action plans are developed with input and collaboration from team members to reduce conflict and misunderstanding of assigned tasks. It is also important to tie the name of the responsible person to job descriptions and personnel performance reviews. It is unfair to assign extra or unfamiliar duties to individuals without proper training and support. The preferred method involves having individuals work in pairs in a collaborative work commitment.

SWOT Analysis

Although Gantt charts or action plans are valuable tools for tracking progress, it is also important to step back, revisit the strategic plan, and assess the big picture. A SWOT analysis (strengths, weaknesses, opportunities, and threats) allows the team members to explore the project from various viewpoints that may be overlooked in the daily routine. The most appropriate time to conduct a SWOT analysis is during a team meeting. After starting the discussion with a broad question (e.g., What is this project trying to accomplish?), the discussion

Tasks	Task	Task lead	Start	End	Duration weeks	% Done	Wrck Days	Days Complete	Days Left
1	1.1	Sue	1/2	1/20	3	100%	15	15	0
2	1.2	Jane	1/9	1/20	2	80%	10	10	0
3	1.3	Rob	1/9	1/20	5	90%	5	5	0
4	1.4	Sue	1/23	3/31	10	40%	50	15	35
5	2.0	Kelly	1/23	2/6	2	80%	10	10	0
6	2.2	Jane	2/13	3/19	5	2%	25	0	25
7	2.3	John	3/5	3/12	2	0%	10	0	10
8	3.0	Sue	3/5	3/12	1	100%	5	0	5
9	4.0	Rob	3/5	3/19	1	0%	5	0	5
10	4.1	Kelly	3/5	3/26	3	0%	15	0	15
11	4.2	Rob	3/5	3/26	3	0%	15	0	15
12	4.3	Sue	3/5	4/2	4	100%	20	0	20
13	4.4	Jane	3/5	4/2	4	0%	20	0	20
14	4.5	John	3/12	4/2	3	50%	15	15	0

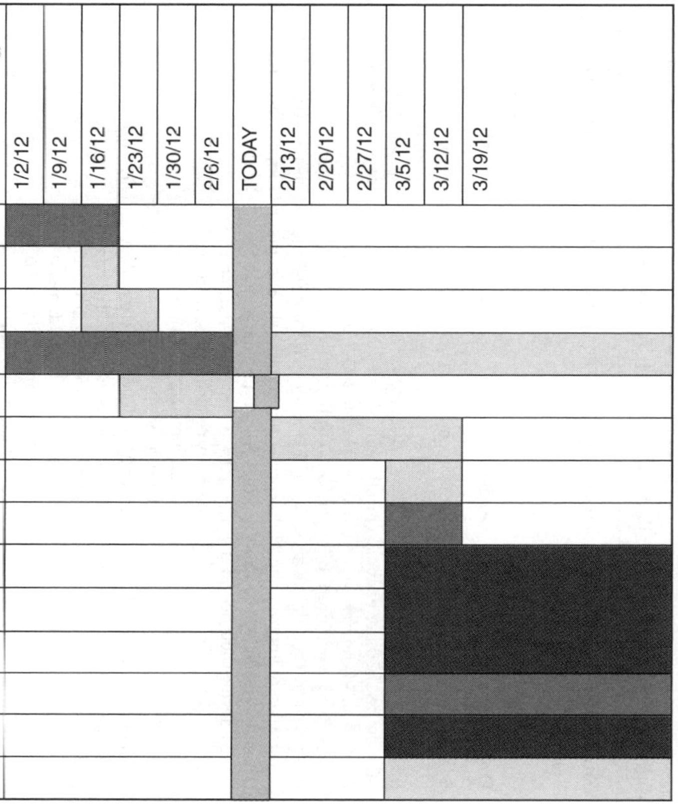

Project Name: ABC — Health

Date columns: 1/2/12, 1/9/12, 1/16/12, 1/23/12, 1/30/12, 2/6/12, TODAY, 2/13/12, 2/20/12, 2/27/12, 3/5/12, 3/12/12, 3/19/12

FIGURE 4-2 Example of a Gantt Chart

Table 4-5   Example of a Detailed Two-Month Action Plan

Goal: Initiate a three-year study to improve the patients' satisfaction of food served during their hospital stay.

Month	Objective	Activity	Responsible Person(s)
March	By the end of the second week of March, form a hospital task force with 40 members (10 per each of the 4 subcommittees) representing a minimum of 8 departments to initiate a 3-year plan to improve the patients' satisfaction of food served during their hospital stay.	Send an email to all hospital employees inviting interested individuals to attend an organizational meeting on March 29 to form a task force to improve patient satisfaction with hospital food.	Stephen Westin, Administrative Assistant for Hospital Services
		Assign 4 managers from different hospital units to chair 4 subcommittees (secondary data, qualitative data, quantitative data, and feasibility) within the task force, plus administrative support for each subcommittee.	Lilly Knowles, MBA, Human Resource Director Stephen Westin
	By the end of March, hire 2 graduate nursing students to work on this initiative as part of their theses.	Contact the local nursing college; place an advertisement; review applications; interview at least 3 graduate nursing students; hire 2 students; complete paperwork for their salary and tuition payments.	Lilly Knowles Stephen Westin
	By the end of March, a minimum of 60 interested hospital employees attend the first task force meeting.	Make attendee name tags including department and job title; have laptop and screen, colored markers, and large white paper tablets on easels available; order nutritious food for meeting; prepare PowerPoint slides for introductory remarks to describe the goals and objectives of the task force.	Lilly Knowles Stephen Westin
		Have each participant sign up on the white tablets for their first and second choices of the 4 subcommittees. If interested employees were not able to attend the meeting due to work conflicts, they were invited to email their subcommittee choices to Stephen within 3 days.	Stephen Westin
		Assign participants to subcommittees based on their choices so each subcommittee represents a variety of departments, job descriptions, pay grades, and expertise. Each subcommittee is overpopulated with members in anticipation of attrition and work schedule conflicts.	Lilly Knowles Stephen Westin

continues

Table 4-5　Example of a Detailed Two-Month Action Plan *continued*

Month	Objective	Activity	Responsible Person(s)
		Arrange date, time, and location for meetings of each of the 4 sub-committees; email participants with their subcommittee assignments and other pertinent information.	Stephen Westin
April	By the end of the fourth week in April, the secondary data task force subcommittee meets with the chair and a minimum of 7 hospital employees.	Agree upon goals and objectives and most convenient time, date, and location for future meetings. For example, a subcommittee goal may be gathering existing secondary data, such as average food cost per patient over the last year.	Janet Johnson, RD, Food Service Manager Evelyn Schwenzer, Administrative Assistant for Food Service Manager
	By the end of the fourth week in April, the qualitative data task force subcommittee meets with the chair and a minimum of 7 hospital employees.	Agree upon goals and objectives and most convenient time, date, and location for future meetings. For example, a subcommittee goal may be interviewing patients (qualitative data) prior to discharge about food choices during hospital stay.	Mark Kendall, MSN, Continuing Education Manager Margaret Riley, Administrative Assistant for Continuing Education Manager
	By the end of the fourth week in April, the quantitative data task force subcommittee meets with the chair and a minimum of 7 hospital employees.	Agree upon goals and objectives and most convenient time, date, and location for future meetings. For example, a subcommittee goal may be adding a few more questions (quantitative data) to the existing mailed patient satisfaction survey.	Chris Mitchell, MS, Information Technology Director Bradley Hanson, Intern, Information Technology
	By the end of the fourth week in April, the feasibility task force subcommittee meets with the chair and a minimum of 7 hospital employees.	Agree upon goals and objectives and most convenient time, date, and location for future meetings. For example, a subcommittee goal may be investigating long-term contracts with food service vendors (feasibility data) to determine ability to change supplier.	Davis March, MBA, Financial Services Coordinator Simon Patel, Administrative Assistant for Financial Services Coordinator

moves to the SWOT analysis. **Table 4-6** shows examples of questions to begin a SWOT analysis.[29] As more questions and responses are added to each box, the big picture emerges for further discussion. The discussion is not a time for finger-pointing, complaints, or criticism, but it is a collective way to improve what is working and to reduce any problems.

Table 4-6   Sample SWOT Analysis

Strengths	Weaknesses
What is working?	Are there problems that could be minimized?
Even if the internal team effort is strong, how can it be improved?	Where are the problems?
	Are the community stakeholders involved?

Opportunities	Threats
Are we missing something that would improve the project?	Are we overlooking a problem?
	How can we eliminate a possible funding cut?
Are there additional grants or funding opportunities that we are overlooking?	Is any agency providing the same type of program or services?

Summary

This chapter covers a variety of theories and models. The application of theories and models as a framework for designing programs and research includes universal theories, system theories, ecological models, community and organization theories and models, social networks and social support theories, and individual behavior theories and models. The chapter ends with a description of strategic planning models including Gantt charts, action plans, and SWOT analysis.

Case Study

At the recent clinic strategic planning meeting, the team members (administrators, healthcare providers, clinic staff, and community members) decided it was time to upgrade the patient management system to include a comprehensive electronic medical record (EMR) system, including converting all paper medical records to e-records, implementing patient exam room e-charting, and installing an e-patient communication system for making appointments, requesting prescription refills,

continues

CASE STUDY *continued*

and making payments. Fortunately, the clinic had enough money in its reserve account to pay for this system upgrade. It was decided that the project would begin with establishing a training computer lab so every employee would be trained on the mock computer software prior to any clinic implementation.

Because Ms. Hill, the training administrator, was familiar with behavioral theories, she used the Social Learning Theory to evaluate the training process instead of merely implementing the training without any evaluation plans. Ms. Hill wanted to make the training a positive experience, so she used the Diffusion of Innovations Theory and let employees volunteer to attend the training sessions. She selected this theory instead of conducting the training by department because she knew that the innovators would seek out the training first and their positive comments would encourage the early adopters to sign up next. After word spread through the clinic, the early majority employees completed the training. Lastly, Ms. Hill had to get a bit creative with a small incentive to get the late majority and laggards to attend the last training session. After each group of employees received 20 hours of computer training, she conducted a satisfaction survey. The categories of survey questions followed the constructs of the Social Learning Theory (see **Table 4-7**).

Table 4-7   How Social Learning Theory Constructs Guide Research Questions

Construct	Question
Behavioral capability	Did the staff leave the training with enough knowledge and skills to perform the specific EMR system that affects their clinic duties?
Expectations	At the training, did the staff receive an overview of how the EMR system benefits the overall clinic operation as well as expectations for specific outcomes in their areas of the clinic?
Self-efficacy	Did the staff experience enough hands-on computer time during the training to feel confident in implementing specific behavioral changes with the new EMR system?
Environment	Is the clinic environment changing to accommodate individual staff needs, for example, location of new computers, online screen viewing, and so on, to implement the EMR system in the patient exam rooms and staff work areas?
Reinforcement	What type of reinforcement is planned within the clinic to influence the staff to continue to make individual behavioral changes related to how the EMR system affects their daily routine?

continues

CASE STUDY *continued*

After the survey data were analyzed, Ms. Hill realized that the training was well received among all levels of clinic staff. Her next step was to move the EMR system from the training classroom to full operation. For this phase, she formed a staff implementation team to minimize any clinic disruption during the EMR training and implementation. After seven months, the EMR system was fully operational with the clinic staff. Ms. Hill began the patient education side of the EMR system by conducting focus groups with clinic patients and presenting the results to her implementation team to plan the next step.

Case Study Discussion Questions

1. What other theories could have been used?
2. How should Ms. Hill form the staff implementation team?

Student Activities

1. Write two research questions related to improving the appointment scheduling and patient flow for an outpatient clinic. Select a theory and write a description about how this theory serves as the framework for designing the clinic intervention.
2. Describe a personal behavior that you would like to change. Select an individual behavior change theory and write how you could apply the principles of the theory to your personal behavior change.
3. Using a Gantt chart, plot the calendar of assignments for a course that you are taking this semester. Be sure to include a vertical line indicating the current week of the course.
4. Describe a group or organization in which you are a member. Using a SWOT analysis, describe how the group or organization might be improved.

References

1. Kerlinger FN. *Foundations of Behavioral Research*, 3rd ed. New York, NY: Holt, Rinehart and Winston; 1986.
2. Research Methods Knowledge Base. Deduction and Induction. Available at: http://www.socialresearchmethods.net/kb/dedind.php. Accessed January 17, 2012.
3. Centers for Disease Control and Prevention. A cluster of Kaposi's sarcoma and *Pneumocystis carinii* pneumonia among homosexual male residents of Los Angeles and Orange Counties, California. *MMWR*. 1982;31(23):305–307. Available at: http://www.cdc.gov/mmwr/preview/mmwrhtml/00001114.htm. Accessed January 17, 2012.
4. Friedman-Kien AE. Disseminated Kaposi's sarcoma syndrome in young homosexual men. *J Am Acad Dermatol*. 1981;5(4):468–471.
5. Hymes KB, Cheung T, Greene JB, et al. Kaposi's sarcoma in homosexual men: A report of eight cases. *Lancet*. 1981;2(8247):598–600.
6. Barre-Sinoussi F, Chermann J, Rey F, et al. Isolation of a T lymphotropic retrovirus from a patient at risk for acquired immune deficiency syndrome (AIDS). *Science*. 1983;220(4599):868–871.
7. Halliday D, Resnick R, Krane K. *Physics*, vol. 1. New York, NY: John Wiley & Sons; 2001.
8. King IM. *A Theory for Nursing: Systems, Concepts, and Process*. New York, NY: Wiley; 1981.
9. Alligood MR. Family healthcare with King's theory of goal attainment. *Nurs Sci Q*. 2010;23(2):99–104.
10. McLeroy KR, Bibeau D, Steckler A, Glanz K. An ecological perspective on health promotion programs. *Health Educ Q*. 1988;15(4):351–377.
11. Bronfenbrenner U. *The Ecology of Human Development: Experiments by Nature and Design*. Cambridge, MA: Harvard University Press; 1979.
12. Seiloff CL. Measuring nursing power within organizations. *J Nurs Schlarsh*. 1991;35(2):183–187.
13. Greenfield EA. Using ecological frameworks to advance a field of research, practice, and policy on aging-in-place initiatives. *The Gerontologist*. 2011;(52)1:1–12.
14. Gottlieb BH. Social networks and social support: An overview of research, practice, and policy implications. *Health Educ Behav*. 1985;12:5–22.
15. Rogers EM, Shoemaker FF. *Communication of Innovations: A Cross-Cultural Approach*. New York, NY: The Free Press; 1971.
16. Glasgow RE, Vogt TM, Boles SM. Evaluating the public health impact of health promotion interventions: The RE-AIM framework. *Am J Public Health*. 1999;89(9):1322–1327.
17. Benson PR. Network characteristics, perceived social support and psychological adjustment in mothers of children with autism spectrum disorder. *J Autism Dev Disord*. 2012;42:2597–2610.
18. George S, Hamilton A, Baker RS. How do low-income urban African Americans and Latinos feel about telemedicine? A diffusion of innovation analysis. *International Journal of Telemedicine and Applications*. 2012;(1)
19. Rosenstock IM. Historical origins of the health belief model. *Health Educ Quart*. 1974;15(2):175–183.

20. Prochaska JO, DiClemente CC. Stages and processes of self-change of smoking: Toward an integrative model of change. *J Consult Clin Psychol.* 1983;51(3):390–395.

21. Fishbein M, Ajzen I. *Belief, Attitude, Intention and Behavior: An Introduction to Theory and Research Reading.* Reading, MA: Addison-Wesley; 1975.

22. Bandura A. *Social Learning Theory.* Englewood Cliffs, NJ: Prentice Hall; 1977.

23. Bandura A. Self-efficacy: Toward a unifying theory of behavioral change. *Psychol Rev.* 1977;84(2):191–215.

24. James DC, Pobee JW, Oxidine D, Brown L, Joshi G. Using the health belief model to develop culturally appropriate weight management materials for African American women. *J Acad Nutr Diet.* 2012;112(5):664–670.

25. Rotter JB. *Social Learning and Clinical Psychology.* New York, NY: Prentice Hall; 1954.

26. Craciun C, Schuz N, Lippke S, Schwarzer R. Enhancing planning strategies for sunscreen use at different stages of change. *Health Educ Res.* 2012;27(5):857–867.

27. Jonsson B, Baker SR, Lindberg P, Oscarson N, Ohrn K. Factors influencing oral hygiene behavior and gingival outcomes 3 and 12 months after initial periodontal treatment: An exploratory test of an extended Theory of Reasoned Action. *J Clin Periodontol.* 2012;39:138–144.

28. Armstrong N. The importance of extended families in the African American community: A qualitative analysis using social learning theory. Proceedings of the National Conference on Undergraduate Research (NCUR), 2012. Weber State University, Ogden, Utah.

29. Piercy WG. Making SWOT analysis work. *Marketing Intelligence and Planning.* 1989;7(5/6):5–7.

CHAPTER 5

Reliability and Validity

CHAPTER OBJECTIVES

By the end of this chapter, students will be able to:

- Explain the concepts of stability and internal consistency as related to reliability
- Demonstrate how reliability and validity are related to each other
- Describe the four types of validity
- Explain the difference between internal and external threats to validity
- Define random errors and systematic errors
- Justify the steps needed to conduct a pilot study

KEY TERMS

External validity	Reliability
Internal validity	Systematic errors
Pilot testing	Validity
Random errors	

Introduction

This chapter introduces the concepts of *reliability* and *validity*. Briefly, in quantitative and qualitative research, reliability refers to consistency. The two different forms of reliability discussed include stability and internal consistency. Next, the chapter defines validity and discusses the types of validity as well as threats to internal and external validity. It is essential to remember that it is more important to be valid than reliable. Validity is defined as the extent to which a test measures what it purports to measure. Therefore, if the test does not measure the correct concept, it does not matter if it is reliable. Lastly, the chapter ends with a detailed description of how to conduct a pilot test.

Reliability

If you are asked to describe the word *reliable*, you might think of dependability or trustworthiness (e.g., a dependable car or trustworthy friend). In research and evaluation, reliability is focused on consistency of the instrument or survey being used, not the respondents. Reliability is related to consistency or the ability to repeat results.[1] For example, if you weigh a package on your bathroom scale several times in two hours, you are likely to get the same weight of 2.6 pounds each time. This exercise shows that your bathroom scale is reliable and consistent. Next you take the same package to the post office. The package weighs 2.1 pounds on the official post office scale, which determines the cost of postage of mailing the package. Because the post office scale is frequently calibrated for accuracy, the scale at the post office is reliable (consistent in reporting the same weight each time) and valid (measures what it purports to measure).

Investigators know that a test is reliable if the results are the same each time it is used with the same individuals. Let's explore why reliability is important. If the test results are not approximately the same each time an individual completes the test, investigators have no way of determining which of the scores is correct. If the results are different each time the test is used, the test is deemed faulty or unreliable.[2] For example, when physicians order a blood lab test, they expect that the machine used to test the blood is reliable. If the machine is not reliable, physicians may fail to prescribe the correct medications, which may result in complications for their patients' health. Physicians count on the reliability of their tests in order to protect the health of those they serve. In another example, if standardized exams are not reliable and an individual obtains a professional licensure because of those test scores, how can we be certain that he *really* has the knowledge necessary for performing his job accurately and safely? From an investigator standpoint, unreliable tests lead to inaccurate conclusions. Other researchers may try to duplicate the study or build on the faulty results. Time and resources are unnecessarily wasted until the lack of reliability is discovered.

This section introduces two ways to establish reliability: stability and internal consistency. Because it is not possible to calculate reliability, researchers and evaluators can only estimate it. Reliability measurement is beyond the scope of this chapter, so definitions are provided for greater understanding, but without calculations.

Stability

Stability is when the results of a survey or instrument are consistent over time. You can check the stability of an instrument by giving it to an individual and then giving it to her again after a certain period of time; this is called the test-retest technique. Test-retest involves two assumptions. First, the item or observation does not change over time. For example, survey questions are not changed between the first and second administrations. Second, the time between the first and second administrations is long enough (e.g., several days or weeks, depending on the instrument) that participating individuals do not remember their responses. If the results remain stable, then the test is reliable. For example, if students take the Graduate Record Exam the first Saturday of each month for three consecutive months, their scores remain somewhat consistent. Another example is the Myers-Briggs Type Indicator of personality types. This instrument claims to remain stable over a person's adult life.[3] However, it should be noted that there are also instruments that are specifically designed to show change over time, such as the Hassles and Uplifts Scales (HSUP). This scale measures attitudes about daily situations instead of focusing on major life events.[4]

Internal Consistency

Internal consistency is defined as the extent to which each question in a survey is related to the same topic. Internal consistency is also called *homogeneity*. In quantitative research, researchers use a split-half technique to measure homogeneity. This technique is done by dividing the entire test or survey into two equal halves (e.g., odd-numbered and even-numbered questions). The two forms are administered to the same individuals. If the odd-numbered questions yield the same results as the even-numbered, the entire test is deemed reliable. For example, instructors write 40 questions about information provided in Chapter 26 of a human anatomy textbook. The even-numbered questions are used for Test A and the odd-numbered questions are used for Test B. Both sets of questions for Tests A and B are printed on one form and distributed to the students. Investigators grade Test A questions to obtain one score, and then grade Test B questions to obtain another, separate score. If the whole exam has internal reliability, the Test A and Test B scores should be approximately equal, with all questions measuring concepts related to material covered in Chapter 26. If questions draw from topics in other chapters, the exam lacks internal reliability.[5]

Related to the discussion of internal consistency, readers may see the term *coefficient alpha* or *Cronbach's alpha* used in the literature.[6] Cronbach's alpha is defined as a measurement of internal consistency among a group of items (e.g., survey, test, or interview questions). This measurement allows researchers to determine how well the items measure different aspects of the same topic.[7] Although the statistical formula to calculate coefficient alpha or Cronbach's alpha is beyond the scope of this chapter, readers should note the range of reliability scores. Cronbach's alpha values range from zero to one. Values closer to one indicate a higher internal consistency than values closer to zero (see **Table 5-1**).[8]

For qualitative data, internal consistency is called *inter-rater reliability* or *inter-observational reliability*. These terms mean that the scoring or observations remain consistent regardless of the person who is doing it. For example, instructors participate in training on how to score essay exams. Following training, instructors receive identical essay exams from 10 different students. When instructors have reliable grading skills, each student grade is consistent among all instructors. If instructors have very different scores on identical students essay exams, their skills are unreliable and more training is required. For inter-observations, investigators use a checklist to standardize and increase reliability. For example, evaluators observing patients and family use a checklist to record the number and duration of conversation interactions, the number of

Table 5-1   Range of Reliability Scores

Reliability Score	Rating
Equal to or greater than 0.9	Excellent
Equal to or greater than 0.8	Good
Equal to or greater than 0.7	Acceptable
Equal to or greater than 0.6	Questionable
Equal to or greater than 0.5	Poor
Less than 0.5	Unacceptable

family members present, the language spoken, the individuals who initiate conversations, and distractions (television, cell phone, eating, etc.) used by patient and family to pass time while waiting. Checklists ensure that evaluators are collecting the same type of observational data. Evaluators use the following formula to calculate an inter-rater reliability score:

Number of concurrences / number of opportunities for concurrence × 100

For example, two investigators use a predetermined checklist to observe 80 patients in the clinic waiting room. According to their checklist, they agree on 68 out of the 80 ratings. The calculation is 68/80 = 0.85 × 100 = 85%. Therefore, the investigators agree 85% of the time, or their observations have a reliability of 85%.[9] There is an acceptable range of reliability scores for qualitative research, with 90% being excellent and less than 50% being unacceptable. Of the two ways to estimate reliability, each one has advantages and disadvantages.[10] See **Table 5-2**, then practice your skills using **Box 5-1**.

Table 5-2   Estimating Reliability: Advantages and Disadvantages

Ways to Establish Reliability	Type	Advantages	Disadvantages
Stability	Test-retest	Single rater is adequate	Often difficult to recruit same respondents to respond twice
		No need to train teams of raters	Individuals may not respond as seriously the second time
		Less expensive and time consuming	
Internal consistency	Quantitative: Split-half forms	Respondents take both surveys at the same time	Need to create a large pool of items
		No need to recruit respondents twice	
	Qualitative: Inter-rater or inter-observation reliability	Best for observational research, especially when video recording is used	Expensive
			Time consuming
		Possible option: One rater reviewing video at two different times	Requires team of raters for best results

Data from Trochim MK. Types of Reliability. Research Methods Knowledge Base. Available at: http://www.socialresearchmethods.net/kb/reltypes.php

BOX 5-1

Evaluation Practice: Reliability

The College of Pharmacy at State University offers two sections each semester of Pharmacology I, which is required for all newly admitted pharmacy students during their first year. Each semester, professors rotate this teaching assignment. In the fall semester, Dr. Nice taught one section and Dr. Stern taught the other section. Over the years, whenever Dr. Nice teaches, students earn higher final grades than when other professors teach the same course. The administrators are concerned that Dr. Nice is teaching students the test questions rather than teaching the broad application of concepts related to pharmacology. Administrators also note that professors are responsible for creating their own exams. Because the administrators did not have time to investigate their concerns, they hired Acme Evaluation Team to investigate the situation. The Acme Evaluation Team began by investigating the internal consistency of the tests offered in Pharmacology I classes. They obtained copies of the midterm exams from Dr. Nice, Dr. Stern, and several other professors from previous semesters. Using the split-half technique, the Acme Evaluation Team concluded that the midterm exams were not internally consistent. Some professors emphasized certain topics while other professors highlighted different topics on the midterm exams. Once this result was known, the Acme Evaluation Team developed a checklist for observing professors' lectures. The checklist was based on the general concepts from a few specific chapters from the textbook. During the second half of the fall semester, Dr. Nice's lectures and Dr. Stern's lectures were observed by two Acme Evaluation Team members. Based on the checklist, it was apparent that Dr. Nice stressed some textbook materials in particular whereas Dr. Stern covered each area equally. The inter-rater reliability score of 96% showed consistency on the part of the Acme Evaluation Team. Based on the results of reliability research, the Acme Evaluation Team made the following recommendations to administrators:

1. Standardize the Pharmacology I course syllabus so the course remains the same every semester for all professors teaching the course and all first-year pharmacy students enrolled in the course.

continues

BOX 5-1 *continued*

2. Update course as needed to stay current with knowledge.
3. Have professors develop a commonly shared test bank based on the major points from each chapter of the textbook.
4. Have all students take online exams in the computer lab during the regularly scheduled class period; exam questions would be randomly generated by the computer from the commonly developed test bank so that teaching the test would be prohibited.

Using these recommendations would mean that students would learn the same material regardless of the professor teaching each section, and professors would save time by not having to develop and grade exams. The administrators incorporated the recommendations, and everyone agreed that the Acme Evaluation Team solved the problem for the College of Pharmacy.

As we move from reliability to validity, it is important to understand the relationship between the two concepts. If a scale is valid, the results should be the same if the same person is tested on it over and over. However, the reverse is not always true. Reliability is about consistency and repeatability. Validity is determined by whether the scale measures what it was intended to measure and whether the results are generalizable to other populations.[11] **Figure 5-1** illustrates relationships between reliability and validity.[12] Keep in mind that the center of the target is the concept that you are trying to measure. Each dot represents one individual who is completing a survey or interview.

Validity

Let's begin the discussion of validity by looking at how reliability and validity are related. As noted in Figure 5-1, it is possible for a test to have low reliability and low validity, high reliability and low validity, and high reliability and high validity. For example, a depression test appears to be consistent and reliable. However, after analyzing the data, researchers discover that it is actually measuring self-esteem rather than depression. In this case, the scale is reliable, but not valid, because it is consistently measuring the wrong construct (self-esteem). It is more important for a test to be valid than to be reliable.

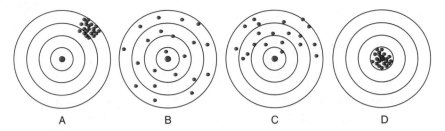

A: Reliable but not valid: Dots are consistently measuring the wrong concept.
B: Low reliability and low validity: Dots are spread across the target; low consistency and low measurement of concept.
C: Neither reliable nor valid: Dots are inconsistent, measuring the wrong concept and missing the target.
D: Both reliable and valid: Dots are packed closely in the center; consistently measures the correct concept.

FIGURE 5-1   Comparing Reliability and Validity
http://www.socialresearchmethods.net/kb/relandval.php. Reprinted by permission of William M.K. Trochim.

Types of Validity

Validity is defined as the extent to which a test measures what it purports to measure, whereas reliability is focused on consistency. There are two types of validity: internal and external.

Internal Validity

Internal validity focuses on the rigor of the study, while external validity deals with generalizability.[13] There are several types of internal validity: face validity, criterion-related validity, construct validity, and content validity.

Face Validity

Face validity examines how the test appears. Does the test look reasonable? Does it appear to be well designed? Is the test appealing? Face validity is not based on theory, but merely the appearance of the test (e.g., potential ease of completion, comprehension, and readability). Researchers and evaluators strive for excellent face validity. Even though the test may not be reliable, it at least looks good. Think of face validity as "showing up in the correct outfit." The individual looks good at the job interview, but there may or may not be enough experience to back up the good looks to land the job. However, keep in mind that first impressions are important, and without the right outfit, the interview may begin poorly. The same is true with evaluation and research; if the survey does not "show up in the right outfit" (i.e., look appealing), then individuals are less likely to complete it.[14] Face validity also refers to the logical sense of the survey. For example, if respondents are told that the survey they are about to complete concerns their level of satisfaction of clinic services, but the survey questions are all related to utilization of clinic services, the survey would lack face validity.

Criterion-Related Validity

Criterion-related validity measures one topic in two different ways. In other words, just because students pass the written test does not mean they can perform a specific skill. For example, suppose researchers are establishing criterion-related validity for intravenous (IV) placement technique among nursing students. First, the nursing students complete a written test related to proper procedures for IV placement techniques. Next, investigators use a checklist while observing nursing students during the step-by-step procedure as they insert IV catheters into the patient's forearm. The written test is validated by using the criterion-related strategy of the observation checklist. It is essential that the nursing students know the didactic information, but they must also know how to perform the required skill.

Construct Validity

Construct validity is used to measure a concept that is not actually observable. For example, although heart rate may actually be observed and felt, something like memory or intelligence cannot.[15] Investigators establish construct validity by exploring relationships with similar measures, experimental measures, and comparison scores among defined groups.

Relationship with Similar Measures   Researchers are interested in developing a shorter depression scale for adolescents. Adolescents are asked to complete both the older, longer depression scale with established validity and the newly developed, shorter depression scale. If the measurements of the established depression scale are similar to the measurements of the new scale, then researchers conclude evidence of construct validity.

Relationship with Experimental Measures   Researchers create a controlled environment that increases anxiety among patients in a rehabilitation facility by turning off the air-conditioning in the unit. After one hour, the patient rooms are uncomfortable, and patients are asked to complete two anxiety scales: one with established validity and a newly developed scale. In the midst of potential anxiety, patients should score higher on both scales. If both scales show similar levels of anxiety, researchers conclude evidence of construct validity.

Comparison Scores Among Defined Groups Researchers create a new dexterity aptitude test with the hypothesis that adults have varying degrees of dexterity. More than 1,000 adults complete the new dexterity aptitude test. If results show that adults in specific fields (e.g., surgeons, dentists, musicians, chefs, hairstylists) score higher on the new dexterity aptitude test than adults in nondexterity occupations (e.g., lawyers, truck drivers, writers, accountants), then there is evidence of construct validity.[16]

Content Validity

Content validity is defined as how well a test measures the specific content it is intended to measure.[11,17] For example, if researchers wish to study how first-year medical students learn about commonly used cardiac medications, they design a test. If the test includes questions about hypertensive pharmacological agents and no other types of cardiac drugs, their test fails content validity. An example of a test that has content validity is the National Council Licensure Examination for Registered Nurses (NCLEX-RN). This exam purports to measure competencies and skills needed for safe, effective nursing practice.[18]

Threats to Internal Validity

Threats to internal validity are defined as those things that confuse or confound test and survey results and overall findings. Researchers and evaluators need to consider threats to internal validity as an alternative explanation for some results. The following discussion explains the nine threats to internal validity. These threats include history, maturation, testing, instrumentation, regression, ceiling and floor effects, attrition, selection, and the Hawthorne effect.

- *History:* History is when an event happens during research that influences the behavior of participating individuals. For example, researchers are conducting research on gun violence. They collect pretest surveys among undergraduates and offer three weeks' worth of gun violence seminars in all resident halls on campus. Prior to collecting posttest surveys, a campus shooting that receives wide media attention happens at another university. This campus shooting completely changes posttest results.
- *Maturation:* Maturation is defined as the natural changes that occur over time with individuals. For example, in an evaluation to determine reading comprehension changes from August to May among third-grade students, results show improvement in reading comprehension skills. Evaluators need to ask themselves if scores improved because of the natural maturation of

students and their improved ability to sit still and focus on test questions as they age or if their reading comprehension improved over the school year.

- *Testing:* Testing refers to differences noted from pretest to posttest that can be attributed to students becoming familiar with the test. Changes may not occur because of the intervention, but rather because respondents are familiar with the test. For example, researchers conduct a food choice seminar for newly diagnosed type 2 diabetic patients and their families. A pretest is conducted at the beginning of the seminar and again at the end. Because the time frame between pretest and posttest collection is less than three hours, posttest responses are influenced by familiarity with the survey, perhaps even more so than retention of presented information.

- *Instrumentation:* Instrumentation measures changes in respondent performance that cannot be credited to the treatment or intervention. For example, observers get bored and record data less accurately after two hours then they did at the beginning of the observation. Respondents experience fatigue when completing long surveys, so questions at the end are less accurate than questions near the beginning.

- *Regression:* Regression may be defined as some respondents performing well on pretests and poorly on posttests, or vice versa, merely by chance. This widespread performance for some respondents may have no explanation other than chance. Data from these high-pretest/low-posttest performances cancel each other, and the overall score is similar to the average mean scores for all participants. This effect is called "regression to the mean." For example, an individual has an upper respiratory infection and is taking medication during the posttest, but did not have an infection when the pretest was collected. Generally, it is impossible to know what factors influenced the very high or very low test scores.

- *Ceiling effect and floor effect:* These are two subsets of this threat to internal validity. Ceiling effect is when all participating individuals perform extremely well on a pretest and posttest, therefore making it difficult to determine any changes the intervention may have had. Investigators need to consider whether scores are artificially inflated by observer and not related to treatment. Floor effect occurs when individual performance starts out low and remains low. This effect leads investigators to think that individuals are unresponsive to treatment, when in fact the low performance may be caused by a factor outside the intervention or treatment altogether. For example, patients are so ill that neither standard-of-care medication nor new Drug A will achieve therapeutic improvements.

- *Attrition:* Attrition refers to individuals lost from the study. Researchers match demographics of participating individuals, and then randomly assign individuals to treatment or control groups. If a large number of individuals leave the study for a variety of reasons, results may reflect more about the individuals who stayed in the study than the treatment conditions of the study. For example, researchers conduct a 10-year study to document the benefits of communal living among senior citizens over 70 years of age. Researchers match individuals living in the community with individuals living in a retirement community. Many participants are lost for follow-up because of natural changes (e.g., illness, disabilities, and death). Results are inconclusive because of the remaining participants rather than the living conditions.

- *Selection:* Selection is when participating individuals are different at the onset of the study. Therefore, results are inconclusive based on differences rather than treatment. For example, researchers are exploring the effectiveness of two different breast cancer chemotherapy treatments. They recruit women to participate in the clinical trial for six months. When results are inconclusive, researchers realize that most women in Group A treatment had one type of breast cancer and most women in Group B had another type of cancer. Therefore, it is not possible to know whether the breast cancer type or the treatment used influenced the results.

- *Hawthorne effect:* The Hawthorne effect gets its name from the workers at the Western Electric Company in Hawthorne, Illinois, who improved their performance when they knew they were being watched. For example, individuals working on an assembly line perform better when they know their annual salary increase is based on the number of widgets they make during a given period. The Hawthorne effect does not take place only in research settings.[19]

Before moving on to the next section, it is important to remember that threats to internal validity should be considered prior to finalizing any research results, and plans should be made as to how they will be avoided during survey creation, data collection, and data analysis.[20-22]

External Validity

External validity is defined as the generalizability of results. In other words, if evaluation or research is repeated with different populations, situations, time, or environments, the results are expected to be the same. A threat to external validity might explain how generalizations are incorrect.[23] Repeating evaluation methods and research in different populations is the best way to access generalizability.

This section explores factors that influence generalizability including population, environment, temporal/sequential factors, participants, testing and treatment interaction, reactive arrangements, and multiple treatment conditions.

Generalizability is linked to independent variables. As a quick review, there are independent and dependent variables. Independent variables are those that researchers manipulate and control. Dependent variables are fixed and not manipulated. For example, if researchers are interested in how the amount of sleep affects blood pressure, the research question could be "Does consistent lack of sleep affect blood pressure readings taken at noon?" The independent variable is sleep, and the dependent variable is blood pressure; the amount of sleep can be manipulated (e.g., 4 hours, 6 hours, 8 hours, and 10 hours). Researchers control the number of hours of sleep by having participants stay in a sleep lab at night and waking them up after 4, 6, 8, and 10 hours of sleep. They give each participant an electronic blood pressure monitor and ask them to record their blood pressure at 8:00 a.m., noon, and 8:00 p.m. Now let's apply this example to factors that influence generalizability, or threats to external validity.

Threats to External Validity

- *Population (also known as selection and treatment):* When population selection is too specific, treatment is matched to a specific sample and is not applicable to a wider population. For example, the sleep study was conducted with a specific age group, so the researchers need to repeat the study with another group. If the sleep study was conducted with young adults and showed that lack of sleep had minimal effect on blood pressure, researchers would need to repeat the study with older adults to determine if results are statistically similar or different. If blood pressure readings were more affected for older adults, then results would reflect lack of external validity. Given these results, researchers would have a new research question: Why does lack of sleep affect blood pressure in older adults more than in younger adults?

- *Environment:* The sleep study was conducted in a controlled university sleep lab. If it were repeated by having participants stay home and set their alarm clocks so that their sleep was still limited to 4, 6, 8, and 10 hours, how would changing the environment affect the blood pressure results for young and older adults? It is possible that (1) both age groups sleep better in their own beds than in a university sleep lab, (2) one group sleeps better in their own beds, or (3) both groups sleep better in the university sleep lab. Regardless, these results would always reflect the possible lack of external validity.

- *Temporal/sequential factors:* The sleep study was conducted during the winter months in a northern geographical area. If the study were conducted during summer months in a southern geographical location, would results be any different? It is possible that the increase or decrease in sun exposure during daytime hours might affect sleep patterns.
- *Participants:* The following factors regarding participating individuals are linked to threats of external validity:
  - *Animal-to-human links:* When researchers use rats or other animals to test specific drugs, it is questionable whether humans will react to the new drug in the same way as rats.
  - *Human-to-human links:* Researchers use college students for many studies because the students are a convenient sample. However, results are questioned because data gathered from college students may not be generalizable to other groups of young adults not attending college.
  - *Gender bias:* Research including only men or only women is not generalizable to the nonrepresented gender group. The same is true for studies that include only heterosexual individuals and fail to recognize lesbian, gay, bisexual, and transgender (LGBT) individuals.
  - *Racial bias:* Research conducted on only African Americans, for example, does not yield generalizable results to other racial groups. In today's world of linking genetics to health conditions, issues of racial inclusion are more important than ever.
  - *Cultural and ethnocentric bias:* Research conducted on one specific cultural group is not generalizable to other cultures. For example, researchers studying the Mexican Hispanic population in Texas may not generalize to other Hispanic groups in the United States. Spanish-speaking individuals do not share the same cultural background (i.e., there are differences among the cultures in Puerto Rico, Mexico, Nicaragua, Honduras, Venezuela, and Spain). Also keep in mind that some religions contribute to cultural differences among various populations.
- *Testing and treatment interaction:* If participants learn from the pretest, then they may be less likely to learn as much from treatment. For example, a pretest is given at the beginning of a "new to dialysis" cooking class. If participants are sure that they received a perfect score on the pretest, they are less likely to listen intently during the class, because they already know the information. When researchers split the sample into two groups—one receiving pretest, treatment (cooking class), and posttest, the other

receiving treatment (cooking class) and posttest—researchers can calculate the differences.

- *Reactive arrangements (also called Hawthorne effect):* The Hawthorne effect was described under threats to internal validity, and it also applies to external validity. If individuals change their behavior when observed (threat to internal validity), results are not generalizable to real-world conditions (threat to external validity).

- *Multiple treatment conditions:* In some research, the same individuals are exposed to multiple treatments. Because multiple treatments may create an artificial setting that does not exist in the real world, results may not be generalizable. For example, if the sleep study is conducted in the university sleep lab, individuals sleep alone (space) in a cool (temperature), quiet (sound) room with soft pillows and luxurious sheets (environment). The setting is artificial, exposing individuals to multiple treatments not linked to real-world bedrooms. At home, they may have a hot bedroom, an uncomfortable bed with old sheets, lumpy pillows, a snoring spouse, and loud neighbors. Results from multiple treatments in the sleep lab are not generalizable to populations trying to sleep in less-than-ideal conditions.

Lastly, researchers and evaluators need awareness of all possible threats to external validity that affect independent variables. Results reporting threats to external validity are not regarded as a weakness in research, but rather an opportunity to develop new research questions. For example, if season and geographical location affect sleep study results, researchers have the opportunity to develop new research questions to explore this newly identified issue. It is possible that lack of generalizability from threats to external validity could lead to exciting and groundbreaking lines of new research.

Relationship Between Internal and External Validity

Researchers remain aware of threats to both internal and external validity, but they know that internal validity is more critical than external. Without internal validity, research is not testing what it reports to measure. However, it is important to keep in mind that as the study inclusion criteria become more selective, the results become less generalizable. For example, researchers wish to study a new hypertension drug. Their selection criteria are limited to African American males over 60 years of age. Although this target population is at high risk for hypertension, limiting the sample criteria limits the generalizability of results.[21]

Measurement Errors

There are two types of errors that influence the results, surveys, tests, and instruments: random errors and systematic errors.

Random Errors

Random errors occur by chance and are inconsistent across the respondents. These errors increase or decrease results in an unpredictable manner; therefore, researchers and evaluators have no control over the occurrence of random errors. Keep in mind that reliability is influenced by random errors because reliability is concerned with the degree of consistency of the measurement.

Random errors influence consistency in various ways. First, participating individuals may change from day 1 to day 2. For example, they get more or less sleep, take or stop taking cough medicine, or forget or remember to bring their reading glasses. Second, tasks change between day 1 and day 2. For example, the day 1 observer may not be available to observe on day 2, or on day 1 the participants mark their responses on the survey and on day 2 participants are asked to mark their responses on a separate answer sheet. Third, if there is a small sample of participating individuals, outside forces have a greater effect on the outcome. For example, if there are only 10 individuals completing a survey and 3 did not get enough sleep, then 30% of the scores might be affected. However, if 25 individuals complete the survey and 3 did not get enough sleep, only 12% of the responses will be affected. Let's put these three sources of random errors into an example for greater comprehension. See **Box 5-2**.

From the example, it is easy to see how one, two, or three random errors occur by chance during research. Each random error alters the reliability of knowing whether a 10-week course was reliable in teaching adolescents how to provide safe self-care for their newly diagnosed medical condition.

Fourth, random errors occur in written tests. There are three examples under this source of random errors:

1. If the test is too short, individual scores are based more on chance and luck than on knowledge. If the exam covers all human bones, but there are only 10 questions, there is a chance that some students know only the bones asked about on the test and some students know all of the bones

BOX 5-2

Random Errors Case Study

Researchers want to verify that adolescents with newly diagnosed type 1 diabetes know the correct procedure for testing their blood glucose levels, determining the correct amount of insulin needed, and injecting the insulin. The adolescents are enrolled in a 10-week health education program sponsored by the local hospital. The researchers observe the adolescents during the week 7 class and again during week 8 class.

- First, the adolescents may change between week 7 and week 8. If they performed the task poorly in week 7, they may have received extra practice at home while their parents watched and critiqued their insulin techniques.
- Second, the task may change slightly from week 7 to week 8 because the instructor has different glucose monitors during week 8, so the adolescents are not as familiar with the equipment. Also, two different researchers observe during week 7 and week 8, and their observation techniques are slightly different.
- Third, there are five adolescents in class during week 7 and only three adolescents attending during week 8.

All three of the random errors occurred by chance, and all three random errors influenced the reliability of the diabetes class outcome data.

except for the ones asked about on the test. Either way, random error occurs because of the inconsistency of the exam.

2. If the test is not graded precisely the same way for each student, random errors cause inconsistent reliability. For example, if a professor does not follow an objective grading rubric, student scores are compromised due to subjective and indefensible grading procedures.

3. If the test is not administered consistently, random errors occur. For example, when students take a makeup exam, professors should provide an environment similar to the classroom (e.g., lighting, sound level, environment, vibration, time allotment) provided to the other students.

Random errors are often the result of the researcher's ability to repeat the items (e.g., measurements, tests, surveys, and observations) the same way to obtain the same results. One way to minimize random errors is to collect data from a larger sample size. The random errors in either direction are less influential on the overall data with a large sample size. Lastly, random errors are reduced through statistical methods by averaging scores over a larger sample size.

Systematic Errors

Systematic errors are consistent in the same direction, so that no matter how many times the experiment is repeated, the same error occurs. Validity is influenced by systematic errors. Systematic errors introduce inaccuracy to the measurement, cause a bias in data, and diminish the extent to which the test is measuring what it purports to measure.[24] Systematic errors are problematic to detect and eliminate. Unlike random errors, it is not possible to reduce the effect of systematic errors through statistical methods.[25] If researchers or evaluators suspect bias in their data, they investigate possible systematic errors.[26]

There are three areas to investigate when searching for systematic errors: environment, observation, and drift. Environment refers to how the setting changes over the course of the research. For example, if the research was conducted outside, the temperature, humidity, wind speed, or heat index may have caused variations in data and results that are difficult to pinpoint. Observation may change due to observer fatigue, time of day, room temperature, training of different observers, attitude of participants, and various other human behavior variables. Lastly, drift is when evidence suggests that the data is slowly moving in one direction.[27] For example, drift may occur if the machine used for lab results is not calibrated each day prior to running complete blood count (CBC) samples. The problem with each type of error is that even when the error is recognized, it is difficult to determine when it began in the data collection process and how much the systematic error influenced the actual results.

Let's explore one example to illustrate how validity is affected by systematic errors. Physical therapy students are studying for a practicum exam on range of motion (ROM) exercises for elderly patients. Because ROM skills are essential to physical therapy, a perfect score is required on this practicum exam to move to the next phase of training. On the day of the exam, two professors decide to set up a hospital room with a mannequin in the bed so students can demonstrate their ROM practice skills. The students arrive at their usual classroom and are told to complete a worksheet while they wait. The two professors call each student, one at a time, alphabetically, to come to the simulated hospital room. They use a checklist to observe each student's skill in taking the mannequin through an ROM exercise series. After completing the skills test, students are told to return to the classroom without being given their exam scores. As the exam continues for three hours, the students at the end of the alphabet become more anxious, because they see the stress of the returning students. The increased anxiety is likely to affect their test performance. This testing technique diminishes the validity of the practicum exam. As an evaluator of this exam, how would you suggest changing the format so that the practicum exam remains valid? There are numerous possible answers, but one solution is presented here. The professors could arrange exam stations in five classrooms, each equipped with a third-year student lying on a padded table with a quilt for comfort and attended by one professor observing the same activity with a prescribed checklist. All students would begin the practicum exam at the same time and rotate to each of the five classrooms. The standardized process would be complete in one hour with high validity.

With the awareness of measurement errors, how do researchers and evaluators reduce the chance of creating them? The following discusses ways to reduce measurement errors:

- *Pilot test:* Whether investigators are conducting quantitative or qualitative studies, pilot testing is essential. Pilot testing is a complete dress rehearsal before data collection. Spending money on pilot testing is always a good investment and worth every cent. Later in this chapter, pilot testing is presented in detail.

- *Data collection training:* Researchers and evaluators train data collectors for consistency (e.g., detailed checklists, machine measurement calibration checks, inter-rater comparisons to avoid creating errors). For example, data collectors read from a script for consistency in instructions prior to having an individual complete a survey.

- *Double data entry:* Evaluators and researchers enter a portion of the data twice and then compare the two entries. If there are multiple errors, investigators go back to the original data and determine why the errors are occurring.

- *Statistical consultation:* Investigators consult with statisticians to seek assistance with entering data and to determine ways to reduce and/or measure data errors.

- *Triangulate data collection:* To increase reliability and validity, researchers and evaluators choose to collect similar data using more than one method. For example, during the first week of the month, investigators conduct interviews about diabetes knowledge related to preferred food choices with patients. With the same patients, investigators conduct survey data on the same topic. Interview and survey responses are compared for consistency.[28]

Reliable and Valid Research

Before leaving the discussion on reliability and validity, it is beneficial to step back and examine a broad view of research. Frequently, evening news programs reveal Food and Drug Administration (FDA) reports recalling specific medications for numerous reasons. Even though drug testing is intensely scrutinized during the research and development phase, FDA recalls are usually linked to research (see **Box 5-3**).[29] Researchers need to know how to distinguish between dependable and undependable research. Researchers build their study protocols on the previous research of colleagues in similar fields of study because it is more efficient and economical. However, if previous original research is proven to be faulty, the entire line of research is built on flawed assumptions and results. Reliable research is based on several basic assumptions, including randomized controlled trial designs and adequate sample sizes, and is free of known bias.

Randomized Controlled Trial Designs

The gold standard of research design is called randomized controlled trials (RCTs). Let's define the terms. When a study is randomized, it means that the research participants are randomly assigned to either a treatment group or a non-treatment group (placebo group). Some clinical trials can study more than one treatment group (e.g., Drug A, Drug B, and Drug C groups). Participants in each group have similar characteristics, such as age, gender, or length of diagnosis at the beginning of study. Random assignment technique allows researchers to draw conclusions with confidence if one group is significantly different at the end of the study.[30] A controlled study is defined as one group receiving treatment while another, similar group receives no treatment. Control groups may be randomized from original groups of participants, or control groups may be similar groups at a different location. For example, colon cancer patients over 50 years of age at University Cancer Center are randomized into two groups: Drug A and no treatment. In another study, colon cancer patients over 50 years of age at University Cancer Center are randomized into two groups: Drug A and Drug B. The control groups are similar colon cancer patients over 50 years of age receiving the standard of care (nonexperimental treatment) at St. Mary's Cancer Hospital located in the adjacent county. Researchers compare similar patients receiving treatment to patients receiving either no treatment (placebo) or non-research-related standard-of-care treatment. Data explore variables such as reduction in tumor size, patient reaction to treatment, length of hospital stay, or time in remission. Even though RCTs offer the ideal design, such studies are

BOX 5-3

A Few Examples of MedWatch Safety Alerts, January 1–December 31, 2012

This box shows a few examples of how the U.S. Food and Drug Administration notify healthcare providers and consumers about medical equipment and products that have been identified as unsafe for the general population. Keep in mind that these medical products underwent extensive research prior to being released for use. However, after use among thousands of people, unknown risks were identified, so the product or equipment must be recalled. This list illustrates that even after extensive research, results may lack sufficient reliability and validity to remain safe for general usage.

Accutron, Inc., Ultra PC% Cabinet Mount Flowmeters for Nitrous Oxide–Oxygen Sedation Systems: Class I recall	When not mixed with oxygen, inhaling nitrous oxide can lead to temporary and permanent brain damage and death.	Posted 10/16/2012
Hospira Lactated Ringers and 5% Dextrose Injection, 1,000 ml, Flexible Containers: Recalled for mold contamination	Voluntary nationwide recall of one lot. Injections of mold could potentially lead to septicemia; in a worst-case scenario, septicemia may have the potential to progress to septic shock, which may be life threatening.	Posted 10/06/2012
Mirapex (pramipexole): Drug safety communication, ongoing safety review, possible risk of heart failure	FDA currently evaluating analysis of randomized clinical trials and epidemiologic studies.	Posted 09/19/2012
I-Flow ON-Q Pump with ONDEMAND Bolus Button: Class I recall, risk of continuous infusion at a rate greater than expected	Bolus button may not lock in the down position when depressed, and/or the orange bolus refill indicator may stay in the lowest position, which can lead to serious adverse health consequences, including death.	Posted 08/31/2012
Reumofan Plus: Recall, undeclared drug ingredient	The FDA has received dozens of additional adverse event reports, including death and stroke, associated with the use of Reumofan Plus since the agency issued its first warning about the product.	UPDATED 08/28/2012; originally posted 06/01/2012
Synthes Hemostatic Bone Putty: Class I recall, potential for putty to ignite	Medical facilities should examine their inventory and immediately stop using the recalled product.	Posted 08/21/2012

continues

BOX 5-3 *continued*

Hospira Propofol Injectable Emulsion: Recall, glass vial defect	Risks associated with this defect could include tissue necrosis in one or more organs that could result in stroke, myocardial infarction, respiratory failure, and loss of renal and hepatic function.	Posted 08/16/2012
Cataplex ACP, Cataplex C, and Pancreatrophin PMG Dietary Supplements: Recall, potential for contamination with salmonella	Risk of serious and sometimes fatal infections, especially in young children, frail or elderly people, and others with weakened immune systems.	Posted 06/29/2012

U.S. Food and Drug Administration. MedWatch Safety Alerts, January 01–December 31, 2012. Available at: http://www.fda.gov/Safety/MedWatch/ucm287881.htm.

not exempt from data collection, measurement, and analysis errors that influence the reliability and validity of overall study results.

Adequate Sample Size

Researchers seek an appropriate sample size for their studies. When a sample is too small, results are inconclusive and significant differences among groups are statistically harder to determine. On the other hand, when a sample is too large, cost, feasibility, and time become problematic. Researchers strive for an ideal sample size to adequately represent the target population. However, a large sample is preferred over a small sample because of the increased precision and accuracy of the study.

Free of Bias

Bias occurs in research and evaluations from numerous causes including selection, measurement, and intervention bias. Selection bias occurs if specific individuals or groups are purposely omitted from the investigation. Measurement bias happens during data collection by researchers or subjects because of systematic errors in measurement. Investigators may influence individual responses by their body language during an interview, or a subject may provide socially desirable responses, such as telling interviewers they smoke a smaller number of cigarettes a day than they actually do or increasing the time and amount of physical activity achieved per week. Lastly, intervention bias involves how intervention groups are treated differently than control groups if the researchers involved know which group is which.[31]

Pilot Testing

Pilot testing is the same idea as a dress rehearsal for a theatrical performance. Pilot tests involve every aspect including environment, data collection, content, and outcomes of a study. Pilot tests involve conducting a preliminary test of data collection tools and procedures to identify and eliminate problems. When investigators execute pilot tests correctly, they save time and resources during the actual data collection process. When investigators fail to conduct a rigorous pilot test, they risk collecting unusable data for a high price. Let's explore how to conduct a pilot study by categories.

Sample of Respondents

Recruit a small number (< 10) of individuals with characteristics similar to the actual sample to test the method of recruitment, such as email, telephone, postal mail, or waiting room recruitment. If it is difficult to recruit individuals for the pilot test, then the recruitment methods for the actual study need revision (see **Box 5-4**).

BOX 5-4

Participant Recruitment for Pilot Test

Use the same method of participant recruitment:

Phone Interviews

Are landlines or cell phones going to be called?

How are phone numbers going to be obtained?

Will random digit dialing be used?

What is the cost incurred to obtain the phone numbers?

What time of the day is ideal for reaching participants?

Are the participants anonymous, or are the names known to researchers?

Mailed or Online Surveys

How are postal or email addresses going to be obtained?

What is the cost incurred to obtain the postal or email addresses?

If email, are listserv lists available?

In-Person Interviews or Surveys

How will participants be recruited?

Will incentives be used?

Are participants anonymous or known to researchers?

Data Collection for Pilot Tests

Pilot tests allow researchers the opportunity to determine if revisions are needed in the actual instrument or in the data collection procedures (see **Box 5-5**).

BOX 5-5

Data Collection for Pilot Test

Use the same method of data collection:

1. Create the exact environment that will be used for the actual data collection (e.g., location and time of day).
   a. If a certain meeting room is the intended site for participants to complete surveys, conduct the pilot test in the exact meeting room. Will the meeting room always be available during the actual data collection? Is the room quiet?
   b. If phone interviews will be conducted, verify that the digital sound recording devices work properly during the pilot test.
   c. If an online survey will be conducted, verify that the links are working and that the survey responses are sent to a secure data collection site.
2. When possible, observe participants while they complete surveys during the pilot test.
   a. How long did it take most participants to complete the survey or interview?
   b. Are they distracted by the environment or digital voice recording device?
   c. Are there enough tables and chairs in the intended location?
   d. Are clipboards needed to provide a writing surface?
   e. Are sharpened pencils or pens available to complete the survey?
   f. Do respondents appear to be annoyed, fatigued, or bored near the end of the survey or interview?

continues

BOX 5-5 *continued*

      g. Do participants ask for erasers to change their responses?

      h. Did respondents skip questions or look forward by skipping pages?

3. After the surveys or interviews are complete, ask the participants a few questions.

      a. What was the purpose of the survey or interview?

      b. Were the directions clear?

      c. Were the questions easy to understand? Do any questions need clarification?

      d. Did any of the questions make them uncomfortable?

      e. Did the response choices allow the participants to enter their intended responses?

      f. Was the survey or interview too long?

      g. Were there any questions that they did not understand?

      h. Were there any questions that they would change or reword?

      i. Did they skip any questions? Why?

      j. Would they tell their friends to participate in this study and complete the survey or interview?

Data Analysis

After the pilot test data are collected, investigators enter the data and conduct a pilot test of the data analysis procedures (see **Box 5-6**).

Outcome

Following the pilot testing and modification phase, researchers and evaluators move forward with conducting the actual study. Some investigators may think that pilot testing is too labor intensive or too expensive to justify the results. These individuals are mistaken. Taking the time to conduct a thorough pilot test is always worth the time and money, because once data are collected, it is too late to fix mistakes that could prove to be fatal flaws for the entire study. Lastly, when reporting results, investigators document the pilot study and revisions made based on results. This notation adds to the authenticity of the study.[32,33]

BOX 5-6

Data Analysis Pilot Test

Begin the data analysis:

1. Prior to entering the data, read through the responses or interviews. Did participants interpret the question as investigators intended?
2. Enter survey data as intended for actual research or evaluation. Although the sample size is limited in a pilot test, investigators calculate mean, median, and mode for each question to determine the range of each question. For interviews, investigators read responses for each question to obtain a general sense of answers from participants.
3. If paper surveys are going to be scanned, verify that the scanning machine is operating properly for scanning the completed surveys from the pilot test.
4. After viewing data, investigators verify whether the results provided the information needed to adequately address research questions or evaluation objectives.
5. Modify survey or interview questions as needed to clarify questions, response choices, or data results.

Summary

This chapter introduced the concepts of reliability and validity. To briefly review, reliability refers to consistency, and validity is the extent to which a test measures what it purports to measure. The two different forms of reliability discussed include stability and internal consistency. The validity discussion included the types of validity, internal threats to validity, and external threats to validity. It is essential to remember that it is more important to be valid than reliable. Lastly, the chapter ended with a detailed description of how to conduct a pilot test.

Case Study

The healthcare providers at the Glenville County Health Department pregnancy clinic have been using the same survey to screen patients for risk of family violence for several years. Only a small percentage of the women who take the survey obtain a score that would indicate that they are at risk for family violence. However, during the course of prenatal visits, when healthcare providers inquire if the women feel safe at home, it is not uncommon for women to disclose living with fear of violence. Because the survey results did not appear to be accurate, the clinic administrators decided it was time for a change. With a limited budget, the administrator decided to form a team composed of four clinic staff, led by Dr. Williams, director of Quality Management for the Glenville County Health Department.

Let's review the steps used by the team.

Step 1: Review Existing Survey Data

Before making any changes, the team reviewed the current survey. Immediately, they realized that the collected data had never been entered into a spreadsheet for analysis. The anonymous paper surveys were merely reviewed by a clinic nurse and placed in a large box for storage. There was no connection between the survey results and the discussion in the exam rooms, nor was there evidence to confirm or refute the presumed percentage of women whose scores indicated that they were at risk. Dr. Williams determined that instead of taking the time to analyze the existing anonymous surveys, the clinic nurses would score each completed survey and enter the score in the woman's electronic medical records (EMR) under the assessment tab. The midwives would continue to ask the women about their perceived level of safety at home and enter the women's comments under the assessment tab. Because the midwives are unaware of the scoring for the current survey, they are not influenced by the score entered by the nurse. For example, if the nurse enters a score of 17, the midwife does not know what that value means

continues

and therefore is not influenced to change her behavior related to inquiring about home safety. This process continued for three months. Using the EMR database, Dr. Williams was able to provide evidence that survey results were not linked to what the women reported to the midwives.

Step 2: Reliability of Existing Survey

The team needed to determine the reliability of the existing survey before developing a completely new survey. One team member suggested using the test-retest technique to see if the survey is stable. Because pregnant women have weekly clinic appointments near the end of their pregnancy, the team decided to ask 20 women to complete the survey for two consecutive weeks. The results showed that the survey was stable, because the responses remained the same from one week to the next week. Next, the team decided to test the internal consistency of the survey. Using the existing 40-question survey responses, they analyzed the entire survey using the split-half technique. The even-numbered questions became Survey A, and the odd-numbered questions became Survey B. Dr. Williams used the statistical measurement called Cronbach's alpha to determine how well the survey questions measured different aspects of the same topic. The Cronbach's alpha score was 0.62, which is low but acceptable.

Step 3: Validity of Existing Survey

Dr. Williams reminded the team that the survey may be reliable, but that does not mean that it is valid. She stated that the problem with the existing survey may be that it is not valid; in other words, it does not measure what it was intended to measure. The team decided to focus on content validity and determine if the survey questions are closely related to domestic violence. Because none of the team members was involved in the development of the current survey, they did not have to be concerned about stepping on the toes of their colleagues. After a meeting in which each question was critiqued, it became evident that they had solved the problem. The majority of the survey questions were not related to family

continues

CASE STUDY *continued*

violence, but rather focused on topics such as neighborhood safety and satisfaction with community resources related to safety.

Step 4: Creating a New Survey

Dr. Williams suggested the team begin the process of creating a new survey by searching the literature. After a simple web search, one team member located a valuable website hosted by the Centers for Disease Control and Prevention (CDC). The website provides a free download book titled *Measuring Intimate Partner Violence, Victimization and Perpetration: A Compendium of Assessment Tools*. The book includes eight chapters: (1) Physical Victimization Scales, (2) Sexual Victimization Scales, (3) Psychological/Emotional Victimization Scales, (4) Stalking Victimization Scales, (5) Physical Perpetration Scales, (6) Sexual Perpetration Scales, (7) Psychological/Emotional Perpetration Scales, and (8) Stalking Perpetration Scales. Each chapter includes several scales with an explanation of how each scale has been used, published research using the scale, reliability and validity, and how to score and analyze each scale.[34]

The team was thrilled with the free and valuable information. Immediately, they began to compile the scales of interest to form their new patient survey.

Step 5: Pilot Testing

The team did not assume that they could skip the pilot testing phase and begin to use the new survey. They carefully followed each step of the pilot testing phase: participant recruitment, data collection, and data analysis. Ten pregnant women participated in the pilot test and were eager to provide feedback on the new survey. Some of the suggestions included lowering the literacy level of some questions, rearranging two subscales to improve the flow of the questions, and adding some questions related to their children's safety. The edits were then made based on the pilot test feedback. Because the clinic uses EMR check-in kiosks in the waiting room, it was possible to make the survey a required portion

continues

CASE STUDY *continued*

of the clinic visit at the first prenatal appointment and at the appointments at 25 and 37 weeks' gestation. When the patients completed the electronic survey and hit "submit," their scores appeared on the assessment page with an explanation of patient's risk for the clinic staff to review at that day's appointment. After six months, the team met again to verify that the survey was working. Dr. Williams presented some data confirming that the pregnant women and midwives found the survey information to be valuable and that it facilitated open communication regarding risk of family violence.

Step 6: One Year Later

The prenatal clinic staff presented the family violence survey and results at the annual Glenville County Health Department board of directors meeting. Because the survey questions were not specific to pregnant women, or gender and age for that matter, the decision was made to have all new clinic patients over the age of 18 years complete the survey at their intake appointments and annually after that time.

Case Study Discussion Questions

1. How would you begin to modify the survey questions now that the survey has been used for a while in the clinic?
2. What are some of the possible threats to internal and external validity that might need to be considered?
3. If the clinic decided to conduct a second pilot test, what would you suggest they modify in the procedure?

Student Activity

Below are several questions related to measurement reliability and validity. This student activity will require you to search the internet for answers regarding reliability and validity of several of the questions.

The National Public Health Performance Standards Program (NPHPSP) is an effort by the CDC to create performance standards for state and local public healthcare systems. You can visit the NPHPSP website at http://www.cdc.gov/nphpsp/.

Questions

1. How many instruments are used by the NPHPSP? What do they measure?
2. To ensure that the standards of the NPHPSP measurement fully covered the gamut of public health action needed at state and local levels, the instruments were designed around what?

Complete an internet search for the article titled "Recommendations from Testing of the National Public Health Performance Standards Instruments" by Beaulieu, Scutchfield, and Kelly, published in the *Journal of Public Health Management Practice* in 2003. Read the article and answer these questions regarding their study on the validity of the NPHPSP instruments.

3. What three types of validity did the authors of this article test the NPHPSP instruments on?
4. What two ways did the authors test the criterion validity?
5. Why did the authors say it was difficult to assess criterion validity for public health systems?

The Student Life Department at Northeast University has decided that in order to better support new students, it will give all incoming freshmen a survey about what kind of support they have in their lives to help them with the transition from being high school students living at home with their parents to being college students living on campus. The university hopes that scores from the test will help reveal students who may need extra support. Brad Johnson, the director of Student Life, does some searching at the library and finds four different measures of social support: the Miller Support and Affection Scale, the Latino Community Social Support Inventory, the Young Adult Social Support Scale, and the Cancer Social Support Scale.

6. Of the four measures that Brad found, which is the most likely to be one he should research further?
7. Brad decides to research one of the scales further and finds that it has a Cronbach's alpha of 0.78. Is this score acceptable?

8. Brad reads more information on the Young Adult Social Support Scale and finds out that it has been tested against other social support scales for adults. When the Young Social Support Adult Scale is compared to a social support scale for adults, what kind of validity is represented?

9. After his research, Brad decides that he will use the Young Adult Social Support Scale for his survey of new freshmen. After the initial survey, the Student Life Department identifies 20 students who they feel have low social support. The Student Life Department decides to pair them up with students who have high levels of social support in a "buddy system." At the end of the year, they give the Young Adult Social Support Scale survey again to the 20 students to see if the buddy system worked. All of the students showed improved levels of social support. The improvement in social support levels is an example of what threat to internal validity? Why?

Answers

1. There are three instruments used by the NPHPSP. They measure the state public health system, the local public health system, and the local public health governance.

2. The NPHPSP instruments were designed around the CDC's 10 Essential Public Health Services.

3. Beaulieu, Scutchfield, and Kelly tested the NPHPSP on face, content, and criterion validity.

4. The authors tested the criterion validity first by using documentary evidence through site visits and conference calls. Second, they used external judges to test criterion validity.

5. Beaulieu, Scutchfield, and Kelly state that there is no "gold standard" external criterion measure for public health systems that has been used on the national level before.

6. Brad should research the Young Adult Social Support Scale further. Because we are searching only about social support among college students, we probably do not want to look at the Miller Support and Affection Scale because we do not want to measure affection among the new freshmen students. Furthermore, we would not want to look at the Latino Community Social Support Inventory or the Cancer Social Support Scale because those measures have been made for very specific populations. Although there are surely freshmen of Hispanic ethnicity, not all

the students are. Furthermore, although there may be some freshmen who are dealing with or have dealt with cancer in the past, again, most have not.

7. Cronbach's alpha measures are a measure of internal consistency. A 0.78 Cronbach's alpha score is considered to be between "acceptable" and "good." Therefore, Brad would continue to consider this test for use among freshmen students.

8. This represents criterion-related validity. When we test a new scale using another scale that has recognized reliability and validity properties, this is called criterion-related validity.

9. The most likely source of the threat to internal validity is maturation. We do not know whether the buddy system was the reason the students had higher levels of social support or because they were simply becoming older, becoming more relaxed with being away from home, and making friends in college. We don't know if this would have happened with or without the buddy system, particularly because there is no control group to measure them against.

References

1. Trochim MK. Theory of Reliability. Research Methods Knowledge Base. Available at: http://www.socialresearchmethods.net/kb/reliablt.php. Last updated October 20, 2006. Accessed June 3, 2012.

2. Shuttleworth M. Definition of Reliability. Explorable. Available at: http://www.experiment-resources.com/definition-of-reliability.html. Last updated 2009. Accessed June 3, 2012.

3. MBTI Basics. The Myers and Briggs Foundation. Available at: http://www.myersbriggs.org/my-mbti-personality-type/mbti-basics. Accessed June 3, 2012.

4. Lazarus RS, Folkman S. The Hassles and Uplifts Scales. Mind Garden, Inc. Available at: http://www.mindgarden.com/products/hsups.htm. Accessed June 3, 2012.

5. Types of Reliability. Statsam Blog. Available at: http://statssam.wordpress.com/2012/02/05/types-of-reliability/. Last updated February 5, 2012. Accessed June 3, 2012.

6. Cronbach LJ. Coefficient alpha and the internal structure of tests. *Psychometrika*. 1951;16(3):297–334.

7. Litwin MS. *How to Assess and Interpret Survey Psychometrics*, 2nd ed. Thousand Oaks, CA: Sage; 2003.

8. George D, Mallery P. *SPSS for Windows Step by Step: A Simple Guide and Reference*, 4th ed. Boston, MA: Allyn & Bacon; 2003.

9. Miller MJ. Reliability and Validity. Lecture Notes from Western International University. Available at: www.michaeljmillerphd.com/res500_lecturenotes/Reliability_and_validity.pdf. Accessed June 3, 2012.

10. Trochim MK. Types of Reliability. Research Methods Knowledge Base. Available at: http://www.socialresearchmethods.net/kb/reltypes.php. Last updated October 20, 2006. Accessed June 3, 2012.

11. Howell J, Miller P, Park HH, et al. Reliability and Validity. Writing@CSU. Colorado State University. Available at: http://writing.colostate.edu/guides/research/relval/pop2b.cfm. Last updated 2012. Accessed June 3, 2012.

12. Shuttleworth M. Validity and Reliability. Explorable. Available at: http://www.experiment-resources.com/validity-and-reliability.html. Last updated 2008. Accessed September 4, 2013.

13. Kramer GP, Bernstein DA, Phares V. *Introduction to Clinical Psychology*, 7th ed. Upper Saddle River, NJ: Pearson Prentice Hall; 2009.

14. Fink A, ed. *How to Measure Survey Reliability and Validity*. Thousand Oaks, CA: Sage; 1995.

15. Westen D, Rosenthal R. Quantifying construct validity: Two simple measures. *Journal of Personality and Social Psychology*. 2003;83(3):608–618.

16. Carmines EG, Zeller RA. *Reliability and Validity Assessment*. Newbury Park, CA: Sage; 1991.

17. Trochim MK. Reliability and Validity. Research Methods Knowledge Base. Available at: http://www.socialresearchmethods.net/kb/relandval.php. Last updated October 20, 2006. Accessed June 3, 2012.

18. National Counsel for State Boards of Nursing. National Council Licensure Examination. Available at: www.ncsbn.org/nclex.htm. Accessed on June 3, 2012.

19. Hawthorne Effect. *The Free Dictionary*. Available at: http://medical-dictionary.thefreedictionary.com/Hawthorne+effect. Accessed June 3, 2012.

20. Threats to Internal Validity. Psychometrics. Available at: http://www.psychmet.com/id12.html. Accessed June 3, 2012.

21. White L. Internal and External Validity. Lecture Notes. Southern Utah University. Available at: http://www.suu.edu/faculty/white_l/research%20design/chapter%20notes/chapter%208.pdf. Accessed June 3, 2012.

22. Yu C, Ohlund B. Threats to Validity of Research Design. Creative Wisdom. Available at: http://www.creative-wisdom.com/teaching/WBI/threat.shtml. Accessed June 3, 2012.

23. Mitchell M, Jolley J. *Research Designed Explained*, 4th ed. New York, NY: Harcourt; 2001.

24. Inspection Training—Linear Instrument Characteristics. ToolingU. Available at: http://www.toolingu.com/definition-350115-5902-systematic-error.html. Accessed June 3, 2012.

25. Allain R. Random Error and Systematic Error. Southeastern Louisiana University. Available at: https://www2.southeastern.edu/Academics/Faculty/rallain/plab193/labinfo/Error_Analysis/05_Random_vs_Systematic.html. Accessed on June 3, 2012.

26. Loktik O. Systematic Errors. Physics Laboratory Tutorial. Columbia University. Available at: http://phys.columbia.edu/~tutorial/rand_v_sys/tut_e_5_2.html. Last updated September 1, 2005. Accessed June 3, 2012.

27. False System Errors. European Centre for Medium-Range Weather Forecasts. Available at: http://www.ecmwf.int/products/forecasts/guide/False_systematic_errors.html. Accessed June 3, 2012.

28. Trochim MK. Measurement Error. Research Methods Knowledge Base. Available at: http://www.socialresearchmethods.net/kb/measerr.php. Last updated October 20, 2006. Accessed June 3, 2012.

29. MedWatch. U.S. Food and Drug Administration. Available at: http://www.fda .gov/Safety/MedWatch/SafetyInformation/SafetyAlertsforHumanMedicalProducts /ucm285497.htm. Accessed September 12, 2013.

30. Understanding Research, Preventing Bias. Heart Healthy Women. Available at: http://www.hearthealthywomen.org/news-center/understanding-research-studies /understanding-research-2.html. Accessed June 3, 2012.

31. Nolte S, Elsworth GR, Osborne RH. Absence of social desirability bias in the evaluation of chronic disease self-management interventions. *Health and Quality of Life Outcomes.* 2013;11:114-123. Available at: http://www.hqlo.com/content/pdf/1477-7525-11-114.pdf. Accessed on September 13, 2013.

32. Office of Adolescent Health and Administration on Children, Youth and Family Grantees. United States Department of Health and Human Services. Tips and Recommendations for Successfully Pilot Testing Your Program. Available at: http:// www.hhs.gov/ash/oah/oah-initiatives/teen_pregnancy/training/tip_sheets/pilot-testing-508.pdf. Accessed on September 13, 2013.

33. Taylor-Powell E. Pilot Test Your Questionairre. University of Wisconsin-Extension, Cooperative Extension. https://www.team-psa.com/brfss/2012/pres/K_Trepanier_questionnaire.pdf. Accessed September 4, 2013.

34. Thompson MP, Basile KC, Hertz MF, Sitterle D. *Measuring Intimate Partner Violence Victimization and Perpetration: A Compendium of Assessment Tools.* Atlanta, GA: Centers for Disease Control and Prevention, National Center for Injury Prevention and Control; 2006. Available at: http://www.cdc.gov/ncipc/pub-res/IPV_Compendium.pdf. Accessed September 4, 2013.

Qualitative Data

CHAPTER OBJECTIVES

By the end of this chapter, students will be able to:

- Discuss the advantages and disadvantages of qualitative research
- Evaluate the reliability and validity of qualitative data
- Analyze the differences between the types of qualitative design
- Discuss some examples of ethical issues related to qualitative research
- Conduct a simple analysis of qualitative data including data organization, coding, and data display

KEY TERMS

Coding

Data display

Qualitative data

Validity and reliability of
    qualitative data

Introduction

Qualitative research studies and evaluation projects explore the insight into human behavior and seek information by gaining more experience with a particular topic through unstructured evidence and data. Qualitative investigations explore the *process* of the topic rather than the results. For example, qualitative investigations ask hospitalized patients about the reasons they were unable to take their medications rather than simply noting in the chart the numbers of times the patient refused to ingest the medications. The data include transcripts from interviews, focus groups, media clips or videos, emails, customer service feedback, field notes, open-ended survey questions, and print media. Data analysis does not rely on numbers and statistics as in quantitative studies, but qualitative investigations are an interpretation of the collected words. Quantitative data involve large samples and standardized measures, whereas qualitative data explore smaller samples and unstructured methods. With qualitative data, the investigator gains detail but loses generalizability. Qualitative studies do not assume preconceived notions but rather seek trends and patterns in the data. The techniques are flexible and allow investigators to change the interview script and add probing questions during an interview as needed to gain more in-depth information. Field notes allow the investigators to describe the environment and document changes in the interviewee's facial and body expression, mood, and tone during the interview.[1] Interviewers also note whether the body language matches the response. For example, the patient states approval of new hospital policies during an interview, but he does not look up and nervously taps his leg with his fingers. Qualitative data results are used by researchers to formulate research questions and by evaluators to create goals and objectives. Qualitative data are also used to build new knowledge, design policies, generate hypotheses, and guide the foundation for further research.[2] This chapter introduces types of qualitative data, data collection methods, ethical issues, and data analyses. **Table 6-1** describes the advantages and disadvantages of qualitative investigations.[3]

Table 6-1 Advantages and Disadvantages of Qualitative Research Design

Advantages	Disadvantages
Useful for complex subjects	Not needed for simple hypotheses
In-depth and comprehensive information	Subjective; difficulty establishing reliability and validity
Greater understanding of entire situation	Limited scope because of data collection approaches
Interactions between variables	Possible investigator bias
Generates useful data	Requires detailed planning
Not dependent on large sample sizes	No precise results with mathematical calculations
Unique results	Not able to be replicated; lacks generalizability

The Qualitative-Quantitative Debate

There are advantages and disadvantages to qualitative as well as quantitative methods. The easiest way to remember the difference between qualitative and quantitative methods is that qualitative data focus on mostly words, and quantitative data contain mostly numbers. Instead of trying to have either side win the debate, it is useful to compare the two methods. Qualitative methods focus on subjective, exploratory, and observational techniques and utilize small sample sizes that are not randomly selected. On the other hand, quantitative methods use large random samples that aim for generalizable results. As for data collection, qualitative data involve interviews, focus groups, and observations, whereas quantitative data are derived from objective surveys, scales, and questionnaires. It is important to keep in mind that there is a fair amount of overlap between qualitative and quantitative methods. For example, it is possible for quantitative data to contain some open-ended survey questions, whereas in qualitative studies, investigators may count the various types of responses from interviews.

Some researchers and evaluators use a combination of both qualitative and quantitative data, which is called a mixed methods approach. The term *mixed methods* is also called triangulation. There is value in conducting mixed methods research that uses both qualitative data to tell the story and quantitative data to provide generalizable data. For example, triangulation is used when researchers conduct interviews with 30 physical therapists representing various work environments, such as outpatient clinics, hospitals, and inpatient rehabilitation centers. The interviews focus on work satisfaction, salary, and benefits. From the interview results, the evaluators create survey questions for distribution to all licensed physical therapists in Ohio. This mixed methods approach provides details from the interviews and generalizability from the large sample size of the survey. Other types of triangulation are (1) methods triangulation, involving combining data from multiple data sources on the same topic; and (2) evaluator triangulation, involving the combination of data from multiple evaluators on the same topic.[4] Within triangulation, evaluators corroborate the various types of data. Corroboration does not verify the accuracy of the participants' responses but rather confirms that the findings reflect what the participants were stating during the interview or focus group.[5]

Qualitative Methods: Validity and Reliability

Before jumping to the specifics, let's review basic definitions. Validity is the degree to which the scale, test, or tool measures what it was intended to measure. In qualitative research, validity is obtaining impressions, patterns, or trends of the experience or topic under investigation.[6] It is important to use skilled facilitators and moderators for qualitative research such as interviews, focus groups, or observations. Investigators try to eliminate as much personal bias as possible so that they do not hear or see what they want to see because of their bias. Investigators verify that the interview questions ask about the specific topic to ensure validity. For example, if the interview questions focus on patient satisfaction, the interview questions need to relate to the satisfaction of the patient's current clinic visit. Also, qualitative investigators address validity throughout the data collection process. As more and more cases are reviewed, patterns, themes, and emerging hypotheses confirm the validity.[7] Another way to increase validity is to seek alternative explanations for the emerging patterns. For example, are the respondents providing honest responses, or are they giving the types of answers they think the interviewer wants to hear? This type of response is called *social desirability*. Or perhaps the respondents are trying to please the interviewer to ensure access to the incentive. Lastly, validity is increased when researchers and evaluators reach a point of saturation, which is defined as when each additional interview, focus group, or observation does not yield any new information. For example, respondents keep stating approximately the same issues related to dissatisfaction with the clinic check-in process. The types of validity in qualitative methods include the following:

- *Construct validity:* To what degree do the interview questions match the concepts and operational definitions in the research or evaluation? For example, do the interview questions about workplace stress match the investigator's definition of workplace stress?
- *Content validity:* Does the design method match what is expected to be measured? For example, are the investigators observing behavior when interviewing would be a more appropriate research design to address the research questions or evaluation objectives?
- *Face validity:* Does the method used show common sense? For example, if the investigators want to know about quality of hospital cafeteria food, did they conduct a taste test with employees, patients, and visitors?[8]

The validity of qualitative methods is criticized for several reasons. First, because investigators are present during interviews or observations, the participant's behavior may change. This is called *reactivity*. For example, children act differently during playtime if they know they are being observed by an adult. Second, investigators may use selection bias when recruiting participants. Third, investigators may inadvertently influence or bias the participants' responses during the interview. Fourth, investigators may not observe all factors in the situation or event under investigation. Fifth, investigators' bias may influence the data analysis.[9,10] For example, if investigators have strong positive or negative opinions about an interview topic, such as abortion, their body language and facial expressions may influence how the respondents answer the interview questions.

Reliability is defined as the ability to yield the same results in repeated studies.[11] The use of qualitative methods is criticized because it is difficult to replicate observations, patterns, and trends with the same phenomenon time after time.[6] Because it is not possible to use the same participants over and over, qualitative investigators address this criticism by using purposive participant sampling based on previous knowledge of the topic from literature reviews. To address investigator bias, investigators work in teams and read from scripted basic interview guides. During observations, research or evaluation teams construct basic checklists and add field notes for additional details. Because interviews and focus groups are digitally recorded, research or evaluation teams verify the reliability of the basic content of each interview. Although quantitative investigators can conduct test-retest procedures to verify reliability, it is possible for qualitative investigators to do the same by repeating observations under varying conditions to verify emergence of similar findings.[12]

Lastly, the use of triangulation methods improves reliability and validity. By using different strategies to study the same topic, investigators gain different perspectives, for example, by making observations under various conditions; interviewing comparison groups, such as staff and patients, to get different perspectives; and having several investigators analyze the same data independently.[13,14]

Types of Qualitative Design

For this chapter, the types of qualitative design include interviews, observational research, case studies, phenomenology, content analysis, ethnography, historical document analysis, and grounded theory.

Interviews

Structured interviews involve asking an agreed-upon set of questions. After conducting a review of the professional literature related to the topic, investigators create a list of structured open-ended interview questions. For example, an open-ended question is "Describe what you did at work today" whereas a closed question is "On a scale of 1 to 10, with 10 being 'I feel great,' how would you rate your health today?" All types of interviews are audiotaped for transcription purposes, and the interviewer also takes notes during the session. Following each interview, interviewers write field notes about observations made during the interview.

Unstructured interviews are different from structured interviews, because the interviewer has guidelines rather than a set of questions and the interview is more like a conversation. The interviewer moves the conversation in different directions to fully explore the topic of interest.[15] For example, if the research topic is physician-assisted suicide, the interviewer may move the conversation from religious beliefs, to legal aspects, to personal desires about end-of-life decisions, depending on what the participant says.

Focus groups are best defined as a group interview. Like interviews, focus groups have a predetermined set of questions, but interviewers also have the leeway to explore comments as desired to gain a deeper understanding of the topic. There are advantages and disadvantages to both interviews and focus groups. Interviewers are allowed to explore questions in depth with each respondent, whereas focus groups allow a group-thinking process, with several individuals sharing their opinions at the same time. Interviews are more time consuming, and focus groups are faster. The cost is approximately the same, because respondents are paid for their time to participate in either an interview or a focus group.

When recruiting focus group participants, it is important that each focus group is composed of six to eight similar individuals. For example, it is not appropriate to host a focus group from a specific department in the clinic, because this configuration would have supervisors and staff in the same focus group. Instead, it would be appropriate to have a focus group with only administrative assistants from across the clinic. When hosting focus groups, it is useful to have individuals with similar characteristics related to the topic of interest. For example, evaluators studying the issues related to workplace injury programs with an emphasis on back pain would recruit individuals receiving physical therapy for a work-related injury.

When conducting focus groups, there should be at least two trained interviewers in the room. One person asks the predetermined questions followed by additional questions or probes to gain more details. For example, if the predetermined question is "How would you describe your level of satisfaction with your last visit to this clinic?" the additional question or probe is "Tell me more about your frustration with the patient check-in process." The probe questions are the researchers' opportunities to listen to the participants' answers to the predetermined questions and gain more details by asking about one area of concern. A second person attends the focus group to take field notes and make sure that the audio recording devices are working and that the participants are comfortable. It is advisable to have one recording device at each end of the table. Each participant's name is written on a table tent so the researchers can address individuals by their first names. It is important that the interviewers receive responses from each participant for each question to ensure the broadest range of responses. As with individual interviews, extensive training is required prior to conducting an interview or focus group (see **Box 6-1**).

Observations

There are various types of observations. Let's look at **Figure 6-1** to see the broad view, then read the following descriptions of each type. In the descriptions of the observation types, it becomes evident that there is overlap. For example, investigators may combine participant and contrived observation for data collection. Keep in mind that observations are filled with potential ethical issues and deceptive practices.

Participant and Nonparticipant Observation

Evaluators and researchers either participate in the activity or observe without involvement as a nonparticipant observer. There are two types of participant observations. First, some participant observation involves a quick turnaround

---

BOX 6-1

Tips for Interviewing

1. Practice interviewing how to ask unbiased questions without reacting to the responses.
2. Select a comfortable location so participants feel at ease.
3. Avoid interview questions with possible "yes" or "no" responses.
4. Maintain a flexible approach by asking questions to receive broad responses and perceptions.
5. Ask repetitive but reworded questions to validate responses.

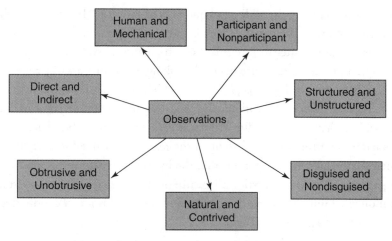

FIGURE 6-1 Types of Observational Research

experience, while immersed in the situation for a brief period of time. For example, a secret shopper has a brief interaction at a fast food restaurant. The entire interaction could be less than five minutes. Second, other participant observations are more demanding and time consuming, because the researcher becomes a member of the group, setting, or community. This investigation requires months or years of emersion into the culture, so that the observation is the natural environment. The investigator writes volumes of field notes and collects documents, photos, and other pertinent data. Some researchers believe that participant observation with total immersion is the only way to gain insights into the setting (see **Box 6-2**).[16] For example, the study involves watching family members in the emergency department (nonparticipant) or acting like a family member in the emergency department (participant).

Obtrusive and Unobtrusive Observation

Evaluators trace or create physical evidence. For example, evaluators use hidden cameras to collect data from individuals or collect data observing what type of food is left on hospital cafeteria trays.

Natural and Contrived Observation

When researchers observe behavior in normal and ordinary settings, it may take a long time for the event to occur. In contrived observations, the setting is staged. Researchers collect the data faster because they do not have to wait for the event

BOX 6-2   Observation

The evaluation team is hired to improve the waiting room environment and the efficiency of the hospital's emergency room, so a direct observation study is an appropriate qualitative research design. Approval by the hospital's institutional review board (IRB) is required prior to initiating this evaluation. Direct observation includes sitting in the waiting room and taking copious field notes on patients, family members, cleanliness, availability of restrooms, walking patterns, food brought in and food purchased from vending machines, placement of furniture and television screens, samples of nonidentifiable conversations, and other pertinent information and events. Observations would also include patient flow from parking options, signage to main entrance, check-in procedures and forms, total wait time and wait time between each phase, involvement of family, attitude of staff, availability of Wi-Fi, and cell phone usage.

to occur. For example, researchers wish to observe how fathers alone interact with their children at an indoor shopping mall playground. They must wait until father/child dyads enter the playground without the mother or another adult. However, in contrived observations, father/child dyads are invited to come and try out new outdoor toys at a staged indoor playground. Contrived observation may lead to ethical issues of deception during recruitment of individuals.

Disguised and Nondisguised Observation

Researchers observe behavior by posing as one of the group members. Nondisguised researchers inform individuals that they are conducting research. Both observations create ethical dilemmas. Disguised observations are deceitful, whereas nondisguised observations yield inaccurate data because individuals act differently when watched.

Structured and Unstructured Observation

To standardize data collection, researchers use checklists when conducting structured observations. With unstructured observations, researchers record field notes for data collection. For example, researchers utilize a checklist when observing the first three minutes of the patient–nurse interaction in the emergency department.

Direct and Indirect Observation

Researchers collect direct observations in real time, whereas indirect observations are collected after the event (secondary data). For example, direct observation is recording the time as well as procedures used by nurses to administer patient medications, whereas indirect observation is reviewing the digital medical administration record (MAR) to record only when medications were administered.[16]

Human and Mechanical Observation

Human observation involves collecting data (e.g., field notes and checklists), whereas mechanical observation uses audio and/or video recorders to collect data. For example, researchers are in the room with the physician when a cancer diagnosis is presented to a patient versus using digital cameras to record the physician–patient interaction. Digital recordings are more accurate for this type of data collection.[17]

Case Studies

A case study is defined as thorough exploration on a specific topic. A case study is an analysis of narrow and detailed variables describing individuals, groups, social units, or situations.[18] Case studies focus on the individual unit rather than the population. Case studies are not generalizable but concentrate on greater understanding of specific topics.[19] For example, if healthcare providers see a patient with extremely unusual symptoms, they could publish a case study describing the presenting symptoms, disease course, treatment, and outcome. Once the manuscript is published, other healthcare providers have the opportunity to share similar experiences in their patient populations (see **Box 6-3**).[15,20,21]

Phenomenology

Phenomenology is the study of human experiences and interpretations of an occurrence within a population. Unlike a case study, phenomenology explores an event or situation within a study population. Researchers wish to understand how the event is viewed or constructed by others. For example, a phenomenological study of the September 11, 2001, attacks would yield a wide variety of perceptions of the events. Individual perceptions may not be accurate, but researchers are not searching for accuracy but rather perceptions of events.

Historical Documents

Relying on inductive reasoning, researchers conduct historical research to study the details of past events. Possible source materials to study include newspapers,

BOX 6-3

Case Study of AIDS: June 5, 1981

On June 5, 1981, *Morbidity and Mortality Weekly Report* (MMWR) published a report of five cases of *Pneumocystis carinii* pneumonia (PCP) among previously healthy young men in Los Angeles. The men were described as "homosexuals"; two died. The Los Angeles County Department of Public Health prepared a case study suggesting an immune deficiency disease with possible sexual contact. The report prompted additional case studies from health departments in New York City, San Francisco, and other cities. In June 1981, the Centers for Disease Control and Prevention (CDC) in Atlanta created an investigative team to identify risk factors and to develop a case definition for national surveillance. Within 18 months, epidemiologists conducted studies to identify the major risk factors for Acquired Immunodeficiency Syndrome (AIDS). In 1983, the CDC reported recommendations for prevention of sexual, drug-related, and occupational transmission.

The Centers for Disease Control and Prevention *Morbidity and Mortality Weekly Report* available at: http://www.cdc.gov/mmwr/preview/mmwrhtml/mm5021a1.htm.

magazines, legal and medical documents, textbooks, periodicals, training manuals, photographs, and so on. This information is useful in planning future events. As with any study, the first step is formulating the research question. For example, how was the polio vaccine distributed to the U.S. population in a short period during the 1950s? Is this historical model useful in planning the dissemination of vaccines for a newly emerging virus, such as H1N1 influenza? Prior to starting historical research, researchers establish the historical data to include in the study collection. Keep in mind that there are specific procedures to follow when seeking the authenticity of historical documents, but this discussion is beyond the scope of this chapter.[22]

Content Analysis

A content analysis is a collection of existing documents on a specific topic. Examples include the following:

- One type of document over time, such as all Seaside Hospital annual reports for the past 10 years

- Different types of documents on a specific topic during a specific period, such as 1 year of identified health magazine articles and medical websites related to cervical cancer information for the layperson audience or media transcripts on a specific topic, such as television health news coverage about cardiovascular disease that emphasizes lifestyle changes (e.g., maintaining healthy weight, adequate daily exercise, and smoking cessation) or emphasizes the latest research on cardiovascular drug therapies and surgical procedures
- Various personal documents on a specific topic, such as diaries, transcripts of videos, journals, or social media entries from patients receiving cancer treatment

Each document collection is analyzed to get an in-depth view of the media reporting, public reaction, personal insight, and trends related to the topic of interest. For example, if hospital administrators are seeking a Certificate of Need from the county in order to build a new hospital, they would hire health researchers to conduct a content analysis related to the press coverage, newspaper editorials, emergency room overcrowding reports, and documentation of public opinion. The analysis of whole collections of documents would paint a positive or negative picture of the need to build an additional hospital in the county.

Ethnography

Ethnography is a combination of interviews, observations, and case studies with an emphasis on the relationship between behavior and culture.[23] A researcher team studies a particular location or population to gain greater understanding to address researcher questions. As with other types of qualitative data, researcher teams observe a setting, collect field notes, conduct interviews, and collect artifacts (e.g., unofficial and official documents). If case studies are used, researchers conduct life stories with specific individuals. Ethnographic research is labor intensive, involves extensive time on location, and is generally not used for evaluations.

Grounded Theory

Grounded theory is qualitative research used to generate new theory based on a process of comparison. The first step is to develop a hypothesis, and then the researcher begins to collect data about the topic from a variety of sources, such as literature reviews, public records, interviews, observation, and surveys.[24,25] By using the technique of grounded theory, researchers select published research or other documentation and make constant comparisons. Researchers compare the first two documents to each other. If the documents yield similar results, researchers continue the process with the third document, and so on. With each additional document, researchers are searching for a bit of novel information that is new but similar to their existing information. If the comparative document yields conflicting or dissimilar results, that document is put aside for further review. As each document is compared to the others, it is either accepted or rejected. Throughout the process, the proposed hypothesis gains strength, or it is determined that it needs further modification. The process is repeated over and over until all known documents are compared and either accepted or rejected. There is no clear end point. Researchers stop when it appears that no new information is available. This end point is called *saturation*.[26,27] The "rejected" documents are revisited to determine if there are any unexplored patterns or situations that need further consideration.

Ethical Issues in Qualitative Research

Some types of qualitative data collection require the consideration of possible ethical issues. In all situations, researchers and evaluators assure participants of confidentiality as stated on the informed consent document that was approved by the appropriate IRB. Regardless of what participants reveal in an interview or on a survey, the investigator's obligation is to maintain confidentiality of the information. To protect participant identity, researchers use pseudonyms and codebooks.

In addition to protecting the confidentiality of the content, investigators are obligated to protect the actual storage of the data. This legal obligation involves protecting files in a locked cabinet or office, establishing computer password protection for digital files, determining the credentials of other investigators with access to the protected files, storage of paper copies of filed notes, and various other data storage issues. Lastly, there are issues related to who owns the data. This issue gets problematic when the agency funding the research or evaluation wants access to confidential data held by the investigators.[28]

Lastly, some argue that researchers conducting participant observation must assume a deceptive role for full immersion into a community. For example, if the study involves documenting the quality of health care in a jail, the researcher would work with the legal system to become an inmate for a year to actually experience the quality of health care. Some researchers argue that this method is deceptive and unethical. Other researchers argue that it is the only way to gain reliable information, because they believe that individuals change their behavior if they know they are being watched.[29] Lastly, some researchers believe that unethical studies yield poor quality results.[30] Generally, all agree that research is only as ethical as the researchers conducting the study, regardless of whether it is qualitative or quantitative research.

Analyses of Qualitative Data

The qualitative investigator analyzes data continually from the initial research phase to the final report. This constant process was labeled *analysis and interpretation* by Goetz and LeCompte.[23] There are several approaches to overall analysis, starting with the research questions (or objectives in an evaluation) and choice of data collection involving (1) broad holistic or big-picture view of the data, (2) collaborative partnerships from various and opposing viewpoints, and (3) detailed descriptions of the studied topic across multiple data sources to seek regular patterns or trends. All approaches involve sifting through data, coding data, and sorting data over and over again as each observation or interview is added to the data collection. Each round of data analysis clarifies patterns and trends while attempting to interpret ongoing observations and interviews to refine conclusions. This section describes each level of qualitative data analysis.

Data Organization

Because qualitative data analysis requires a constant process of examining, sorting, and reexamining data, investigators need to precisely organize the data. There are two basic ways to organize the large quantities of data: manually and by computer.

Manual

Although computers are more commonly used to store data, investigators continue to find notebooks and boxes a useful way to organize the data. First, investigators copy the original documents and then store the original documents in a safe. Second, the copied documents are coded, cut apart, recoded, stored with notes in the margins, and continually resorted throughout the analysis process. In each reiteration, investigators add more extensive notes in the margins. In the beginning the notes are general, but later the notes focus on specific concepts.

Computers

Computers are increasingly the tool of choice for gathering, entering, retrieving, managing, and analyzing qualitative data. There are numerous qualitative software programs available. Despite the advantages of using a qualitative software program, qualitative investigators still are required to explore the data for patterns and trends leading to theory construction, because computers cannot analyze the complex meanings and perceptions explored in qualitative research and evaluations (see **Box 6-4**).[31]

Coding Data

Data Reduction

Interview questions and responses are typically tape-recorded and then transcribed verbatim before analysis is begun. Transcription is extremely time consuming.[32] Because of the large amount of data that can be generated in qualitative research, a data reduction process must be used to aid analysis. This procedure includes organizing the data; identifying emerging themes, categories, and patterns; and testing hypotheses against the data.[29]

There are two types of codes: preassigned or a priori codes and exploratory codes. A priori codes are described by investigators prior to starting data analyses.

BOX 6-4

Examples of Qualitative Software Programs

There are both open source (free) and proprietary (for pay) computer-assisted qualitative data analysis programs. Both have their advantages and disadvantages. Below are examples of both kinds.

Open Source

Coding Analysis Toolkit (CAT): A web-based program developed by the Qualitative Data Analysis Program of the University of Pittsburgh. Able to import data from other programs, CAT uses keystrokes and automation instead of a mouse to speed up activities.[33]

Compendium: A computer program that facilitates the mapping and management of ideas and arguments, allowing people to record and structure collaboration.[34]

Proprietary

ATLAS.ti: A computer program that assists researchers in uncovering and systematically analyzing data hidden in text and multimedia, allowing users to code and annotate.[35]

NVivo: Helps people to manage, shape, and make sense of unstructured information in text and multimedia formats.[36]

For example, if the evaluation focuses on the efficiency of the hospital outpatient admissions process, a priori codes include courtesy of staff, wait time, cleanliness, paper documents versus paperless electronic medical records, and scheduling. Exploratory codes are added to the a priori codes as data are collected and analyzed once new themes emerge. For example, using the previous example, evaluators may discover that temperature of the waiting room and long wait times for valet parking are frequently mentioned patient complaints yet were not on the a priori code list.

As the data are collected, researchers and evaluators store two electronic copies of the original document, in case one document is damaged or lost. These stored files are not analyzed. Before starting to code any data, researchers read a third copy of the documents several times to improve familiarity. They begin coding into the a priori code files. Researchers start to file any portion of the document that does not fit into one of the a priori codes for the "leftover" files. These files are revisited later, and new exploratory codes are created. In addition to the a priori codes, researchers may slice the data codes into general categories, such as activities, personnel, methods, events, and location; or into taxonomic codes, such as who, what, when, and how. Researchers code and recode data several times and into several different categories until the data begin to take shape as patterns and trends emerge. In all coding situations, each segment is labeled with an appropriate code related to the research questions or evaluation objectives. When complete data files contain multiple collections, such as interviews, focus groups, and observations, coding categories become more and more complex.[37] It is then necessary to create subfiles and segmented subfiles, so that every data fragment is analyzed and considered in the results.

There are three coding strategies.[38] First, open coding is the simplest form and is used first to sort the data into a priori or exploratory code categories. Second, axial coding is the intermediate step. This coding allows the investigator to begin to link the data into logical connections between categories. Third, selective coding is the last step and involves establishing the patterns and trends in the data. At this point, the categories are further refined for theory development and validation. All three steps are repeated over and over as the data are revisited in the process of data collection and analyses.

During the coding process, investigators work both individually and in teams to determine if the coding strategies are appropriate. Sometimes the a priori codes are merged together to form new, broader code categories, and other times the codes are split into subcategories. Coding is time consuming and only ends when investigators agree that sufficient patterns and trends are identified to address the research questions. At this point, investigators have the option to quantify the responses in each code category. For example, researchers state that 18 respondents (62%) stated that the staff was friendly and efficient in completing the necessary paperwork for admission. This process is not an attempt to transform qualitative data into quantitative data or to remove the individual richness, but rather it is used to add description to code lists. Lastly, qualitative investigators provide direct quotes to illustrate examples and emphasize noteworthy findings.

Data Display

When displaying qualitative results, it is useful to use graphics. Qualitative data are displayed using tables, diagrams, charts, and graphs. Frequency tables are used to describe categorical data, such as demographics (see **Table 6-2**).

Unlike paragraphs of description, diagrams provide a visual depiction of volumes of data. Data used for **Figure 6-2** were the key words taken from interview data of university students with chronic health challenges.[39] The font size illustrates the number of times the word appears in the interview transcripts. Obviously, the words *independent*, *control*, *family*, *parents*, and *support* comprise the key themes. Further analyses of the interviews showed the struggles between the students' desire to be independent and in control of their chronic health challenges, but still needing support from parents and family.

Charts and graphs show chronological order or categories, and there are advantages to using charts and graphs over writing a descriptive paragraph. In **Figure 6-3**, it is easy to see that the number of auto fatalities decreased for pediatrics and increased for the elderly in Highland County from 2010 to 2013.

Table 6-2   Frequency Table for Demographic Data

Demographic Variable (*n* = 25)	
Gender	
Female	15 (60%)
Male	10 (30%)
Geographic Place of Residence	
Urban	13 (52%)
Rural	12 (48%)
Employment Status	
Unemployed	2 (8%)
Part-time employment	2 (8%)
Full-time employment	20 (80%)
Retired	1 (4%)

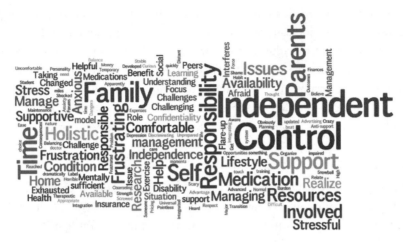

FIGURE 6-2 Word Cloud
Diagram was made using Wordle, which is available at: www.wordle.net.

With this small sample size, investigators can interview family members to gain more information about this trend. This chart also displays trend data that can be used to justify community education for the elderly population. The pie chart of **Figure 6-4** shows the data for 1 year.

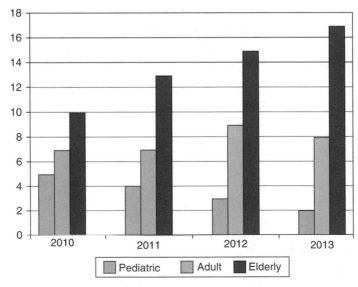

FIGURE 6-3 Number of Auto Fatalities in Highland County: 2010–2013

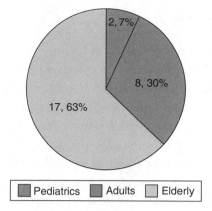

FIGURE 6-4   Auto Fatalities by Age Group in 2013

Summary

This chapter focuses on all aspects of qualitative design. The chapter begins with a discussion of the differences between qualitative and quantitative designs, including the advantages and disadvantages of each design. The topic of reliability and validity of qualitative data is presented, followed by a description of each type of qualitative design. After a discussion of possible ethical issues in qualitative methods, the chapter concludes with a description of how to conduct a simple analysis of qualitative data including data organization, coding, and data display.

Case Study

Research question: Among Medicaid recipients, why do some women receive mammograms in a timely manner and other women never receive mammograms?

The results of this study will be used to design a brochure to encourage women receiving Medicaid to receive mammograms. Drs. Jackson and Graham design a qualitative study to answer the research question. After receiving approval from the IRB, they begin the recruitment process.

continues

CASE STUDY *continued*

They decide to conduct a series of focus groups with two types of women: Group One includes women receiving Medicaid between the ages of 50 and 65 who have received at least two mammograms, and Group Two includes women receiving Medicaid between the ages of 50 and 65 who have never received a mammogram. Researchers wish to recruit a diverse group of women, so they post recruitment advertisements on social media sites as well as in local newspapers. They place brightly colored brochures in clinic waiting rooms, church bulletins, neighborhood laundromats, and local cafes with bulletin boards. The incentive is $50 plus a taxi voucher for participating in a 90-minute focus group. The focus groups are scheduled for 90 minutes to give women a chance to arrive, locate the room, and get comfortable. However, the actual focus group takes only 1 hour. Focus groups are held at 10:00 a.m. and 6:30 p.m. on Tuesday, Thursday, and Saturday in the community rooms at two centrally located neighborhood libraries. From the flyer or advertisement, women are instructed to call an 800 number to schedule a convenient time to participate in the focus group nearest to their home. When women call, the scheduler asks them a few questions to determine their eligibility for Group One or Group Two. After the scheduler confirms each woman's current Medicaid status, age, ethnicity, and home address, a taxi voucher is mailed to each participant. The scheduler reminds each woman that she may not bring children or other family members to the focus group. Focus groups consist of 6 to 8 women of similar demographics and convenient focus group location. In some cases, two focus groups are conducted at the same time in two different community rooms at the same library for Group One women and Group Two women. The day before each focus group, the scheduler calls to remind each woman of the time, date, and location of the focus group and to verify that her taxi voucher was received.

To avoid personal bias, Drs. Jackson and Graham hire six experienced qualitative researchers to conduct the focus groups. In each focus group, one researcher serves as facilitator and the second researcher serves as moderator. After each focus group, researchers swap roles to avoid exhaustion. By using paper table tents for each participant, the researchers are able to state each woman's name. As women enter the

continues

CASE STUDY *continued*

community room, they are served a beverage and snack, are given a pre-printed name table tent, and are asked to take a seat at the table. After the digital recording devices are checked at both ends of the table, the focus group begins with an explanation of the informed consent document, followed by the opportunity to ask questions. Each woman signs the informed consent document and gives the researchers one copy, keeping the other copy for future reference. Any woman not comfortable with the procedure is invited to leave at this time and still receive the $50 incentive.

As the focus group begins, the researcher asks each woman to respond to the following question: "When I say mammogram, what is the first thing that comes to mind?" After receiving a response from each participant, the researcher asks the next question on the predetermined interview guide. For the Group One women, the next question is "How would you describe a mammogram to a woman who had never had a mammogram?" For the Group Two women, the next question is "Because you have not had a mammogram, what would you like to ask a woman who has had a mammogram about the procedure?" Researchers have the flexibility of asking additional probing questions to gain further detail on any specific question. Each interview question requires a response from each participant, but the probing questions are directed at one or a few women. The process continues until each interview question is answered by each participant. The digital recording devices remain on until the women are paid their $50 incentives and leave the room.

After each focus group, digital recordings are transcribed. Drs. Jackson and Graham review the transcriptions in a timely manner. If one question is consistently misunderstood by participants, they change the wording to improve clarity for future focus groups. Major revisions are allowed but require submitting an amendment to the IRB. Drs. Jackson and Graham, along with their graduate students, continue to review the transcripts and discuss possible emerging patterns and themes. Once some themes begin to emerge, the research team decides approximately how many more focus groups to convene. Ideally, they want to reach a point of saturation where no new data are noted in the transcripts;

continues

CASE STUDY *continued*

however, each focus group is expensive and their funding is limited (see **Table 6-3**).

Table 6-3 Budget for One Focus Group

			Total
Facilitator and moderator	Two researchers for two hours each	$150 per hour	$600
Beverages and snacks			$30
Room rental fee			$100
Incentives	Eight women	$50	$400
Taxi vouchers	Eight women	$30	$240
Supplies			$20
Transcriptionist	Three hours of typing for every hour of recording	$60 per hour	$180
Total			$1,570

Fortunately, Drs. Jackson and Graham budgeted $35,000 for conducting the focus groups. After 16 focus groups are conducted and analyzed, the research team agrees that saturation is achieved and key themes have emerged. The challenging aspect of qualitative data analyses is that the actual words of the themes may or may not ever be stated by the focus group participants. For example, after reading and rereading the Group One responses to the first question, the emerging theme was labeled "peace of mind." The women never stated that getting a mammogram gave them peace of mind, but the collective responses were items like, "I like to know that I'm ok"; "I get a mammogram, because breast cancer runs in my family. I need to get checked each year"; "I do it as an example for my daughters"; "It is just good to get checked out once in a while"; "I never know if I'm doing the breast self-exam correctly. I like the pros to tell me I'm ok for another year." Researchers agree that all of these quotes, as well as many more, illustrate a "peace of mind" theme as to why women receive periodic mammograms. For the Group Two responses to the first question, the emerging theme is labeled "fear of the unknown." The quotes include "You never know what they might find. I'd rather not know"; "I don't want to be exposed to that much radiation. I heard that it might cause breast cancer. I don't know about that"; "There is no cancer in my family, and besides it is a

continues

CASE STUDY *continued*

scary and dangerous procedure anyway"; "I'm not sure that I need to know"; "I do not know what I would do if they found something."

Summary

By looking at only a few quotes from the first question, it is possible to see how researchers are challenged to juggle the data by looking at the big picture while not missing the tiny details. They want to make sure that the comments are unique and not the result of a group-thinking process where everyone agrees with whatever the first respondent said. Researchers do not want to over- or underanalyze data, but they also do not wish to miss a central theme. Qualitative research data are both challenging and intriguing as researchers dig deeper to discover the meaning of and answers to their research questions.

Case Study Discussion Questions

1. Besides focus groups, what other types of qualitative data could have been used to answer the research questions?
2. Describe the process of developing the codebook for retrieving the themes from the focus groups.

Student Activity

For the following case studies, design a qualitative study that addresses the pertinent issues.

Case Study 1

Baxter Hospital plans to open a larger pediatric unit within 2 years. This unit houses a large waiting room with an indoor play area; 2 cafes; 8 operating room suites; outpatient recovery rooms for 1-day stay procedures; 60 private inpatient pediatric rooms with single beds for adults wishing to spend the night; 3 specialty rooms for art, music, and physical therapy; 12 pediatric intensive care beds; and a helicopter rooftop landing site. The hospital administrators wish to market the new pediatric unit as the leading facility in the state. The pediatric design architects know how to utilize the space for efficiency and utility, but they need help with creating a positive, healing atmosphere in the overall space and in the specific units. The space needs to work for children of all ages, parents, family members, nurses, therapists, and healthcare providers. What type of qualitative study would answer the concerns of the design architects?

Case Study 2

Sandersburg is located about 90 miles from a large city and has a population of about 30,000. For the past 5 years, the local community hospital has lost money. Because it is a small, 80-bed hospital, it is not able to offer the extensive services of the two larger regional hospitals. However, the people living in Sandersburg do come to the hospital for minor emergencies and outpatient surgeries. Sandersburg is near a popular ski resort, and tourists utilize the hospital during the winter months. Emergency medical transport teams work out of Sandersburg's emergency department for triage to the regional hospitals. Although the need for the hospital is well documented, financial experts are unable to determine how to make enough profit to justify keeping the hospital open. What type of qualitative study would address how to increase the hospital's profits enough to stay open?

Case Study 3

Greenleaf, a national health insurance company, decided to open a clinic in a busy downtown area near a metro station. It conducted a needs assessment prior to selecting this location. Using GIS mapping, Greenleaf learned that a large percentage of its policyholders worked within a 1-mile radius of the clinic. Over the past year and after an extensive billboard, mail, television, and radio advertising campaign, the clinic continues to be underutilized by nearby workers. What type of qualitative study would address why policyholders are not utilizing the medical services of the nearby clinic?

Case Study 4

After 20 years in service, Serenity Hospice is a well-established facility offering in-home palliative and end-of-life care to the people in Hills County. For the past year, Ms. Hudson, director of nursing, tracked the number of nurses who have left the facility after working there less than 6 months. Because Serenity Hospice knows that this type of nursing is not for everyone, it offers nurses (1) 2 weeks of paid hospice training prior to their first in-home assignment, (2) a buddy nurse with more experience, (3) 48 hours of paid time off after each patient death, and (4) 6 weeks of paid personal time off in the first year of employment. Even with these benefits, nurses are leaving after a few months. Ms. Hudson conducts exit interviews with each nurse, but she does not feel that she is getting enough information to solve the nursing staff problem. What type of qualitative study would address why Serenity Hospice is losing nursing staff after a few months of employment?

References

1. Marshall C, Rossman GB. *Designing Qualitative Research*. Thousand Oaks, CA: Sage; 1998.
2. Lindlof TR, Taylor BC. *Qualitative Communication Research Methods*, 2nd ed. Thousand Oaks, CA: Sage; 2002.
3. Shuttleworth M. Qualitative Research Design. Experiment Resources. Available at: http://www.experiment-resources.com/qualitative-research-design.html. Published September 14, 2008. Accessed May 3, 2012.
4. Denzin NK, Lincoln YS. *The SAGE Handbook of Qualitative Research*, 4th ed. Thousand Oaks, CA: Sage; 2011.
5. Stainback S, Stainback W. *Understanding and Conducting Qualitative Research*. Reston, VA: Council for Exceptional Children; 1988.
6. Rubin A, Babbie E. *Research Methods for Social Work*. Pacific Grove, CA: Brooks/Cole; 1993.
7. Ethical Issues in Conducting Qualitative Research. The Association for Educational Communications and Technology. Available at: http://www.aect.org/edtech/ed1/40/40-05.html. Last updated August 3, 2001. Accessed May 3, 2012.
8. Kirk J, Miller M. *Reliability and Validity in Qualitative Research*. London: Sage; 1986.
9. Maxwell JA. Understanding and validity in qualitative research. *Harvard Educational Review*. 1992;62(3):279–300.
10. Whittemore R, Chase SK, Mandle CL. Validity in qualitative research. *Qual Health Res*. 2001;11(4):522–537.
11. McCall G, Simmons JL. *Issues in Participant Observation*. Reading, MA: Addison-Wesley; 1969.
12. Schaffir WB, Stebbins R. *Experiencing Fieldwork*. Newbury Park, CA: Sage; 1991.
13. Golafshani N. Understanding reliability and validity in qualitative research. *The Qualitative Report*. 2003;8(4):597–607.
14. Wolcott HR. *Qualitative Inquiry in Education: The Continuing Debate*. New York, NY: Teachers College Press; 1990.
15. Adler PA, Adler P. Observational techniques. In: Denzin NX, Lincoln YS, eds. *The SAGE Handbook of Qualitative Research*. Thousand Oaks, CA: Sage; 1994:377–392.
16. Trochim M. Qualitative Methods. Research Methods Knowledge Base. Available at: http://www.socialresearchmethods.net/kb/qualmeth.php. Last updated October 20, 2012. Accessed May 3, 2012.

17. Joppe M. The Research Process: Observation. University of Guelph School of Hospitality and Tourism Management. Available at: http://www.htm.uoguelph.ca /MJResearch/ResearchProcess/Observation.htm. Accessed June 3, 2012.

18. Parasuraman A. *Marketing Research*, 2nd ed. Boston, MA: Addison-Wesley; 1991.

19. Polit D, Hungler BP. *Nursing Research: Principles and Methods*, 2nd ed. Philadelphia, PA: Lippincott; 1983.

20. Stake R. Case study methods in educational research: Seeking sweet water. In: Jaeger RM, ed. *Complementary Methods for Research in Education*. Washington, DC: American Educational Research Association; 1988:251–279.

21. The Centers for Disease Control and Prevention. First Report of AIDS. *MMWR*. 2001;50(21):429. Available at: http://www.cdc.gov/mmwr/preview/mmwrhtml /mm5021a1.htm. Accessed September 5, 2013.

22. Key JP. Research Design in Occupational Education. Oklahoma State University. Available at: http://www.okstate.edu/ag/agedcm4h/academic/aged5980a/5980 /newpage19.htm. Published 1997. Accessed May 3, 2012.

23. Goetz J P, LeCompte MD. *Ethnology and Qualitative Design in Educational Research*. Lexington, MA: D. C. Heath; 1984.

24. Glaser B, Strauss A. *The Discovery of Grounded Theory*. Chicago, IL: Aldine; 1967.

25. Kirk J, Miller M. *Reliability and Validity in Qualitative Research*. London: Sage; 1986.

26. Strauss A, Corbin J. *Basics of Qualitative Research*. Newbury Park, CA: Sage; 1990.

27. Gilgun JF. Steps in the development of theory using a grounded theory approach. *Qualitative Family Research Newsletter*. 1990;4(2):11–12.

28. Gilgun JF. Definitions, methodologies, and methods in qualitative family research. In: Gilgun JF, Daly K, Handel G, eds. *Qualitative Methods in Family Research*. Newbury Park, CA: Sage; 1992:22–40.

29. McRoy RG. Qualitative Research. The University of North Carolina at Pembroke. Available at: http://www.uncp.edu/home/marson/qualitative_research.html. Accessed May 3, 2012.

30. Miles M, Huberman M. *Qualitative Data Analysis: A Sourcebook of New Methods*. Beverly Hills, CA: Sage; 1984.

31. Fielding NG, Lee RM. *Using Computers in Qualitative Research*. London: Sage; 1992.

32. Marlow C. *Research Methods*. Pacific Grove, CA: Brooks/Cole; 1993.

33. Coding Analysis Toolkit. University of Pittsburgh. Available at: http://cat.ucsur.pitt .edu/. Accessed May 3, 2012.

34. Compendium Institute. Available at: http://compendium.open.ac.uk/institute/. Accessed May 3, 2012.

35. ATLAS.ti. Available at: http://www.atlasti.com/index.html. Accessed May 3, 2012.

36. NVivo. Available at: http://www.qsrinternational.com/products_nvivo.aspx. Accessed May 3, 2012.

37. Wolcott H. On seeking—and rejecting—validity in quantitative research. In: Eisner EW, Peshkin A, eds. *Qualitative Inquiry in Education: The Continuing Debate*. New York, NY: Teachers College Press; 1990:121–152.

38. What Is Qualitative Research? QSR International. Available at: http://www .qsrinternational.com/what-is-qualitative-research.aspx. Accessed May 3, 2012.

39. Brunny J, Vazques-Otero C, Curtis T, Perrin K. *Creating Connections Between Adolescent Health and Adult Medicine: Transitions for Undergraduate Students with Health Challenges*. Technical Report. Bringing Science Home Research. University of South Florida, Tampa, FL, 2012.

CHAPTER 7

Elements of Research

CHAPTER OBJECTIVES

By the end of this chapter, students will be able to:

- Explain the differences between basic and applied research
- Develop a list of possible variables and how each is identified in research
- Analyze the advantages and disadvantages of group assignment choices
- Explain the difference between a dictionary definition and an operational definition
- Create a decision tree for the three types of research: true experimental, quasi-experimental, and nonexperimental design.

KEY TERMS

Constructs	Quantitative research design
Operational definition	Variable

Introduction

This chapter introduces quantitative methods. Quantitative methods use numerical data to answer specific questions and are analyzed using statistics. After the research questions or evaluation objectives are developed, it is time to think about various research designs. For this discussion, it is important to understand the elements of research prior to exploring the types of research designs, including non-experimental, quasi-experimental, and true experimental designs. It is important to keep in mind that the purpose directs the design. For example, if patient satisfaction of the clinic services is the purpose of the evaluation, then evaluators design the evaluation to explore the issues that may affect patient satisfaction, including types of services requested and received, unavailable services, appointment scheduling procedures, wait time for an appointment, wait time at the clinic, interaction with clerical staff and healthcare providers, cleanliness of clinic, checkout procedures, and parking services. All aspects of patient satisfaction are considered to evaluate satisfaction of the full experience. On the other hand, if the research question is to determine whether Treatment A is more effective than Treatment B, then the research design reflects an experimental design. In all situations, research questions must guide the design. Without specific research questions, it is not possible to design the correct study. Furthermore, without the correct design, incorrect data collection results in inadequate interpretation. Even with specific research questions and correct design, researchers consider a range of plausible and alternative explanations when reviewing the results. Before exploring types of quantitative research design, it is important to understand the elements of research.

Elements of Research

Basic and Applied Research

There are two types of research: basic and applied. Both types of research are important to the advancement of knowledge, but they work in different ways because of their unique goals. First, basic research is defined as gathering information, discovering knowledge by asking new questions, and building on existing knowledge. It is the fundamental understanding needed to move science forward. Basic research is done first, and then applied research builds on the results. If basic researchers are asked about the meaning of their research, they would state that their research is about learning more with or without direct application. Second, applied research is defined as exploring ways to solve practical problems rather than to acquire knowledge. Often, applied research builds on existing basic research to address and answer problems.[1] For example, basic researchers explore the existence of human genes, whereras applied researchers link specific genes to specific diseases. As stated by George Smoot, "People cannot foresee the future well enough to predict what's going to develop from basic research. If we *only* did applied research, we would still be making better spears."[2] It is important to understand the knowledge gained through basic research prior to utilizing the information in applied research. For example, a nephrologist conducting basic research studies anatomy and physiology of the kidney, whereas a nephrologist involved in applied research explores how diabetes affects kidneys. Always keep in mind that whether the research is basic or applied, research questions determine all aspects of the research project, including the evaluation. There are two kinds of research questions: theoretical and practical. Theoretical questions ask about how a specific theory may be applied to research variables to solve a health-related problem. This is an example of a theoretical question: By applying the Health Belief Model, is it possible to increase mammogram compliance rates among elderly women residing in rural communities? Practical questions are not based on theories, and the questions are more direct. This is an example of a practical question: Is Drug A or Drug B more effective in lowering cholesterol levels over a 6-month period for males over 50 years of age?

Variables

Variables are defined as something that can be changed or manipulated during an experiment or intervention. Variables may also represent an unknown quality or characteristic and are defined by their roles in the evaluation or research. The following list describes the purpose of each variable:

- An independent variable (IV) is what researchers change or manipulate to understand its effect on the dependent or controlled variable. It is the variable believed to cause the change. For example, in medical research, the IV is the new drug for decreasing the side effects of chemotherapy.

- A dependent variable (DV) is affected by or reacts to the independent variable. For example, were the side effects (DV) of the chemotherapy drug decreased after taking the new drug (IV)?

- A mediating variable is defined as an intervening variable because it acts between the IV and the DV. For example, a patient with stage IV cancer may have greater chemotherapy side effects than a patient with stage II cancer because of the degree of tissue involvement.

- A moderating variable is used to show how relationships change with different variables. Using the same example, age is a possible moderating variable. Patients under the age of 60 may have greater tolerance of chemotherapy side effects than elderly patients because of their other comorbidity medical conditions.

- Confounding or extraneous variables interfere with the independent and dependent variables. Sometimes researchers are not aware of confounding variables until late in the study. For example, some of the patients receiving chemotherapy and the drug to reduce side effects may share with each other that a specific type of herbal tea also helps to decrease the side effects. Unbeknownst to the researchers, the patients share this information in the waiting room. This specific herbal tea may be helpful, so the patients report a decrease in side effects, but the reduction has nothing to do with the experimental drug. These types of events are difficult and sometimes impossible to discover for researchers.

- A controlled variable is held constant so relationships among other variables may be analyzed without interference. For example, gender may serve as the control variable while the researchers study the relationship between age and the effectiveness of the drug used to reduce chemotherapy side effects. When holding gender constant, the researchers can study whether the drug works better for one gender than it does for the other.

Without intentionally causing confusion, it is important to note that previously defined variables are also viewed as either categorical or continuous for data analysis. Categorical variables are defined as variables that name groups or categories, such as gender, ethnicity, zip code, employment status, or marital status. Within each group, the choices are independent from or mutually exclusive of the other choices. For example, a survey question asks, "What is your current marital status?" The choices include single, married, divorced, or widowed. Even if a person has experienced several of the listed choices, the question is asking for the respondent's current marital status. He or she can only be one of the choices at any one point in time. Continuous variables are measured over an incremental range and may take on any value within a range, such as age, weight, blood glucose level, annual income, resting heart rate, or cholesterol level. For example, someone is either alive or dead (a categorical variable) but his weight could change over time (a continuous variable). Each respondent provides his current weight, so calculations determine an average weight for all respondents. It is common for an evaluation to include several categorical and continuous variables, such as comparing gender and marital status to weight and blood glucose levels to determine the compliance level among patients with diabetes.

Variables also have attributes. Once investigators determine each type of variable, the next step is to assign attributes to the variables. When gender is asked on a survey, the choices are the following: 1 = *female*, 2 = *male*, 3 = *transgender*,

4 = *other*. It is important that each variable provides an exhaustive list of choices. The choices must also be mutually exclusive, which means that each choice is clearly different from the other choices. For example, the following survey question is an example of *not* being mutually exclusive:

Circle your age bracket. (INCORRECT)
20–30
30–40
40–50
50–60
60–70
70–80
80+

An error occurs when the respondent's age is 30. She could circle 20–30 or 30–40 because the choice selections overlap, causing an error of mutual exclusivity. To avoid this error, the following answers are the correct survey choices:

Circle your age bracket. (CORRECT)
20–29
30–39
40–49
50–59
60–69
70–79
80+

Another example of a variable attribute is agreement. This survey question is asking respondents for their level of agreement:

I feel happy most days. (Circle the choice that best describes you.)
Strongly agree
Agree
Neutral
Disagree
Strongly disagree

The last variable attribute allows respondents to "check all that apply." In the example, it is possible that a respondent is working full-time and seeking a new job, or a respondent is working one steady, part-time job as well as working a seasonal job on the weekends.

Describe your employment status today. (Check all that apply.)
Full-time employment
Part-time employment with steady, regular hours

Part-time with unreliable hours
Seasonal employment
Temporary or day labor
Contract employment, set hours for specific periods
Seeking employment

Observations or Measurements

There are single and multiple observations. Single observations or measurements are individual items such as the following: observing one hour of play therapy, assessing presurgery leg strength for patients having hip replacement surgery, calculating what percentage of each food item is eaten by patients on one hospital unit, and so on. The variable is observed and recorded only once. Multiple measurements involve measuring one variable several times over a defined period of time, such as weighing patients every Monday to determine the effectiveness of a weight loss program. Another multiple measurement involves collecting pretest survey data prior to an intervention and then again after the intervention. For example, patients complete a survey related to depression during their therapy sessions, then take the prescribed antidepression medication for one month, followed by completing the same survey again. The data analysis reveals the effectiveness of medication.

Treatments or Programs

In research and evaluations, a treatment or a program is defined as a single intervention, regardless of the time involved or the number of sessions. A treatment can be one health education class, a 15-week semester of health education classes, a 12-month clinical drug trial for breast cancer, or a hospital-wide training program for the use of electronic medical records. It is common to have one group of individuals participating in the treatment and one control group or nonparticipating group. It is also possible to have individuals or groups of individuals enter the treatment or program in waves. For example, the hospital may train the emergency department staff on the new computer system, and then add the operating room staff, followed by the inpatient units, and lastly the outpatient and auxiliary staff. Everyone receives the training over six months, but the waves allow the trainers to work in smaller groups as the technical issues get resolved over time. Another example would be if patients with type 2 diabetes were assigned to different waves of treatment based on low, medium, or high doses of experimental insulin drugs until the optimal dose is determined through clinical research (see **Box 7-1**).[3]

BOX 7-1

Ethical Issues in Research Design

Researchers conducting true experimental design clinical drug trials face ethical issues regarding treatment. A 12-month, three-arm study design includes the current standard of care, Drug A, and Drug B for patients with chronic obstructive pulmonary disease (COPD). Researchers randomly assign 600 patients with COPD to one of the three treatment options. This is done by assigning the first person to enroll in the study to Group 1, the second person to Group 2, the third person to Group 3, the fourth person to Group 1, and so on. Each group includes 200 patients. After 1 month, it is clear that 70% of the patients in one group have higher pulmonary breathing scores than the other two groups, whereas the other two groups have lower scores and several patients who quit the study because of adverse side effects. Because the researchers are blinded, they do not know which group is showing better pulmonary scores, and they are only 1 month into a 12-month study. Here are a few ethical questions for consideration:

1. Should the researchers stop the study immediately and risk not learning whether the other two groups will improve with longer exposure to the treatment?
2. Is it possible that the improving patients are different from the patients in the other two groups and therefore are improving faster because of the differences rather than the treatment?
3. Is it possible that the improving patients are receiving standard of care and the experimental treatment is harmful?
4. Should the researchers stop the research?
5. How should the researchers proceed?

Group Assignment

Depending on the design, investigators assign each individual to a specific group prior to the beginning of the evaluation or research. There are several ways to make such group assignments, including random group assignment, quota group assignment, and every *n*th group assignment.

Random Group Assignment

Random assignment is conducted using a variety of methods. As an example, first, investigators place different-colored cards in envelopes, with each color representing a different arm of the treatment. For a four-arm study, the red card is for standard of care, the blue card is for Drug A, the yellow card is for Drug B, and the purple card is for Drug C. As a second example, if there are 200 individuals to be enrolled in the study, the numbers 1 through 200 are randomly scrambled. The first enrolled person is assigned the first number on the scrambled list, the second enrolled person is assigned the second number, and so on. Every enrolled individual receives a random number; the researcher assigned participants 1–49 to standard of care, 50–99 to Drug A, 100–149 to Drug B, and 150–200 to Drug C (see **Box 7-2**).

Quota Group Assignment

For quota group assignment, investigators use census data to determine what percentage of individuals is in each group. For example, investigators may wish to represent population diversity in the United States according to the 2010 U.S. census. Using **Table 7-1**, investigators recruit specific individuals based on their ethnicity and other inclusion criteria.[4]

Every nth Group Assignment

In the *n*th group assignment, investigators select individuals or data in a preset and specific pattern, such as every 10th or 20th individual. If for example,

---

BOX 7-2

Sample of Random Group Assignment

Enrollment Order	Randomized Numbers 1–200	Group Assignment 1–49 = Standard of Care; 50–99 = Drug A; 100–149 = Drug B; 150–200 = Drug C
1st person	23	Standard of care
2nd person	138	Drug B
3rd person	14	Standard of care
4th person	57	Drug A
5th person	190	Drug C
6th person	103	Drug B
So on . . . to 200		

Table 7-1   Sample of Quota Group Assignment

	Percentage from 2010 U.S. Census	Study Population: 1,500 Individuals
White	72.4	1,086
Black or African American	12.6	189
American Indian and Alaskan Native	0.9	13.5
Asian	4.8	72
Native Hawaiian and other Pacific Islander	0.2	3
Some other race	6.2	93
Two or more races	2.9	43.5

Data from Humes KR, Jones NA, Ramirez RR. Overview of Race and Hispanic Origin: 2010. The United States Census Bureau. Available at: http://www.census.gov/prod/cen2010/briefs /c2010br-02.pdf

investigators wished to mail a satisfaction survey to a random sample of patients who received outpatient surgery in the last six months from three regional hospitals, they might decide to use *n*th group assignment. After receiving approval from the institutional review board for the study, investigators obtain a list of 1,800 adult patient names and mailing addresses. The investigators select every 5th person to receive the satisfaction survey for a total of 360 mailed surveys. There is a limitation of concern when using this method. If the patient list of names was in alphabetical order, investigators run the risk selecting too many individuals from one common name group, such as Smith, Johnson, Rodriguez, or Patel, depending on the common ethnicity of the geographic area. To resolve this limitation, researchers could arrange the patient list by date of surgery rather than alphabetically prior to selecting every 5th individual to receive the mailed satisfaction survey.

Constructs

A construct is a concept, thought, or notion that is more challenging to measure, such as depression, self-esteem, degree of pain, motivation, or achievement rather than a concrete concept, such as body mass index, height, weight, girth, or blood glucose level. Frequently, investigators group several specific qualities together to form a construct. For example, during first 24 hours after a total hip replacement, a pain-level construct is measured by grouping together the following assessments: the individual's rating of her pain (0 = *none* to 10 = *severe pain*), number of pain medication requests, range of motion, age of individual, and number of other medical conditions. By forming a pain-level construct, healthcare providers determine if individuals are experiencing more or less pain than is typically expected. When defining a concept, it is important to seek agreement from experts on how to describe the terms and determine if the chosen items truly measure the construct. The term used is *construct validity*, and it is defined as the degree to which the construct measures the concept being studied. If the construct has low validity, then the study results yield low generalizability to other study populations. If the construct has high validity, when the construct is used with a different study population, similar results yield high generalizability.[3]

Operational Definitions

Operational definitions are based on constructs as well as the research questions or goals and objectives. It is up to the investigator to provide clear and concise definitions for each construct used. Investigators may select a dictionary definition or provide a more specific definition suited for the evaluation or research. For example, if the study involves interviewing elderly patients, it is necessary to provide an operational age definition for *elderly*. The inclusion criteria may be patients age 60 and over, but others may define elderly as age 65 and over. In cases like this, there is no absolute correct definition for the term *elderly*, so investigators state that for this particular study, the definition of *elderly* will be individuals at or above 65 years of age on the day of the interview. For each construct, it is necessary to provide an operational definition.

Types of Research Design

Now that we have defined some typical terms, let's discuss the types of designs. By thinking of the type of design as a framework or scaffolding, it is necessary to add the elements of observation or measurement, treatments or programs, assignment of groups, and time to complete the framework. Let's explore how each element fits into the structure. Keep in mind that not every element is used in all three types of design.

There are three types of design: true experimental, quasi-experimental, and nonexperimental design. True experimental design is when random assignment is used to determine how participants are assigned to groups. Quasi-experimental design does not use random assignment. Lastly, nonexperimental design is used when there is no need for group assignment. For example, if the investigators wish to know more about patient satisfaction with dietary services, they would place a postcard survey on each patient tray and ask the patients complete the survey after

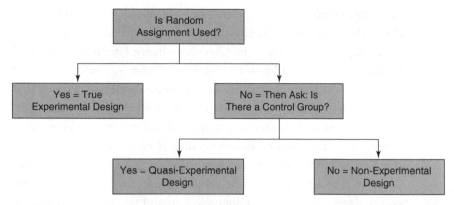

FIGURE 7-1   Choosing a Research Design
Modified from Trochim M. Types of Designs. Research Methods Knowledge Base. Available at: http://www.socialresearchmethods.net/kb/destypes.php. Reprinted by permission of the author.

each meal. In this case, there is no need for a random assignment. Now let's explore each type of design in greater detail (see **Figure 7-1**).[5]

True Experimental Design

True experimental design includes (1) exploring cause-and-effect relationships, (2) manipulating the independent variable, and (3) random assignment of participants to equivalent groups. Let's discuss each of these points in detail.

1. True experimental design allows researchers to determine cause-and-effect relationships. As independent variables are changed, investigators understand the effect on the dependent variable. In addition, investigators must control the other types of variables as much as possible to strengthen the cause-and-effect relationship. Because it is not possible to prove an absolute cause-and-effect relationship, investigators use statistical calculations to determine that the results are due to actual findings rather than probability due to random chance.[6]

2. With a causal relationship in the research question or evaluation objectives, the manipulation of the treatment variable, also called the independent variable, produces different outcomes in the dependent variable. Any differences in the dependent variable are because of the applied treatment conditions or manipulation of the treatment. For example, if investigators wanted to verify which type of blanket is more effective in reducing chills and shaking among postoperative patients 30 minutes after surgery,

the independent variable is the type of blanket and the dependent variable is the reduction in the amount of chills and shaking experienced by the postoperative patients 30 minutes after surgery. Fifty patients received blankets from the traditional warmer unit, and 50 patients received constant-temperature electric blankets. If nurse investigators found that blankets from the warming unit were just as effective as the constant-temperature electric blankets, the hospital would save money by not purchasing the expensive constant-temperature electric blankets.

3. Random assignment determines how participants are assigned to a minimum of two equal groups: one experimental group and one control group. Keep in mind that random selection and random assignment are not the same. Random selection is a sample chosen from a population, whereas random assignment is used in true experimental design.

Another aspect of random assignment is called *research blinding*. When individuals are not told which treatment they are receiving, it is a blinded study. For example, after the patient enrolls in the study, they are asked to select one of three envelopes. Each envelope contains either a blue, yellow, or red card. Researchers open the envelope and write down the individual's name and the color of the card selected. In this case, researchers know which treatment the individual will receive, but the individual is not aware that the blue card is for standard of care, the red card is for Drug A, and the yellow card is for Drug B. When the random assignment is not conducted by the study researchers, it is called a double-blinded study because neither the individual nor the researchers are aware of which drug the individual will receive. In this situation, a researcher not involved in the study would assign the colored cards to the drug treatment options. The individual still selects an envelope, but the study researcher is not aware what each colored card represents. This option is the strongest research design and reduces researcher bias.

For example, take this research question: Does the anti-inflammatory Drug A, Drug B, or Drug C (standard of care) decrease swelling and improve tolerance of physical therapy for individuals recovering from knee replacement surgery? Individuals scheduled for knee replacement surgery are evaluated by a physical therapist to document their presurgery leg strength levels and other physical conditions. After the surgery, 75 individuals recovering from knee replacement surgery are recruited for a true experimental randomized clinical trial. After signing the informed consent documents, each individual selects an envelope with an enclosed colored card, assigning them to Drug A, Drug B, or Drug C.

Twenty-five individuals are assigned to each group. An outside researcher records the individual's name and card color for a double-blinded study technique. All recruited individuals are similar on a specific number of characteristics, such as age range, type of surgery technique, other health conditions, presurgical body mass index, surgeon, and hospital. After adequate healing postsurgery, individuals receive Drug A, B, or C. After six weeks of physical therapy, researchers receive data from the physical therapy records to determine if there are statistical differences between the swelling and physical therapy tolerance of the patients receiving Drug A, B, or C. In this example, the independent variable is the anti-inflammatory drug and the dependent variable is the swelling and physical therapy tolerance. Because other variables (such as gender) were held constant, the cause-and-effect relationship is strong (see **Box 7-3**).[7]

Although randomized controlled trials are considered the gold standard of research, it is worth noting some limitations of true experimental designs before moving to the next type of research design. One limitation is that individuals in the control group may inadvertently be exposed to the treatment; for example, individuals share experiences in a common waiting room. Also, because of logistical and feasibility constraints, it is not always possible to use randomized assignment techniques. When the research setting is a school or a residential facility, it is not feasible to randomly assign each student or resident to various treatment options, especially when the differences are noticeable. In this situation, investigators would use quasi-experimental design.

BOX 7-3

Diagram of True Experimental Research Design

Pretest (leg strength)	Treatment	Posttest (leg strength)
A_1	$X_{E \text{ Drug A}}$	B_2
A_1	$X_{E \text{ Drug B}}$	B_2
A_1	$X_{C \text{ Standard of care}}$	B_2

E = Experimental group
C = Control group

Data from Gribbons B, Herman J. True and quasi-experimental designs. *Practical Assessment, Research & Evaluation*. 1997;5(14). http://PAREonline.net/getvn.asp?v=5&n=14.

Quasi-Experimental Design

Quasi-experimental design is also thought of as a "sort of" experimental design. The two key distinctions are the independent variable is manipulated but lacks random assignment, OR the independent variable is not manipulated but includes random assignment (Figure 7-1). Research results yield limited generalizable conclusions. In quasi-experimental design, the assignment is based on factors such as cost, convenience, feasibility, or some other criteria. Investigators may or may not have control over which individuals or groups are assigned to each treatment group. Also, if the design involves using multiple waves of enrollment, it is quasi-experimental design (see **Box 7-4**).

With fewer restrictions, quasi-experimental design is mainly used in applied research, for example, community-based participatory research, rather than true experimental design. A few of the limitations of quasi-experimental design are that it cannot determine cause-and-effect relationships and cannot exclude *all* the reasons why a relationship does exist, including the lack of definitive causal inference and possible confounding bias caused by the dissimilarity among groups.[8]

Nonexperimental Design

Nonexperimental design is the most common design and involves variables that are not manipulated. Nonexperimental variables are not manipulated because they involve a single attribute such as gender, socioeconomic status, learning style, or any other personal characteristic that cannot be reasonably changed by the investigators. A single attribute can also be built of multidimensional events. For example, the single topic of "patient flow in the clinic" is multidimensional from entry to exit, but remains a single idea. Another example would involve one survey related to the single topic of depression, but the survey is composed of 35 questions. The last example would be the single topic of the median income of the U.S. population over the last 20 years. The topic remains a single attribute, but the investigator reviews numerous entries of previously collected data in the U.S. census. Unlike true and quasi-experimental research, nonexperimental research involves (1) no cause-and-effect conclusions caused by alternative explanations, (2) no manipulation of the independent variable, and (3) no random assignment of participants. This type of design uses mostly descriptive statistical analysis. For example, if evaluators were hired by the hospital administrator to evaluate the job satisfaction of nursing staff in the three critical care units, the evaluators would conduct a nonexperimental design including (1) a one-time job satisfaction survey among the currently employed nursing staff; (2) a review of employment records to explore the differences between the nurses currently

BOX 7-4

Sample of a Quasi-Experimental Design

Research question: The evaluators are implementing and evaluating a new post–myocardial infarction regimen program at Mountainside Hospital, so a quasi-experimental design was chosen. Over the next nine months, all post–myocardial infarction patients were invited to join the study. If they agreed, they signed the informed consent documents. Because of the number of myocardial infarction patients, evaluators decided it would be most effective to enroll patients in one of three different intervention groups: Group One, patients recovering from myocardial infarction in January, February, and March; Group Two, patients recovering from myocardial infarction in April, May, and June; or Group Three, patients recovering from myocardial infarction in July, August, and September. Evaluators made the assumption that the patients recovering in each group have approximately the same demographic variables given the overall demographic characteristics for all patients receiving care at Mountainside Hospital.

Group One: In January, February, and March at Mountainside Hospital, all myocardial infarction patients between 60 and 70 years of age receive one hour of health education related to their medication adherence regimen plus four weeks of cardiac nutrition counseling and cardiovascular exercise instruction. Group Two: In April, May, and June at Mountainside Hospital, all myocardial infarction patients between 60 and 70 years of age receive one hour of health education related to their medication regimen plus two weeks of cardiac nutrition counseling and cardiovascular exercise instruction. Group Three: In July, August, and September at Mountainside Hospital, all myocardial infarction patients between 60 and 70 years of age receive the hospital's standard of care—one hour with the health educator to answer questions about diet and medication and two weeks of cardiovascular exercise instruction.

Following group interventions, evaluators collect data from the medical charts of the participating patients to determine three-month, six-month, and nine-month recovery status. The medical chart review and data collection continued until the Group Three patients were nine months post-intervention. Following the data analyses, evaluators would recommend the type of intervention that yielded the best recovery results for the post–myocardial infarction patients.

working in the critical care units and the nurses who left the critical care units, such as ascertaining the average length of time working in the critical care units prior to leaving, the type of shifts (12 hour, 10 hour, 8 hour), education background, and years and type of nursing experience; and (3) an assessment of nurses leaving the critical care units but remaining employed at the hospital and moving to different units versus resigning from the hospital. These data reveal critical care nursing job satisfaction using a nonexperimental design. However, it is noted that nonexperimental design does not assess cause-and-effect relationships, but rather focuses on descriptive data, considers alternative explanations, and poses conclusions without causal relationships.[9]

Summary

This chapter focuses on an introduction to quantitative data methods and design. As discussed, quantitative research and evaluations use numerical data to answer specific research questions or evaluation objectives and is analyzed using statistics. The discussion moved to defining various research designs including true experimental, quasi-experimental, and nonexperimental design. It is important to remember that the purpose of the research or goals of the evaluation direct the design.

Case Study

Research Question

At North Central University, researchers are conducting a study to determine which of the following three interventions is best at lowering hypertension: Group One receives Drug A (standard of care), Group Two receives Drug A (standard of care) and must self-report walking two miles three times per week, and Group Three receives Drug A (standard of care) and must self-report 30 minutes of yoga practice three times per week. Individuals in all three groups are encouraged to maintain their usual exercise routine and only add walking or yoga per their random assignments.

continues

CASE STUDY *continued*

Operational Definitions

For this study, *hypertension* is defined as a clinical blood pressure reading of 140/90 mm Hg or higher during one clinic visit. Blood pressure is taken three times per visit (beginning, middle, and end) to verify blood pressure readings. The individual may not be taking any hypertension medication at the time of study recruitment.

For this study, a *patient* is defined as any adult between 45 and 60 years of age, employed 40 hours per week at North Central University. All participating patients have the same health insurance plan offered by the university.

Recruitment

Patients are recruited from two university-based clinics located on the main university campus and the midtown university campus. A total of 300 patients will be recruited over a six-month period from April through September. To receive the monthly $25 incentive (total $150), during the first week of each month, individuals stop by the clinic to turn in their completed exercise log sheets and have their blood pressure taken by the clinic nurse.

Study Design

True experimental design is used for this study, because researchers have a control group (Drug A only) and two intervention groups: Drug A and walking intervention, and Drug A and yoga intervention. The independent variable is exercise, and the dependent variable is blood pressure reading. For six months, each study participant stops by the clinic during the first week of each month to receive the $25 incentive, have their blood pressure taken three times, turn in their medication and exercise log sheets, and receive the month supply of medication.

Random Group Assignment

This study is double-blinded, so neither the healthcare providers nor the patients know if the participating individuals are receiving identical

continues

CASE STUDY *continued*

medications or not or what types of exercise interventions they complete. An outside researcher meets with each individual with a hypertension diagnosis to explain the study, obtain the signed informed consent documents, and, lastly, ask the individual to select a sealed envelope. The researcher opens the sealed envelope, and based on the code, the individual receives a packet of information for Group One, Two, or Three. The outside researcher explains the medication regimen of one tablet taken each morning with food and the exercise log sheets for the participant to record her usual lifestyle routine. If the individual is randomized to Group Two, the packet contains information about walking two miles, three times per week, in addition to his usual routine. If the individual is randomized to Group Three, the packet contains information on viewing yoga on a free website and a yoga DVD for those individuals with a DVD player. If the person does not have computer access or a DVD player, the outside researcher provides portable DVD player.

Data Collection

At the end of the six months of data collection, the researchers will conduct a medical chart review for all participating individuals. The variables include gender, age, baseline blood pressure, monthly blood pressure readings, exercise log sheets, and medication log sheets.

Case Study Discussion Questions

1. What are the possible limitations of this study?
2. How could the study be improved?
3. What are the possible ethical issues?

Student Activity

Read online the following peer-reviewed abstract summaries and answer the questions that follow.

Case Study 1

Robitaille Y, Fournier M, Laforest S, Gauvin L, Filiatrault J, Corriveau H. Effect of a fall prevention program on balance maintenance using a quasi-experimental design in real-world settings. *J Aging Health*. 2012;24(5):827–845. doi: 10.1177/0898264312436713

http://www.ncbi.nlm.nih.gov/pubmed/22422760

Questions

1. Is this basic or applied research?
2. How were participants assigned?
3. What kind of research design did this study use?
4. How many observations were there?
5. What was the independent variable(s)?
6. What was the dependent variable(s)?
7. What are some variables that should be controlled by researchers?
8. What is one possible confounding variable?
9. What could be one possible mediating variable?

Answers

1. Applied. Because they are working in a real-world setting and not in a laboratory, these researchers want to know if a real health program has real effects in a real setting, with people who have a real need.
2. Ten organizations were assigned to receive the program (the experiment) and seven organizations did not receive the program (control) in the first year but would receive it after the study was over.
3. Quasi-experimental design. Subjects were assigned to an experiment but were not randomized into either the experimental or control groups.
4. There were four observations. There was a pretest, a posttest, and two follow-up tests.
5. The Stand Up! program.
6. Balance performance tests and the incidence of self-reported falls.
7. Researchers should be aware of participants' age, sex, education, current frequency of physical activity, and current health information, as they could all possibly affect the outcome of the study. For example, if the intervention group happens to have younger, more active seniors and the control group happens to have seniors with more serious health problems

that affect balance, it may be those factors that affect balance more than the intervention unless they are controlled for in statistical analysis.

8. One possible confounding variable would be the number of people who dropped out of the study. If they left the study because they experienced a fall and hurt themselves, this would have an effect on whether the program was successful, and not just whether people randomly did not complete it. Researchers should always investigate why some people finish interventions and why others do not, to see if the reason they did not would have an effect of the efficacy of the program.

9. Some participants were very excited about the program. Therefore, it is possible that they were very motivated to integrate physical activity into their lifestyle, which had an outcome on intervention.

Case Study 2

Turk V, Khattran S, Kerry S, Corney R, Painter K. Reporting of health problems and pain by adults with an intellectual disability and by their carers. *J Appl Res Intellect Disabil.* 2012;25:155–165. doi: 10.1111/j.1468-3148.2011.00642.x http://www.ncbi.nlm.nih.gov/pubmed/22473967

Questions

1. Is this basic or applied research?
2. How were participants assigned?
3. What kind of research design did this study use?
4. How many observations were there?
5. What were the independent and dependent variables?

Answers

1. Both. This study wanted to simply find out if people with intellectual disabilities reported their health problems differently than their caretakers. However, there are practical applications that could help caretakers better understand the needs of their charges and be more responsive to them.
2. All people who were listed on the learning disability register were eligible for the study as long as their physicians agreed to it.
3. Nonexperimental design. Random assignment was not used in this study, nor was there a control group used for comparison.

4. Even though participants were not interviewed multiple times, there were still multiple observations because several different measures were taken. This is called *triangulation*.

5. There were no independent or dependent variables because no characteristic was being manipulated. This was an exploratory study that looked at different reporting practices among people with intellectual disabilities and their caretakers. If a training intervention was given to one group of caretakers on recognizing health problems and not given to another, then the intervention would be the independent variable, and differences in reported health problems would be the dependent variable.

Case Study 3

Long JA, Jahnle EC, Richardson DM, Loewenstein G, Volpp KG. Peer mentoring and financial incentives to improve glucose control in African American veterans. *Ann Intern Med.* 2012;156:416–424. doi: 10.7326/0003-4819-156-6-201203200-00004
http://www.ncbi.nlm.nih.gov/pubmed/22431674?dopt=Abstract

Questions

1. What was the research question of this study?
2. Was this basic or applied research?
3. How were participants assigned?
4. What kind of research design was this?
5. How many observations were there?
6. What was the independent variable(s)?
7. What was the dependent variable(s)?
8. Were there controlled variables?

Answers

1. Does a peer mentoring or financial incentive lower blood glucose levels among patients with diabetes better than care as usual?
2. Applied. Researchers wanted to know which kind of care helped patients with diabetes lower their blood glucose best.
3. Randomly. Neither the study researchers nor the VA lab staff knew who was in which group.
4. True experimental design. This was a randomized controlled trial, the gold standard of research.

5. Many. There was a pretest and a posttest that looked at blood glucose levels. Additionally, patients were surveyed monthly on whether they had experienced any diabetes symptoms.

6. Peer mentoring or financial incentive group assignment was the independent variable.

7. Blood glucose level at the end of the study was the dependent variable.

8. Yes: all participants were male, of the same age group, and African American. This reduced the likelihood that any difference in the outcomes was confounded by differences in gender, age, or race. Furthermore, in the peer mentoring group, all mentors were of similar gender, age, and racial background, limiting the likelihood that differences between groups were caused by confounding variables.

Case Study 4

Craciun C, Schuz N, Lippke S, Schwarzer R. Facilitating sunscreen use in women by a theory-based online intervention: A randomized controlled trial. *J Health Psychol.* 2012;17:207–216. doi: 10.1177/1359105311414955 http://www.ncbi.nlm.nih.gov/pubmed/21752862

Questions

1. What was the research question of this study?
2. Was this basic or applied research?
3. How were participants assigned?
4. What kind of research design was this?
5. How many observations were there?
6. What was the independent variable(s)?
7. What was the dependent variable(s)?
8. Were there controlled variables?
9. What are some possible confounding variables?
10. What is one mediating variable?

Answers

1. Does a difference in the type of sunscreen promotion affect actual sunscreen use?
2. Applied. Researchers want to know if an intervention will affect the real-world sunscreen use of individuals.

3. Randomly. The computer randomly assigned individuals to different groups upon log-in to the study website. Neither the investigator nor the study participants knew who would be assigned to what intervention.

4. True experimental design. Because there was random assignment to groups with a manipulated characteristic, this study was a true experiment.

5. Three. This study had multiple observations; there was a pretest and two follow-up surveys.

6. The independent variable in this study was the type of sunscreen promotion used.

7. The dependent variable in this study was sunscreen usage.

8. The only controlled variable in this study was gender, as all participants were women. Therefore, if there were differences in the three different groups, they were not because of gender.

9. There are several possible confounding variables. First, participants were recruited from a number of websites, including university websites and blogs. There could be differences in the knowledge about sun exposure risks among these women based on educational differences. Secondly, women were recruited from different countries. There is no way of knowing if differences between the interventions were because of cultural differences. Finally, there was a wide range of ages in this study (18 to 66 years of age). The researchers did not discuss whether perhaps an older participant would be more likely than a younger person to use sunscreen after learning about the risks and benefits.

10. The mediating variable in this research study was planning a sunscreen strategy. Both interventions were given motivational information. However, the added step of creating a plan to use sunscreen resulted in better future use.

References

1. California State University-Fresno. Basic vs. Applied Research. Research Methods by Dummies. Available at: http://psych.csufresno.edu/psy144/Content/Design/Types/appliedvsbasic.html. Accessed May 3, 2012.

2. Hale J. Understanding Research Methodology 5: Applied and Basic Research. Psych Central. Available at: http://psychcentral.com/blog/archives/2011/05/12/understanding-research-methodology-5-applied-and-basic-research/. Accessed on September 15, 2013.

3. Trochim M. Construct Validity. Research Methods Knowledge Base. Available at: http://www.socialresearchmethods.net/kb/constval.php. Last updated October 20, 2012. Accessed May 3, 2012.

4. Humes KR, Jones NA, Ramirez RR. Overview of Race and Hispanic Origin: 2010. The United States Census Bureau. Available at: http://www.census.gov/prod/cen2010/briefs/c2010br-02.pdf. Published March 2011. Accessed May 3, 2012.

5. Trochim M. Types of Designs. Research Methods Knowledge Base. Available at: http://www.socialresearchmethods.net/kb/destypes.php. Last updated on October 20, 2012. Accessed May 3, 2012.

6. Colorado State University. Differences Between Experimental and Quasi-Experimental Research. Available at: http://writing.colostate.edu/guides/research/experiment/pop3e.cfm. Accessed May 3, 2012.

7. Gribbons B, Herman J. True and quasi-experimental designs. *Practical Assessment, Research & Evaluation.* 1997;5(14). http://PAREonline.net/getvn.asp?v=5&n=14. Accessed March 12, 2012.

8. Shadish WR, Cook TD, Campbell DT. *Experimental and Quasi-Experimental Designs for Generalized Causal Inference.* New York, NY: Houghton Mifflin Company; 2002.

9. Crosby RS, DiClemente RJ, Salazar LF. *Research Methods in Health Promotion.* San Francisco, CA: Jossey-Bass; 2006:96–97.

CHAPTER 8

Surveys

CHAPTER OBJECTIVES

By the end of this chapter, students will be able to:

- Analyze the advantages and disadvantages of utilizing an existing survey or developing a new one to address research questions
- Compare and contrast the techniques used for online, mailed, and in-person surveys
- Describe and give examples of the various types of surveys
- Evaluate surveys for possible cultural and diversity issues

KEY TERMS

Achievement tests	Pretest
Aptitude tests	Readability score
Likert scales	Semantic differential scales
Performance tests	Subscales
Pilot test	

Introduction

This chapter introduces survey selection, survey data collection, and types of surveys, as well as the differences among tests, inventories, and scales. Following the quantitative data survey discussion, the chapter moves to qualitative observational research methods and includes a consideration of ethical issues. The chapter ends with an exploration of cultural and diversity issues related to survey design. Lastly, reliability and validity are presented in terms of survey development.

Survey Selection

Let's begin by discussing the differences between selecting an existing survey versus creating a new survey. When investigators determine that they will use a survey for data collection, they can use an existing survey or develop a new survey. It is useful to understand the advantages and disadvantages of using an existing survey (see **Table 8-1**).

If the decision is made to use an existing survey, then the investigator needs to know where to find an existing survey that meets the study. See **Table 8-2** for examples of where to locate a variety of existing surveys.

As with existing surveys, there are advantages and disadvantages to creating surveys. The major advantage is that survey questions created by the research team may more closely answer research questions better than preexisting surveys. Other advantages include the ability to control survey length and literacy level. Disadvantages include the need to conduct several time-consuming pilot tests and revisions to establish reliability and validity and the high cost of development. After considering the advantages and disadvantages of using existing surveys or creating an original survey, some investigators decide to use a

---

Table 8-1   Advantages and Disadvantages of Using Existing Surveys

Advantages	Disadvantages
Saves time	Costly if purchase is required
Saves money if available through open access	Trying to use with a different sample (e.g., adolescents instead of adults)
Pilot tested and revised	Questions do not exactly match research questions
Established reliability	Extraneous questions add length to survey
Established validity	Health literacy is too high or low for population
Previously used in at least one study	Investigator does not have the statistical skills to perform data analysis required; costly to hire statistician
Established data analysis methodology	Must establish data analysis methodology

Table 8-2 Examples of Existing Surveys

Books of surveys	The *Mental Measurements Yearbook*.[1] A valuable resource, the *Mental Measurements Yearbook* is published annually and provides extensive information about numerous existing surveys (e.g., survey questions, reliability, validity, methodology for data analysis, published studies that previously used the survey, how to gain permission to use the survey, and, if applicable, the cost). Some scales have several different subscales. A scale measures and categorizes a variable. A subscale is just a smaller portion of a larger scale. For example, the Youth Risk Behavior Surveillance System (YRBSS) measures several different risk behaviors among youth, including smoking, drinking, drug use, and sexual activity.[2] All of the questions that correspond to a different risk behavior are subscales of the larger YRBSS measure. If investigators use a survey with multiple subscales, they must verify with survey authors whether reliability and validity were established for each subscale or only for the entire survey. If reliability and validity were established for the entire survey, then investigators selecting to use only one subscale need to establish reliability and validity for that one subscale. Some survey questions are available for free, but the score sheets that they use or data analysis that it requires is expensive. Other surveys are completely free.
Publications	While conducting the literature review, investigators review which studies are published on the same topic. Within publications, authors refer to the survey they used for the study. Investigators may decide to use the same study based on their research questions or evaluation objectives and the information provided in the journal article. If the survey is not shown as an appendix to the publication, then investigators contact the authors for more information about how to obtain the survey.
Government websites	The Centers for Disease Control and Prevention offers a variety of surveys that are available at no cost. Many of the surveys that are available through the government have been widely used and have been proven valid and reliable.
	Behavioral Risk Factor Surveillance System (BRFSS) is the world's largest ongoing telephone health survey system. This survey tracks health conditions, risk factors, and health behaviors. The 2011 version can be found at http://www.cdc.gov/brfss/questionnaires/pdf-ques/2011brfss.pdf.
	Measuring Intimate Partner Violence and Victimization and Perpetration is a set of surveys that measure partner violence on 20 different variables. It can be found at http://www.cdc.gov/ncipc/pub-res/IPV_Compendium.pdf.
	Measuring Bullying, Victimization, Perpetration and Bystander Experiences, a growing public health concern, this is set of surveys that measures a range of bullying and intimidation behaviors and can be found at http://www.cdc.gov/ViolencePrevention/pdf/BullyCompendium-a.pdf.
	The YRBSS is a survey similar to the BRFSS survey. The YRBSS measures many different risk behaviors among youth, including smoking, drinking, drug use, and sexual activity. The YRBSS has been used since the 1990s and provides trend data over time among the U.S. youth population. It can be found at http://www.cdc.gov/healthyyouth/yrbs/questionnaire_rationale.htm.

combination—an existing survey to answer a few research questions and creating questions to answer the remaining research questions.

Creating a Survey

This section provides an overview of survey development. Although the steps described are straightforward, new investigators soon realize that each step involves numerous smaller steps to complete the task. The time spent in meticulous survey development is rewarded in high-quality results. Results are only as good as the survey.

Steps to create a survey:

Step 1:   Review the research questions with other research team members. Have each team member write, on 3×5 cards, possible survey questions that answer research questions. For example, if there are four research questions, researchers label one card "Research Question 1," then write a survey question pertaining to the first research question. After all the possible survey questions are written, the cards are sorted into piles—one for each research question. At this point, researchers review and edit the survey questions written for Research Question 1. Keep asking each other, "How does this question answer the research question?" Review and edit again until everyone agrees that each survey question addresses the overall objective of Research Question 1. Repeat this process for each research question. Create the first draft of the survey from the selected questions.

Step 2:   Ask only survey questions that answer the research questions. Extra questions increase survey length and time required for respondents to complete the survey. Long surveys lead to respondent fatigue, which increases the possibility of inaccurate data.

Step 3:   Organize survey questions from easy to difficult. The first question should be nonthreatening, such as "How would you describe your health status today? (1) Excellent, (2) Very good, (3) Good, (4) Fair, (5) Poor." Leave plenty of white spaces, such as wide margins and space between questions, so that the survey is appealing. Dense text is intimidating and confusing.

Step 4:   Write questions in a simple and concise manner. Use a vertical or horizontal format throughout the survey. Ensure that the choices are distributed evenly. For example, uneven choices are (1) Good (2) Fair (3) Poor (4) Very Poor; these choices begin near the middle of the scale without listing Excellent and Very Good. If open-ended questions are used, limit the space on paper surveys or limit the number of characters in textboxes for online surveys. Avoid asking double questions. For example, "How satisfied are you with the level of medical and nursing care at this clinic?" or "Do you like swimming or surfing?" These questions should be two separate questions to lessen confusion. Suppose the survey respondent liked swimming very much, but did not enjoy surfing. How would he answer this question?

Step 5: Group similar questions. For example, all food intake questions are grouped together, and all exercise questions are grouped together. Questions about sensitive issues (e.g., sexual behaviors, substance abuse, or other personal behaviors) are placed in the middle of the survey. Keep in mind that with long surveys, respondents get fatigued. Questions near the end may not receive the same attention from respondents. Place demographic questions at the end of the survey.

Step 6: Avoid skip patterns. Skip patterns on paper-and-pencil surveys are confusing. For example, "If you answer Yes to Question 16, then skip forward to Question 22." Such skip patterns lead to inaccurate responses and missing data. However, if a survey is administered online, skip patterns are invisible because the respondent does not realized they are being skipped based on an answer that they provided.

Step 7: Provide clear instructions for each transition. For example, if questions in one section use a four-point Likert scale about quality of life and the next section is about exercise, then new instructions are needed. (For example, "The next six questions are about your exercise habits. Please select the response that best describes your behavior.")

Step 8: Check the readability score. Most word processing software programs offer the ability to calculate readability scores. Generally, readability scores of seventh- to eighth-grade reading levels are acceptable for adults. Lower reading levels are recommended for surveys completed by adolescents or adults with low literacy levels. A simple rule to remember: Avoid words with three or more syllables. For example, "cardiac symptoms" becomes "chest pain"; "daily medication" becomes "pills taken every day."

Step 9: Proofread the survey several times. Ask colleagues who are not involved in the survey development to proofread it. Remember that spell-check software only recognizes spelling errors, not inappropriate words. For example, "public" and "pubic" are both spelled correctly, but the letter "L" changes the meaning dramatically.

Step 10: Pretest the survey. For example, researchers ask colleagues and students to review the survey and offer suggestions. From these comments, the survey is revised. A pretest differs from a pilot test in that a pretest is not asking individuals from the target population to complete the survey.

Step 11: Pilot test the survey. Recruit 10–20 individuals similar to the target population to complete the survey. Respondents provide feedback to researchers either as a group or individually. Revise the survey based on their comments. A pilot test can also serve as the first step in establishing reliability. By testing and then retesting the same audience, researchers calculate the consistency of the survey. In other words, did the respondents select the same choices for each question on the first and second administration of the survey? If necessary, researchers repeat pilot tests.

Step 12: Finalize the survey format.

Although survey development is time consuming, if done correctly well-designed surveys become valuable tools of research and yield data for addressing research questions. After data are collected, investigators establish methodology for data analysis including reliability, validity, cut-scores (which are discussed later in the chapter), and trends across samples from various target populations.[3,4]

After the survey question format is complete, investigators write a cover letter to potential participants that includes a description of incentives. A short cover letter or opening statement on the computer screen entices the potential respondent and describes the purpose of the research or evaluation. The remaining portion of the letter states how long the survey takes to complete, potential benefits for participation (e.g., gift cards or incentives), and how responses are kept confidential.[4] Keep in mind that investigators are not present when a potential respondent opens the envelope or clicks on the emailed link, so the introduction needs to be concise and easy to read in a few seconds (see **Box 8-1**).

BOX 8-1

Example of a Cover Letter

Name of Company or University
on Official Letterhead

Date

Dear Participant:

You are being invited to participate in a research study called **<insert name of study>**. The study is being conducted by **<researcher's name>** of **<insert institution, company, or university>**. The purpose of this study is to **<insert study purpose>**.

You are being invited to participate in this research study by **<insert survey method (e.g., completing the attached surveys or completing the online survey)>**. This survey has been approved by the institutional review board of **<insert institution name>**. The following questionnaire will require approximately **<insert amount of time>** to complete, and there is no known risk. For completing this survey, you are eligible for **<insert compensation stipulations>**. Although you may not experience any benefits directly, information collected in this study may benefit **<insert possible benefactors**

continues

BOX 8-1 *continued*

(e.g., a certain profession or a certain population)> in the future by better understanding **<insert general purpose>**.

This survey collects no identifying information of any respondent, and responses are anonymous. In order to ensure that all information will remain confidential, please *do not* include your name. Copies of the project will be provided to **<insert appropriate information if applicable>**. If you choose to participate in this project, please answer all questions as honestly as possible and return the completed questionnaires promptly by **<insert method of return, such as interoffice mail, drop box location, or provided stamped envelope>**. Participation is strictly voluntary, and you may refuse to participate at any time.

Completion and return of the questionnaire will indicate your willingness to participate in this study. If you have any questions concerning your rights as a research participant, please contact **<insert IRB name>** at **<insert contact information>**. If you require any additional information or have questions, please contact **<insert researcher's name>** at the number listed below.

Your participation is appreciated.

<Researcher's name>
<Phone number and email address>
<Company/institution name and/or email address>

The closing statement thanks respondents for their participation, describes how incentives are retrieved (if applicable), and reassures them of the confidentiality of their responses. As previously mentioned, researchers need to remember the audience (e.g., age, gender, reading level) when composing the cover letter and closing statement. The appropriateness of incentives is important to entice potential respondents. Gift cards to national discount stores are appreciated by any respondent. If the survey is collected in specific zip codes, such as the catchment area of a clinic, verify that the national discount store is close to the clinic. Lastly, the value of incentives should be appropriate for time and effort. For example, a 25-question survey offers a $5 gift card, whereas a $50 gift card is appropriate for a 90-minute interview.[4]

Survey Data Collection

Whether the survey is conducted online, in person, or by mail, there are some common procedures used with all three methods of survey data collection.

Step 1:   After developing the research questions or evaluation objectives and obtaining approval from the IRB for human subject research, investigators determine which survey data collection technique is appropriate.

Step 2:   It is necessary to obtain access to the sample regardless of the survey data collection choice. First, for mailed surveys, investigators must acquire the addresses, either email or postal, to send the survey. There are several ways to obtain such postal addresses, including purchasing address lists from clearinghouse vendors or from professional organizations. As for email addresses, investigators can contact professional organizations. If the evaluation or research is related to the mission of the professional organization, then email lists may be available for free or, in some cases, for purchase. If investigators wish to email employees or students within a university or organization, then they contact administration for ways to send emails to the entire population of the organization. Second, if investigators wish to conduct in-person surveys, they obtain names and contact information through key informants or snowball techniques. Key informants are individuals known to investigators as being experts in a specific discipline. For example, investigators request to conduct an in-person survey with nurses working in the trauma unit. Snowball techniques involve interviewing one person and then asking if they are willing to give you the name of another person who might be interested in participating in the in-person survey. For example, investigators conduct an in-person survey with a woman who is a breast cancer survivor. Upon completion of the survey, the investigator asks her if she knows another woman who survived breast cancer and who might be willing to answer the same questions. One individual connects to another, and so on. The snowball technique has potential ethical issues if the first individual provides names and contact information without seeking permission from the referred individual.

Step 3:   For in-person data collection, investigators schedule appointments at the convenience of the respondents. If investigators are using online or mailed surveys, they notify the potential respondents that they will be receiving a survey in a few days. According to Dillman, Smyth, and Christian,[5] there are ideally seven days between each segment of the survey data collection. For example, there are seven days between the introduction notification and the receipt of the survey. It is also recommended that online or mailed surveys arrive near the end of the week, when respondents are wrapping up their email or postal mail for the week.

Step 4: Surveys are received by potential respondents seven days after the introduction notification. Mailed surveys are sent with a self-addressed stamped envelope (SASE), and the return address is also written on the survey in case the survey and SASE get separated.

Step 5: Seven days after surveys are received, investigators send (email or postal) a thank you or reminder. If postal mail is used, the thank you or reminder is a postcard. The message is simple: "Thank you for responding to the <title of study> survey that was sent to you last Friday. If you have not had a chance to return it, please do so at your earliest convenience," then signed by the principal investigator.

Step 6: Seven days after the thank you/reminder email or postcard, investigators send a second survey. If postal mail is used, the second survey includes a SASE for return mail.[5]

There are advantages and disadvantages to each of the three (online, mailed, or in-person) survey data collection methods (see **Table 8-3**).

Table 8-3 Advantages and Disadvantages of Online, Mailed, and In-Person Surveys

	Advantages	Disadvantages
Online surveys	Fast way to collect data; inexpensive if email address lists are available for no cost; high number of potential respondents	Impersonal; no way of knowing who completed survey; no way for respondent to obtain clarification on any specific survey questions; no tracking system; no verifiable demographic information on respondents (i.e., not certain if respondent is providing accurate information); unable to predict number of respondents; difficult to receive email addresses for target population; expensive to purchase email addresses
Mailed surveys	Fast way to collect data; tracking system established by matching each survey	Impersonal; no way of knowing who completed survey; no way for respondent to obtain clarification on any specific survey questions; no tracking system; no verifiable demographic information on respondents; unable to predict number of respondents; difficult to receive mailing addresses for target population; expensive to purchase mailing addresses
In-person surveys	Able to clarify questions during survey interview; verify person responding to questions; in-depth information collected	Potentially difficult to recruit participants; expensive; time intensive; data entry is time consuming

Types of Surveys

Tests

Tests are defined as "a set of stimuli presented to an individual in order to elicit responses on the basis of which a numerical score can be assigned."[6] Let's look at each segment of the definition:

> *Set of stimuli:* This set may be written questions on a test (e.g., the American College Testing [ACT] examination); a demonstration of a specific skill, such as each step required to establish an intravenous catheter; an ophthalmic examination to determine visual acuity; or a verbal conversation assessment to verify proficiency in another language.
>
> *Elicit responses:* Responses are verbal, written, or kinetic as in a demonstration of a skill set.
>
> *Assigned numerical score:* Test results are recorded as a standardized number so each individual is assessed using the same criteria.

The following discussion explores three types of tests: achievement, performance, and aptitude.

Achievement Tests

Achievement tests measure the mastery, comprehension, or proficiency of acquired skills by individuals. These tests compare one group of individuals to another group. There are two ways to interpret achievement tests: norm-referenced tests and criterion-referenced tests. Norm-referenced tests compare the test scores of each individual to the test scores of other individuals. For example, the Florida Comprehensive Assessment Test (FCAT) measures knowledge in different areas of education in elementary, middle, and high school.[7] The FCAT allows investigators to calculate the mean or average scores of individuals for each grade level and subject area for all Florida public school students. The mean score becomes the norm by which all schools are compared. By using the norm for comparison, schools and students are ranked at various levels of achievement. In Florida, state funding is allocated by comparing the normative scores to each school. In norm-referenced tests, it is important that the difficulty of each question is close to equal, so the overall test yields consistent results (reliability) and measures what the test claims to measure (validity).[6] A second example is the Medical College Admission Test (MCAT). Investigators calculate the mean or average score for the MCAT nationwide. This mean score becomes the norm by which all colleges and universities compare their premed students' scores. Students are ranked, compared to the norm, at various levels of achievement. Medical school admission committees rank the applicants by comparing their scores to the norm of all students who took the MCAT that year.

Criterion-referenced tests do not compare individuals, but rather describe the performance of one individual based on a set of criterion or level of mastery. In criterion-referenced tests, there is a predetermined required level of mastery used to assess the performance of each individual. For example, a state requires that all first-time drivers score a minimum of 70% on the written driver's license examination. However, even though an individual passes the written driving test, there is no evidence that this individual knows how to drive a car.

Performance Tests

Performance tests measure what an individual can do rather than what an individual knows. Using the driving test example previously discussed, the achievement test determines that an individual knows the state laws pertaining to driving, but the performance test measures an individual's skill at actually operating a vehicle. When investigators construct performance tests, they develop a checklist of skills that are assessed by individual performance. Performance testing has advantages because this type of testing cannot be assessed with paper-and-pencil examinations; however, the disadvantage is that performance testing is time consuming and expensive, and scoring is more subject to error or bias of the grader.[6]

Aptitude Tests

Aptitude tests measure general ability and knowledge, whereas achievement tests focus on specific subjects. It is easier to remember the difference by thinking that aptitude tests measure previously acquired knowledge. However, aptitude tests are not a measure of intelligence. Investigators frequently use aptitude tests to predict future success. For example, the Graduate Record Examination (GRE) measures verbal reasoning, quantitative reasoning, and analytical writing skills acquired over a long period of time, but that can be related to any particular discipline.[8] The GRE measures general knowledge, but it is also used as a predictor of success in graduate school. Most universities use the GRE as one component of the graduate school admissions process along with the undergraduate grade point average, letters of recommendation, and personal statement.

Test performance range refers to the fluctuations in acceptable scores. Individuals in the healthcare field are familiar with this concept. Most laboratory test results show a range of normal that is frequently termed *within normal limits*. For example, the normal lab values range for hematocrit (the percentage of red blood cells in the blood) is 36.1–44.3% for females and 40.7–50.3% for males.[9] The same concept is true for other types of testing. All students know that their performance in a course determines their final grade. However, although students receive a wide range of scores, instructors determine the range of acceptable final scores needed to pass the course.

Personality Inventories

Personality inventories assess certain patterns or trends. For example, the Myers-Briggs explores individuals' personality types and cognitive styles.[10] When investigators select personality inventories, they should pay special attention to validity and reliability. For example, some inventories only measure one personality trait (e.g., having an introverted or extroverted personality), whereas others are more comprehensive but limited in other ways. Generally, investigators administer several personality inventories to determine trends. Administering several inventories strengthens the final inclination or tendency, even if several of the personality inventories have a moderately weak validity. For example, in a criminal court case, investigators administer multiple personality inventories along with interviews to assist in the determination of whether a person is mentally fit to stand trial.

Scales

There are two kinds of scales: response and concept. Response scales assign an answer to a single question.

"How do you feel today?"

1. Excellent
2. Very good
3. Good
4. Fair
5. Poor

On the other hand, a concept scale is a collection of questions that measure a single subject or concept (e.g., self-esteem), whereas other scales measure several subjects. Single-dimension scales are like a number line. If self-esteem is measured, individuals respond to a series of questions related to the one topic. The responses from all questions are combined, so investigators have one score for self-esteem. In the case of multiple subjects, investigators select a scale that measures two or more topics (e.g., relationships between depression and self-esteem).[11] For example, the GRE measures several skills at once (e.g., quantitative, verbal, critical thinking, grammar, and reading comprehension). The following discussion focuses on one-dimension scales including Likert, Thurstone, semantic differential, and knowledge, attitude, and behavior scales.

Likert Scales

In Likert scales, investigators may choose whether to have an even number of possible responses or an odd number of responses. This decision is based on the results of the pilot study and is different for each project. When an even number of responses are selected, the investigator forces the respondent to provide either a positive or a negative opinion, because the option "undecided" is removed. If the investigator selects an odd number of choices, the "undecided" response is available. In either case, each response choice is assigned a numerical value. It is typical that low numbers are assigned to low-level responses (e.g., *strongly disagree* = 1 and *strongly agree* = 5) for ease in understanding data results. Here are examples of each response option:

Rate your level of satisfaction regarding the care you received from your healthcare provider.

1. Very dissatisfied
2. Moderately dissatisfied
3. Dissatisfied
4. Undecided
5. Satisfied
6. Moderately satisfied
7. Very satisfied

Rate your level of satisfaction regarding the care you received from your healthcare provider.

1. Very dissatisfied
2. Dissatisfied
3. Undecided
4. Satisfied
5. Very satisfied

Rate your level of satisfaction regarding the care you received from your healthcare provider.

1. Very dissatisfied
2. Dissatisfied
3. Satisfied
4. Very satisfied

When researchers reverse the wording of the survey questions to vary the selection choices, it is called *item reversal*. In the data analysis, researchers must remember to reverse the coding scheme to achieve the correct results (see **Box 8-2**). Rosenberg's self-esteem scale illustrates a four-point Likert scale and reversal items.[12]

Lastly, Likert scale responses are summed to reach a final score for each responding individual. Researchers develop a cut-score for the scale, or use the cut-score provided for established Likert scales.[13] Think of cut-scores as final grades in a course. If there are 500 possible points in a course, students receiving between 500 and 450 receive an A, 449 to 400 receive a B, 399 to 350 receive a C, and so on. Cut-scores are the same, but related to specific topics. For example, patients diagnosed with fibromyalgia respond to a Likert scale survey related to their self-reported perceived daily degree of pain. Based on the summed scores of 10 questions, investigators determine the cut-scores: patients with a total score of 50 to 41 have severe pain, 40 to 31 have moderate pain, 30 to 21 have mild pain, and 20 to 0 have minimal pain. In this example, healthcare providers might use this type of Likert pain scale to more accurately treat patients with a chronic pain diagnosis. See Box 8-2 again. Note that Rosenberg's self-esteem scale does not offer a cut-score but rather merely states that the higher the score, the higher the respondent's self-esteem.

If investigators decide to create an original Likert scale rather than use an existing scale, it is advisable to seek resources outside this introductory text. The following description provides a brief overview of how scales are developed. Given that advice, the first step is to gather a group of experts to generate ideas related to the topic of interest. One method is to write each idea on a separate 3×5 card. After collecting at least 80 cards, the group sorts the ideas into piles for each subset subject area. From these piles, investigators begin to create survey questions. Once the survey is finalized and approved by the experts in the group, it is time to conduct a pre-pilot test on the survey. A pre-pilot test involves asking other experts to review the survey and provide comments. These comments could indicate that you have left out an important subject area or that something should be left out. Again, changes are made based on suggestions. The next step is to conduct a pilot test with a group of individuals similar to those individuals who would be recruited for the actual study. The pilot test does not include individuals from the actual study sample. It is common for investigators to employ statisticians as consultants to determine whether the survey questions measure what it is intended to measure or, in other words, whether the survey is valid. In the last step, investigators make final edits and then conduct the actual study using a Likert scale.

BOX 8-2

Rosenberg's Self-Esteem Scale

The scale is a 10-item Likert questionnaire with items answered on a 4-point scale ranging from strongly agree to strongly disagree. The original sample for which the scale was developed consisted of 5,024 high school juniors and seniors from 10 randomly selected schools in New York State.

Instructions: Below is a list of statements dealing with your general feelings about yourself. If you strongly agree, circle **SA**. If you agree with the statement, circle **A**. If you disagree, circle **D**. If you strongly disagree, circle **SD**.

1.	On the whole, I am satisfied with myself.	SA	A	D	SD
2.*	At times, I think I am no good at all.	SA	A	D	SD
3.	I feel that I have a number of good qualities.	SA	A	D	SD
4.	I am able to do things as well as most other people.	SA	A	D	SD
5.*	I feel I do not have much to be proud of.	SA	A	D	SD
6.*	I certainly feel useless at times.	SA	A	D	SD
7.	I feel that I'm a person of worth, at least on an equal plane with others.	SA	A	D	SD
8.*	I wish I could have more respect for myself.	SA	A	D	SD
9.*	All in all, I am inclined to feel that I am a failure.	SA	A	D	SD
10.	I take a positive attitude toward myself.	SA	A	D	SD

Scoring: SA = 3, A = 2, D = 1, SD = 0. Items with an asterisk are reverse scored; that is, SA = 0, A = 1, D = 2, SD = 3. Sum the scores for the 10 items. The higher the score, the higher the self-esteem. The scale may be used without explicit permission. The author's family, however, would like to be kept informed of its use:

The Morris Rosenberg Foundation
c/o Department of Sociology, Building 2112
University of Maryland
College Park, MD 20742-1315

Thurstone Scales

Thurstone scales are similar to Likert scales, because both ask respondents about their attitudes. However, Likert scales ask the degree of agreement, whereas Thurstone scales list statements and ask respondents to pick the statements that match their attitudes on the topic.[14] The following discussion presents how Thurston scales are developed.[6]

Step 1: A group of experts make lists of about 50 to 100 statements related to a broad topic (e.g., patients diagnosed as obese).

Step 2: The original list is given to another group of individuals with some knowledge of the broad topic, such as senior nursing students and fourth-year medical students. The student groups read each statement and label it as positive, neutral, or negative. They are not providing their opinion or attitude, but rather their perception of the statement (see **Table 8-4**).[15]

Step 3: For each statement, investigators create a table (see **Table 8-5**). Investigators calculate the middle (median) score for each statement. The median score falls in the middle, with 50% of scores above it and 50% below. Next investigators calculate the first quartile. The first quartile (Q1) is the value below which 25% of the cases fall and above which 75% of the cases fall—in other words, the 25th percentile. The median is the 50th percentile. The third quartile, Q3, is the 75th percentile. The interquartile range is the difference between third and first quartiles, or Q3 − Q1.

Step 4: Investigators select one statement for the median scores ranging from 1 to 11. Notice that in Table 8-5, not all 12 median scores are represented, but there is a representative sample of statements.

Table 8-4   Example of Statement Labels

Negative	• People diagnosed as being obese deserve their health problems. • Obesity controls the population by contributing to premature death. • I will never become obese.
Between negative and neutral	• I won't become obese if all my friends are not obese.
Neutral	• It's easy to become obese. • Because obesity is preventable, resources should focus on preventing instead of curing. • People who are obese are no different from other people I know.
Between neutral and positive	• People who are obese can still have a normal life.
Positive	• Obesity is a disease that anyone can get if they are not careful. • Obesity affects us all. • People diagnosed as obese should be treated just like everybody else.

Table 8-5 Sample of Thurstone Statements

Statement	Median	Quartile 1 (25% below and 75% above)	Quartile 3 (75% below and 25% above)	Interquartile Range = Q3 – Q1
People diagnosed as being obese deserve their health problems.	1	1	2	1
Obesity controls the population by contributing to premature death.	2	1	2.5	1.5
I will never become obese.	3	1.5	5	3.5
I won't become obese if all my friends are not obese.	4	2	4.5	2.5
It's easy to become obese.	5	4	6.5	2.5
Because obesity is preventable, resources should focus on preventing instead of curing.	5	4	6	2
People who are obese are no different from other people I know.	6	5	9.75	4.75
People who are obese can still have a normal life.	8	5.5	11	5.5
Anyone can become obese.	9	5.5	10.5	5
Obesity is a disease that anyone can get if they are not careful.	9	6	10	4
Obesity affects us all.	10	7.5	11	3.5
People diagnosed as obese should be treated just like everybody else.	11	10	11	1

Step 5:   In Table 8-5, look at the statements with median scores of 5 and 9. If several statements have the same median score, researchers select the statement with the smallest interquartile range. The smallest interquartile range shows the least amount of variability among the students ranking the statements.[15] Once all statements are selected, investigators complete the final version of the Thurstone scale and pilot test the scale with a representative sample. As with Likert scales, after the pilot study is complete, a few revisions are made prior to the actual data collection.

Semantic Differential

Semantic differential scales measure an individual's attitude about a specific topic based on opposite adjectives. The middle of the scale is zero, and the ends of the scale are opposites. Some advantages of this scale are that it is simple to design, an inexpensive way to collect data, and easy to adapt to various uses with different age groups, cultures, and literacy levels.[16] As an example, if investigators wanted to know women's attitudes and knowledge about types of birth control, the semantic differential is shown in **Table 8-6**. Once individuals complete each

Table 8-6 Semantic Differential Scale: Attitudes and Knowledge about Birth Control Options

Daily Birth Control Pills

	5	4	3	2	1	0	1	2	3	4	5	
Inexpensive	5	4	3	2	1	0	1	2	3	4	5	Expensive
Inconvenient	5	4	3	2	1	0	1	2	3	4	5	Convenient
Requires clinic visit	5	4	3	2	1	0	1	2	3	4	5	Does not require clinic visit
Not for spontaneous sex	5	4	3	2	1	0	1	2	3	4	5	Good for spontaneous sex
Requires partner cooperation	5	4	3	2	1	0	1	2	3	4	5	Partner cooperation not required
Protects against sexually transmitted infections	5	4	3	2	1	0	1	2	3	4	5	Does not protect against sexually transmitted infections
Not very effective for protection against pregnancy	5	4	3	2	1	0	1	2	3	4	5	Very effective for protection against pregnancy

Long-Term Reversible Contraception (IUDs and Vaginal Rings)

	5	4	3	2	1	0	1	2	3	4	5	
Inexpensive	5	4	3	2	1	0	1	2	3	4	5	Expensive
Inconvenient	5	4	3	2	1	0	1	2	3	4	5	Convenient
Requires clinic visit	5	4	3	2	1	0	1	2	3	4	5	Does not require clinic visit
Not for spontaneous sex	5	4	3	2	1	0	1	2	3	4	5	Good for spontaneous sex
Requires partner cooperation	5	4	3	2	1	0	1	2	3	4	5	Partner cooperation not required
Protects against sexually transmitted infections	5	4	3	2	1	0	1	2	3	4	5	Does not protect against sexually transmitted infections
Unpleasant side effects (e.g., weight gain)	5	4	3	2	1	0	1	2	3	4	5	No unpleasant side effects (e.g., weight gain)
Dangerous side effects for women who smoke	5	4	3	2	1	0	1	2	3	4	5	Safe for women who smoke
Not safe for young women	5	4	3	2	1	0	1	2	3	4	5	Safe for young women
Not safe for older women	5	4	3	2	1	0	1	2	3	4	5	Safe for older women
Protects against HIV/AIDS	5	4	3	2	1	0	1	2	3	4	5	No protection against HIV/AIDS
Messy to use	5	4	3	2	1	0	1	2	3	4	5	Not messy to use
Requires skill to use properly	5	4	3	2	1	0	1	2	3	4	5	Does not require skill to use properly
Not very effective for protection against pregnancy	5	4	3	2	1	0	1	2	3	4	5	Very effective for protection against pregnancy

of the semantic differential scales, investigators analyze data by exploring each topic as well as the collective scores.

Knowledge, Attitude, and Behavior Scales

Scales of knowledge, attitude, and behavior are studied separately and collectively. When investigators study the level of knowledge on a specific topic, results allow investigators to develop health education programs based on the general knowledge known about a particular disease or medical condition. Investigators develop true/false questions or Likert scale–type responses depending on the type of data needed for the analysis. Of course, keep in mind that true/false data are nominal and Likert scales are ordinal. **Box 8-3** shows an example of a scale of knowledge, attitude, and behavior.[17]

BOX 8-3

Example of a Knowledge Survey

The following five questions are a sample test related to diabetes knowledge.

The diabetes diet is:
- a. Not the way most people eat
- b.* A healthy diet
- c. High in carbohydrates
- d. Too high in protein for most people

Which of the following is highest in carbohydrates?
- a. Baked salmon
- b. Cheddar cheese
- c.* Baked potato
- d. Peanut butter

Which of the following is highest in fat?
- a.* Low-fat milk
- b. Apple juice
- c. Baked potato
- d. Honey

Glycosylated hemoglobin (hemoglobin A1C) measures the average blood glucose level for the past:
- a. Day
- b. Week
- c.* 6–10 weeks
- d. 6 months

Infection may be caused by:
- a.* high blood glucose levels
- b. low blood glucose levels
- c. no change in blood glucose levels

* correct response

Modified with permission from Diabetes Knowledge Test. University of Michigan Diabetes Research and Training Center. Available at: http://www.med.umich.edu/mdrtc/profs/survey.html#dkt.

If investigators wished to use the entire Michigan Diabetes Knowledge Test for their study, it would be necessary to obtain permission, use the complete survey, and score the test according to the analysis described by the original authors.

Attitude scales measure opinions, values, attitudes, and other characteristics.[6] As with all studies, the first step is to develop the research question or evaluation objectives, followed by creating operational definitions for each variable. For example, if investigators are studying adolescents, they state the age range as the operational definition (e.g., 13–19 years of age, 12–20 years of age, or another range determined by researchers). At this point, investigators determine whether a scale is needed to answer the research questions or evaluation objectives. This process begins by answering the question "What is being measured?"

Behavior questions ask about specific actions rather than knowledge and attitudes. The following questions change the knowledge questions about diabetes into behavior questions about diabetes.[17]

Since I was diagnosed with diabetes, I follow the diabetes diet as prescribed by my physician.

1. Strongly disagree
2. Disagree
3. Agree
4. Strongly agree

I select baked salmon instead of a baked potato because baked potatoes are high in carbohydrates.

1. Strongly disagree
2. Disagree
3. Agree
4. Strongly agree

I drink water, because some drinks (e.g., low-fat milk) are high in fat.

1. Strongly disagree
2. Disagree
3. Agree
4. Strongly agree

I go to the lab every three months to have my glycosylated hemoglobin (hemoglobin A1C) levels checked, because it measures my average blood glucose level for the past 6 to 10 weeks.

1. Strongly disagree
2. Disagree
3. Agree
4. Strongly agree

I try to avoid letting my blood glucose level get too high, because high blood glucose levels might cause infections.

1. Strongly disagree
2. Disagree
3. Agree
4. Strongly agree

Cultural and Diversity Influences in Data Collection

When developing surveys, it is important to keep in mind cultural and ethnic influences in data collection measurement decisions. Let's go over a few examples of how respondents may feel excluded by the question response choices. If individuals feel that questions or response choices disrespect them, they are less likely to complete the survey or interview. When investigators lack cultural sensitivity in the interview or survey development phase, it results in missing data. In this case, investigators are left wondering why data are missing, but never relate it back to lack of diversity and cultural sensitivity. Here are a few examples from survey questions:

Example 1
What is your race/ethnicity? (Select one)

1. White
2. Black
3. Hispanic
4. Other

This question eliminates many groups, for example, Native Americans, Asians, Pacific Islanders, and so on. It also does not allow multiracial individuals to select several choices. The best solution is to use the ethnicity choices offered on U.S. Census forms (see **Box 8-4**).[18]

Example 2
What is your gender?
1. Female
2. Male

The responses for this question exclude transgender individuals.

Example 3
What is your annual income?
1. Less than $59,999
2. $60,000–$89,999

BOX 8-4

Questions about Ethnicity and Race

What is this person's race? Mark one or more choices.

1. White
2. Black, African American, or Negro
3. American Indian or Alaska Native
4. Asian Indian
5. Japanese
6. Native Hawaiian
7. Chinese
8. Korean
9. Guamanian or Chamorro
10. Filipino
11. Vietnamese
12. Samoan
13. Other Asian
14. Other Pacific Islander
15. Some other race
    Write response: _____

Is this person of Hispanic, Latino, or Spanish origin?

1. No, not of Hispanic, Latino, or Spanish origin
2. Yes, Mexican, Mexican American, Chicano
3. Yes, Puerto Rican
4. Yes, Cuban
5. Yes, another Hispanic, Latino, or Spanish origin
   Write response: _____

Reproduced from The 2010 Census Questionnaire: Seven Questions for Everyone. Population Reference Bureau. Available at: http://www.prb.org/Articles/2009/questionnaire.aspx.

3. $90,000 –$129,999
4. $130,000 or more

The responses for this question classify individuals into a narrow range of choices. Because poverty in the United States for a family of four is set at

$23,050[19] and the median U.S. income is $51,914,[20] the choices classify almost 50% of the population within the lowest choice. These choices limit data accuracy.

Example 4
Do you describe yourself as any of the following choices?
1. Cancer survivor
2. Disabled person
3. Domestic violence victim
4. HIV+ person

All of these choices list the adjective first, followed by the individual. It is always best to describe the individual first followed by the descriptive term: (1) Person who survived cancer, (2) Person with a disability, (3) Survivor of domestic violence, and (4) Person living with HIV+ health status.

These are just a few of many examples where individuals feel excluded and then choose not to complete survey questions.

For interview questions, the way the question is presented influences the honesty of the response. Here are two examples:

1. "You don't smoke, do you?" versus "About how many cigarettes do you smoke each day?"
2. "Have you had more than 10 sexual partners in the last 30 days?" versus "How many sexual partners would you estimate that you have had in the last 30 days?"

Whether investigators develop survey questions or interview questions, the level of cultural and diversity awareness influences the data collection process. Pilot testing is critical in the development of culturally appropriate data collection. Investigators ask a representative sample to read questions and provide honest feedback to ensure suitability of questions and response choices.

Survey: Reliability and Validity

Before closing the discussion about surveys, it is essential to remind readers to review the concepts of reliability and validity. These two concepts are fundamental regardless of whether investigators select an existing survey or develop a new survey. As a brief review, reliability is defined as the consistency of what is measured. For example, if an individual's blood glucose level is measured using Brand A monitor and then measured again using Brand B monitor, the results should be the same if the monitors are reliable. The same is true with data collection.

If physical therapy students are given a muscle anatomy exam on Wednesday and the same exam on Friday, the scores should be nearly the same if the exam is reliable. Validity concerns whether the test measures what it was intended to measure. There is external and internal validity. External validity deals with generalizability to other groups. Internal validity focuses on the rigor of the research, for example, study design, precision in data collection, and consideration of all possible explanations for results. It is more important for a survey to be valid than reliable.

Summary

This chapter covers survey selection, including whether researchers decide to use an existing survey or develop a new survey. There are advantages and disadvantages to both existing and new surveys, but decisions are made based on research questions. Survey data collection introduced online, mailed, and in-person surveys. The next section investigated various types of quantitative surveys, including tests, inventories, and scales. Lastly, at the end of the chapter, there was a discussion of cultural and diversity issues related to surveys.

Case Study

Research Questions

Researchers desired to study how adult children cope with the stress of caring for a hospitalized elderly parent. For this study, researchers developed three research questions:

1. Is there a difference in coping with stress between male and female adult children serving as caregivers for their elderly parents?
2. Is there a difference in coping with stress if the hospitalized elderly parent is male or female?
3. Is there a difference in coping with stress if the hospitalized elderly parent is the caregiver's parent or the parent of a spouse or significant other?

continues

CASE STUDY *continued*

Operational Definitions

Adult caregiver is defined as an adult, age 21 or older, spending a minimum of four hours per day at the bedside of the elderly patient who is a parent, or stepparent, or the parent of the caregiver's spouse or significant other. *Stress* is measured by survey responses for the Perceived Stress Scale.[21] *Coping* is measured by survey responses for the Brief COPE scale.[22]

Survey Development

After researchers develop a final draft (see **Box 8-5**), the survey is pretested with colleagues of the research team and then revised as needed. After receiving approval from the IRB, the researchers pilot test the revised survey at a small community hospital near campus with 20 respondents.

Example of Survey Instructions

Thank you for participating in this survey. We appreciate you taking the time to complete this survey. There are three sections to complete. The person who gave you the survey will come back to pick it up in about 15 minutes.

< Perceived Stress Scale[21] >

< Brief COPE Scale[22] >

Data Collection Training

Undergraduate and graduate students are invited to participate in data collection. Each student completes a four-hour hospital volunteer course to obtain a hospital access volunteer badge. In addition, students receive data collection and data entry training provided by the researchers. Data collection training includes instructions on how to (1) enter a patient's room politely, (2) introduce the study to visitors and patients, (3) obtain informed consent signatures, (4) answer questions about the study and/or survey, and (5) thank respondents and collect completed surveys. Data entry training includes tracking data, entering data, and basic data analysis (e.g., frequencies and histograms).

continues

CASE STUDY *continued*

BOX 8-5

Demographics

Now a few questions about you.

Your gender:

　Female

　Male

　Transgender

Your age:

　20–29 years

　30–39 years

　40–49 years

　50–59 years

　60–69 years

　70–79 years

　80–89 years

　90+ years

Describe your relationship to the person for whom you are providing care:

　Parent

　Parent of spouse

　Parent of significant other

Describe the gender of the person for whom you are providing care:

　Female

　Male

　Transgender

While in the hospital, how many hours per day do you provide care for this person?

　0–3 hours per day

　4–6 hours per day

　7–9 hours per day

　10 or more hours per day

When not in the hospital, how many hours per day do you provide care for this person?

　0–3 hours per day

　4–6 hours per day

continues

CASE STUDY *continued*

BOX 8-5 *continued*

7–9 hours per day
10 or more hours per day
When not in the hospital, where does this person live?
Alone at home
My home
Retirement community (independent living)
Assisted living facility
Nursing home
Hospice facility
Are you the primary caregiver for this person?
Yes, I am the primary caregiver; I have no one to help me
Yes, I am the primary caregiver, but home healthcare aides help me
Yes, I am the primary caregiver, but other family members help me
No, I am not the primary caregiver; this person lives in a residential facility

Thank you for completing this survey. You will be given a gift card when the survey is collected.

Data Collection

Data collection takes place at one large (more than 1,000-bed) hospital in a metropolitan area. Researchers collect survey data in three two-hour time intervals during the day: morning (9:00–11:00 a.m.), afternoon (1:00–3:00 p.m.), and evening (6:00–8:00 p.m.). Each week, researchers randomly select 10 units from the 6 patient care floors. Each floor has 3 units (East, West, and Central) with 24 total units. Because there is a mix of double and private patient rooms, there is not a set number of rooms per unit. Within the randomly selected unit, trained students walk from room to room. If the patient has a visitor, the student introduces

continues

CASE STUDY *continued*

the study and invites the visitor to complete the survey. The first page of the survey is the informed consent form. Students answer any questions, provide a pencil, leave the survey, and state that they will return in about 15 minutes to collect the survey. It is common for visitors to wait in unit-designated waiting rooms while patients have procedures. Students also approach visitors in designated waiting rooms because they are likely to have free time for survey completion. After 15 minutes, students collect surveys and provide a $5 gift card to each respondent. The completed surveys are placed in an envelope, which is labeled by the date, time, location of unit, and number of surveys enclosed; then the envelope is sealed and delivered to researchers that day.

Data Entry

When students are not collecting data, they enter data into a spreadsheet. Information on the outside of the envelope is entered prior to entering survey data to ensure that tracking data are not separated from completed surveys.

Data Analysis

Upon entering survey data, researchers analyze the data. For the Perceived Stress Scale, the score for items 4, 5, 7, and 8 are reversed (0 = 4, 1 = 3, 2 = 2, 3 = 1, and 4 = 0). After the scoring is reversed, the scores are summed for a final perceived stress score. According to the Perceived Stress Scale, the mean score for females is 13.7 and for males is 12.1.[21] For the Brief COPE, there is no reverse coding required. The scale includes questions that reflect the following categories (item numbers shown on survey): self-distraction (1 and 19), active coping (2 and 7), denial (3 and 8), substance use (4 and 11), use of emotional support (5 and 15), use of instrumental support (10 and 23), behavioral disengagement (6 and 16), venting (9 and 21), positive reframing (12 and 17), planning (14 and 25), humor (18 and 28), acceptance (20 and 24), religion (22 and 27), and self-blame (13 and 26). Beyond scoring

continues

CASE STUDY *continued*

the Perceived Stress Scale,[21] Brief COPE scale,[22] and demographics, researchers seek the guidance of biostatisticians for the remainder of the data analysis. The final report for the study includes frequencies, histograms, and statistical analysis required to answer the research questions.

Case Study Discussion Questions

1. Discuss the strengths and weaknesses of this proposed study.
2. Discuss whether the survey questions answer the research questions. How would you suggest improving the survey questions?

Student Activity

Charlottesburg is a medium-sized college town in the Midwest. Historically, the town was a farming community. At the turn of the century, the town opened an agricultural college that steadily gained in size and importance. Now a four-year state-supported school, the college is one of the major public universities in the state. Many of the town's citizens work at the university and live within a couple miles of it. Recently, the issue of obesity became a topic of interest to the president of the college, Ms. Delcomb. Ms. Delcomb noticed that many of the students, staff, and faculty are less active than in the past and have a variety of unhealthy habits, such as smoking and eating fast food. After talking with local doctors, Ms. Delcomb has decided that Charlottesburg is just one more town that must face the obesity epidemic. In order to help the town, Ms. Delcomb wants to start encouraging healthy practices at the college among the students, staff, and faculty.

Ms. Delcomb thinks it would be a good idea to see what the current situation is at the college in Charlottesburg before she goes forward with plans for a health campaign. Because diet and exercise are important parts of preventing obesity, Ms. Delcomb wants to ask a sample of students, staff, and faculty about their habits. She has prepared a list of questions she would like you, a work study student who works in her office, to help her turn into a survey.

Here are the questions that Ms. Delcomb gives you:

Question 1:   Do you consider yourself to be overweight, underweight, or "just about right"?

Question 2:   Are you an unhealthy eater?

Question 3:   Do you exercise regularly? (*Exercise* means any physical activity where you are moving your body for at least 30 minutes; *regularly* means most days a week.)

Question 4:   What makes it hard for you to eat healthily?

Question 5:   What makes it hard for you to exercise regularly?

Question 6:   How many servings of vegetables and whole grains did you eat last week?

Question 7:   How would a program that helped you eat better and exercise more make you happier in the future?

After looking at the questions, you think they can be improved somewhat. Answer the following questions about what you would do to make this survey better, and explain your answers.

Questions

1. You want to make sure all of the questions that Ms. Delcomb gave you answer the research question. In this case, the research question is "What are the current diet and exercise habits of students, staff, and faculty at the college in Charlottesburg?"
2. Is Question 1 the best question to start the survey?
3. Are there any questions that are "double-barreled," meaning they ask about more than one thing?
4. Which question is most likely to elicit an untrue response?
5. Question 3 seems very long. Should we shorten it and just ask people if they exercise regularly?
6. Questions 5, 6, and 7 are open ended. Should we keep these?

Answers

1. Although knowing if a program to help people make better food choices and exercise more would make them happier is a great idea, it doesn't answer our research question, which is to determine current diet and exercise habits. Question 7 will have to go.
2. Question 1 is probably not the best question to start the survey because some people may be sensitive about their weight. Placing it near the end of the survey might be a better idea.

3. Yes. Question 6 is a double-barreled question because it asks about vegetables and whole grains. Although vegetables and whole grains are both foods, they are very different types of foods. If somebody answered "five servings," would we know if they were all vegetables, all whole grains, or some combination of the two?

4. Question 2 is probably most likely to illicit an untrue response because it implies some judgment about the answer that is likely to be given. If healthy is good, then unhealthy is bad. Most people don't want to be seen as bad, so they might be inclined to answer the question in a socially desirable way. You might consider changing this question to ask how many times a week they eat certain foods such as fast food, sugary drinks, salty snacks, and so on. This way, you are the one who can ascertain the healthiness of each respondent's diet.

5. You should not shorten Question 3. This question provides an operational definition of "regular exercise." If you didn't have this definition, someone who walks to the end of their driveway once a day might consider it regular exercise when it really isn't. Furthermore, someone who went walking for half an hour every evening might not consider it exercise because it is not physically intense, when in fact it should be counted.

6. This is a trick question. The real answer is that it depends on what you want to know, how many people you are surveying, how many other questions there are, the environment in which you are surveying them, and so on. However, we might consider leaving them in because open-ended questions can give us valuable information. If we were to have respondents check predetermined boxes, it might limit some very important impediments to healthy eating and exercise that we failed to consider.

References

1. Spies RA, Carlson JF, Geisinger KF, eds. *Mental Measurements Yearbook*, 18th ed. Lincoln, NE: Buros Institute of Mental Measurements; 2010.

2. Centers for Disease Control and Prevention. Questionnaires and Item Rationales. Available at: http://www.cdc.gov/healthyyouth/yrbs/questionnaire_rationale.htm. Accessed June 3, 2012.

3. U.S. Department of Justice, Office of Juvenile Justice and Delinquency Prevention. *Evaluating Juvenile Justice Programs: A Design Monograph for State Planner.* Washington, DC: Community Research Associates. Available at: https://www.bja .gov/evaluation/guide/documents/basic_guidelines_for_the_develop.htm. Published 1989. Accessed September 7, 2013.

4. Questionnaire Development. Survey Pro. Available at: http://www.esurveyspro.com /article-questionnaire-development.aspx. Accessed June 3, 2012.

5. Dillman D, Smyth J, Christian L. *Internet, Mail, and Mixed-Mode Surveys: The Tailored Design Method*, 3rd ed. Hoboken, NJ: Wiley Publications; 2009.

6. Ary D, Jacobs L, Razavieh A, Sorenson C. *Introduction to Research in Education*, 8th ed. Belmont, CA: Wadsworth/Cengage Learning; 2010.

7. The Florida Comprehensive Assessment Test. Florida Department of Education. Available at: http://fcat.fldoe.org/fcat/. Accessed June 3, 2012.

8. About the GRE Revised General Test. Educational Testing Services. Available at: http://www.ets.org/gre/revised_general/about/. Accessed June 3, 2012.

9. Hematocrit. Medline Plus. Available at: http://www.nlm.nih.gov/medlineplus/ency /article/003646.htm. Last updated February 8, 2012. Accessed June 3, 2012.

10. Myers Briggs Test: What Is Your Personality Type? Personality Pathways. Available at: http://www.personalitypathways.com/type_inventory.html. Accessed June 3, 2012.

11. Trochim MK. General Issues in Scaling. Research Methods Knowledge Base. Available at: http://www.socialresearchmethods.net/kb/scalgen.php. Last updated October 10, 2006. Accessed June 3, 2012.

12. Rosenberg M. *Society and the Adolescent Self-Image*. Princeton, NJ: Princeton University Press; 1965.

13. Trochim MK. Likert Scaling. Research Knowledge Base. Available at: http://www .socialresearchmethods.net/kb/scallik.php. Last updated October 10, 2006. Accessed June 3, 2012.

14. Thurstone LL. Attitudes can be measured. *Am J Sociol*. 1928;33:529–554.

15. Attitude Scales: Rating Scales to Measure Data. Management Study Guide. Available at: http://www.managementstudyguide.com/attitude-scales.htm. Accessed June 3, 2012.

16. Heise, DR. The semantic differential and attitude research. In: Summers F, ed. *Attitude Measurement*. Chicago, IL: Rand McNally; 1970:235–253. Available at: http://www .indiana.edu/~socpsy/papers/AttMeasure/attitude.htm. Accessed September 7, 2013.

17. Diabetes Knowledge Test. University of Michigan Diabetes Research and Training Center. Available at: http://www.med.umich.edu/mdrtc/profs/survey.html#dkt. Accessed June 3, 2012.

18. The 2010 Census Questionnaire: Seven Questions for Everyone. Population Reference Bureau. Available at: http://www.prb.org/Articles/2009/questionnaire .aspx. Published April 2009. Accessed June 3, 2012.

19. 2012 Annual Federal Poverty Guidelines. Families USA. Available at: http://www .familiesusa.org/resources/tools-for-advocates/guides/federal-poverty-guidelines .html. Accessed on June 3, 2012.

20. USA People QuickFacts. The United States Census Bureau. Available at: http:// quickfacts.census.gov/qfd/states/00000.html. Accessed June 3, 2012.

21. Cohen S, Kamarck T, Mermelstein R. A global measure of perceived stress. *J Health Soc Behav*. 1983;24:386–396.

22. Carver CS. You want to measure coping but your protocol's too long: Consider the Brief COPE. *Int J Behav Med*. 1997;4:92–100; Available at: http://www.psy.miami .edu/faculty/ccarver/sclBrCOPE.html. Accessed September 7, 2013.

9

Data Tools

CHAPTER OBJECTIVES

By the end of this chapter, students will be able to:

- Evaluate the differences between categorical and continuous data
- Apply data organization skills to present data
- Describe measures of central tendency
- Describe standard deviation

KEY TERMS

Categorical data	Measure of central tendency
Continuous data	Normal curve
Frequency distributions	Standard deviation

Introduction

Research tools are used by evaluators as well as researchers. This chapter describes how data are classified by scales of measurement including categorical data using nominal and ordinal scales and continuous data using interval and ratio scales. Next there is a discussion about how data are organized using frequency distributions and graphic presentations. The chapter concludes with a detailed explanation of the measures of central tendency (mean, median, and mode), the normal curve, and the concepts of variance and standard deviation. The information learned in this chapter serves as the foundation of understanding the basic concepts of inferential statistics.

Data Classification

There are numerous ways to classify data, so this discussion begins with the most basic way and then moves into more detailed descriptions. As seen in **Figure 9-1**, the first way to classify data is as either categorical or continuous data.

Categorical Data

Categorical data are defined as variables that are named and placed into groups, classification, or categories. For example, if you wanted to group zoo animals by type, you could put them in different categories (e.g., mammals, birds, fish, reptiles, amphibians). Each animal belongs to only one category and not any other. There are two types of categorical data: nominal and ordinal.

Nominal Data

Nominal data are best remembered when you think of naming variables. For nominal data, there is no particular order and the codes are arbitrary. One example is if the investigator wishes to know the residential zip code of the responding

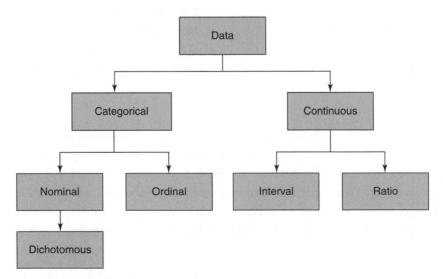

FIGURE 9-1   Classifications of Data

individual. Investigators code the zip codes with arbitrary numbers: 1 = 33610, 2 = 33612, 3 = 33479, 4 = 33481, and 5 = 33509. It does not mean that individuals marking 5 have "more zip code" than individuals marking 1 on the survey. Each code number is merely an alternate code given to the zip codes (see **Table 9-1**).

Other examples of nominal data include ethnicity, place of employment, and geographic location. A subset of nominal data is dichotomous data. Dichotomous data consist of only two choices. For example, a survey question could ask, "Are you a current resident of Hillsborough County, Florida?" The choices are "Yes" or "No," and no other choices are available.

Ordinal Data

Ordinal data are best remembered by thinking about a marathon race. The winners are ranked as first, second, and third place in the order they cross the finish line. However, ordinal data do not assume that the distance between runners as they cross the finish line is equal. There might be 3 seconds between the first-place runner and the second-place runner, but there might be 20 seconds between the second-place runner and the third-place runner. For example, the survey question asks:

Which choice describes your age?
1 = 20–29 years old
2 = 30–39 years old
3 = 40–49 years old
4 = 50–59 years old
5 = 60–69 years old
6 = 70–79 years old
7 = 80–89 years old
8 = 90 years old or more

Table 9-1   Sample of Nominal Data

Case Number	Zip Code	Codebook
1	2	33612
2	3	33479
3	4	33481
4	1	33610
5	2	33612
6	5	33509
7	1	33610
8	2	33612
9	2	33612
10	5	33509

These choices allow the respondents to select a category of age rather than providing information about their exact ages.

Ordinal data are also represented in satisfaction scales. A range from 0 (no satisfaction) to 10 (high satisfaction) allows satisfaction to vary among respondents (see **Table 9-2**). The ordinal data for satisfaction scale in Table 9-2 can be arranged from lowest to highest: 0, 1, 2, 3, 4, 5, 6, 6, 8, 9. Each respondent ranks his or her amount of satisfaction based on their perspective of satisfaction.

Continuous Data

Continuous data are defined as data that have equal space between each variable, much like a ruler or yardstick. A continuous variable is any variable between the two values. For example, height and weight are continuous variables. There are two common types of continuous data: interval and ratio.

Interval Data

Interval data are in rank order, like ordinal data, except that the space or intervals between the data are always equal. Think of a measuring tape. There is an equal distance of 1 inch between 10 and 11 inches and between 18 and 19 inches. One example is when an investigator involves adolescents in a clinic, and the survey question asks:

What is the month and year of your birthday?
Month: _____
Year: _____

From this information, investigators calculate the exact age in months for each respondent. This information is more accurate than asking adolescents their ages in years because one might be 13 years and 1 month, whereas another might be 13 years and 11 months. This additional information is valuable because adolescents mature at different rates.

Table 9-2 Sample Ordinal Data: Satisfaction Scale

Case Number	Satisfaction Scale
1	2
2	8
3	1
4	6
5	4
6	5
7	0
8	6
9	9
10	3

Table 9-3   Sample Interval Data: Length of Hospitalization

Case Number	Weeks	Days	Length of Stay in Days
1	3	4	25
2	0	1	1
3	0	2	2
4	1	4	11
5	0	5	5
6	2	3	17
7	4	1	29
8	0	6	6
9	0	4	4
10	1	2	9

Another example is when individuals are asked, on a survey, to report their length of hospitalization in weeks and days. Again, investigators calculate their exact length of hospitalization in days (see **Table 9-3**).

Ratio Data

Ratio data are like interval data with equal intervals, except that ratio data have an absolute zero point. Absolute zero is defined as the absence of the variable measured. For example, when measuring height, the absolute zero is 0 inches, because you can't have a negative height. What about temperature? The absolute zero in temperature does not mean that there is no temperature below zero. Of course, temperatures drop below zero in very cold places. The absolute zero on the Celsius scale is the temperature at which water freezes at sea level. It is an agreed-upon, but arbitrary, number of zero temperature. Because there is an absolute zero point, investigators may calculate ratios. For example, in currency, a ratio is calculated to say that $20 is four times as much as $5. Ratios are also used to calculate election results, when announcers state that the winner received twice as many votes as the losing candidate. In health, investigators use ratios to calculate the number of people in the population with a specific disease; for example, there are 195.2 deaths due to heart disease in the United States per 100,000 population per year.[1] An example survey question for ratio data is the following:

> What was the cost of your copayment for today's visit in the clinic?
>
> 1 = I did not pay a copayment for today's visit.   7 = $30
> 2 = $5   8 = $35
> 3 = $10   9 = $40
> 4 = $15
> 5 = $20
> 6 = $25

Table 9-4 Sample of Ratio Data: Weight

Case Number	Weight (in Pounds)
1	132
2	91
3	167
4	253
5	152
6	129
7	231
8	189
9	274
10	173

Investigators list these choices after investigating the amount of copayments collected prior to clinic visits. In this clinic, the copayments fall into $5 increments up to $40.

Another example of gathering ratio data is when investigators record an individual's weight in the electronic medical record (EMR) at each clinic visit (see **Table 9-4**).

Now let's summarize the four types of data and explore how investigators analyze and report data (see **Table 9-5**).

Next, practice your skills using **Table 9-6**.

With an understanding of the four types of data, let's explore how investigators can analyze and report data.

Table 9-5 Summary of Four Types of Data

Case Number	Zip Code	Satisfaction Scale	Length of Hospitalization			Weight (in Pounds)
			Weeks	Days	Length	
1	33601	2	3	4	25	132
2	33612	8	0	1	1	91
3	33613	1	0	2	2	167
4	33601	6	1	4	11	253
5	33612	4	0	5	5	152
6	33611	5	2	3	17	129
7	33612	0	4	1	29	231
8	33601	6	0	6	6	189
9	33613	9	0	4	4	274
10	33601	3	1	2	9	173

Table 9-6   Evaluation Practice: Data Classification

When investigators develop surveys, they are aware of data created from each question. For the questions below, select the data classification that each response yields.

Question	Nominal (a)	Ordinal (b)	Interval (c)	Ratio (d)
1. How old are you today?				
2. What is the highest level of education you have achieved? • High school diploma or GED • Trade or vocational training • Some college—no diploma • Associate degree • Bachelor degree • Graduate degree or higher				
3. Rate your health today: • Excellent • Very good • Good • Fair • Poor				
4. How many points did you receive on your midterm exam in Biology I?				
5. What letter grade did you receive on your Biology I midterm exam? • A • B • C • D • F				
6. What was the temperature this morning when you stepped outside your home?				
7. How did you acquire a clinic appointment today? • I had a walk-in appointment • I went online to schedule an appointment • I called to schedule an appointment • I received a postcard with the appointment date and time				
8. How many minutes did you wait in the clinic waiting room today?				
9. Did you exercise for 60 minutes yesterday? • Yes • No				
10. What was the rank of your clinic softball team in the community? • First place • Second place • Third place • Fourth place • Fifth place				

Answers: 1c, 2b, 3b, 4c, 5c, 6d, 7a, 8c, 9a, 10b

Data Organization

Investigators organize data in a variety of ways depending on the purpose of reporting. This section includes discussions of descriptive data, graphic presentations, univariate data, measures of central tendency, the normal curve, and lastly, standard deviation and variability.

Descriptive Data

After investigators collect their data, they enter the data into a spreadsheet (e.g., Microsoft Excel) or directly into a statistical software program (e.g., SPSS or SAS). The first step allows investigators view the data and to identify missing data. For example, in **Figure 9-2**, Case 5 has missing data for the age of the respondent, and Case 16 has "7" entered under satisfaction, which is not a valid

	A	B	C
1	Age	Gender	Satisfaction
2	50	1	3
3	57	1	4
4	56	1	2
5		2	3
6	71	1	2
7	73	1	1
8	61	2	2
9	67	1	3
10	59	2	4
11	78	1	2
12	81	1	3
13	90	1	4
14	58	2	5
15	68	2	1
16	83	2	7
17	94	1	3
18	57	2	2
19	72	1	4
20	78	2	3
21	62	1	2
22			

FIGURE 9-2 Sample of Excel Data Spreadsheet
Used with permission from Microsoft

choice (1 = low and 5 = high). Because each survey was numbered when collected, investigators locate surveys with errors and enter the corrected or missing data. In addition, investigators randomly select 10% of the surveys and reenter the responses to verify the accuracy of the data entry process. *Data cleaning* is the term used for the process of checking the data for accuracy and correcting errors.

Once descriptive data are cleaned, investigators organize the data to answer simple research questions or evaluation objectives. For example, take the research question: "What is the distribution of ages of the adults over 50 responding to the clinic satisfaction survey?" Investigators use Excel to sort data and report concise results.

Step 1: Highlight all three columns.
Step 2: Click on the Data tab and click on "A to Z."
Yield the spreadsheet seen in **Figure 9-3**.

	A	B	C
1	Age	Gender	Satisfaction
2	50	1	3
3	56	1	2
4	57	1	4
5	57	2	2
6	58	2	5
7	59	2	4
8	61	2	2
9	62	2	3
10	62	1	2
11	67	1	3
12	68	2	1
13	71	1	2
14	72	1	4
15	73	1	1
16	78	1	2
17	78	2	3
18	81	1	3
19	83	2	4
20	90	1	4
21	94	1	3

FIGURE 9-3   Sample of Sorting Excel Data Spreadsheet
Used with permission from Microsoft

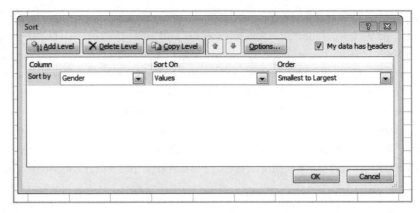

FIGURE 9-4 Sorting by Level
Used with permission from Microsoft

Report: Of the 20 responding adults, the age distribution is 6 (30%) 50–59 years, 5 (25%) 60–69 years, 5 (25%) 70–79 years, 2 (10%) 80–89 years, and 2 (10%) 90+ years.

To sort by gender, highlight all three columns, click the Data tab, click Sort, and add one level (see **Figure 9-4**). This results in the information noted in **Figure 9-5.**

Because there are only 20 respondents, investigators calculate results by hand. However, Excel can be used for calculations on larger datasets.

Report: Of the 20 responding adults, the gender distribution is 12 (60%) females and 8 (40%) males.

The same sorting process is used if investigators wish to report clinic satisfaction of survey respondents.

Report: Of the 20 responding adults, the clinic satisfaction is 2 (10%) poor, 6 (30%) fair, 6 (30%) good, 5 (25%) very good, and 1 (5%) excellent.

Graphic Presentation

Although descriptive data are useful to organize information, investigators usually use histogram and frequency polygons to provide a visual depiction of data. Histograms are generally used to display nominal data, whereas frequency polygons display continuous data (see **Figure 9-6**).

Figure 9-7 shows a frequency polygon of continuous data collected on three patients who participated in a 12-week weight loss program. Data show that Patient A lost the most weight. Patient B and Patient C fluctuated weight, but overall had the same weight in Week 1 as in Week 12.

Now it is time to practice your skills using **Table 9-7**.

	A	B	C
1	Age	Gender	Satisfaction
2	50	1	3
3	56	1	2
4	57	1	4
5	62	1	2
6	67	1	3
7	71	1	2
8	72	1	4
9	73	1	1
10	78	1	2
11	81	1	3
12	90	1	4
13	94	1	3
14	57	2	2
15	58	2	5
16	59	2	4
17	61	2	2
18	62	2	3
19	68	2	1
20	78	2	3
21	83	2	4

FIGURE 9-5   Sample of Advanced Sorting of Excel Data Spreadsheet
Used with permission from Microsoft

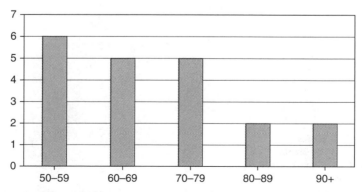

FIGURE 9-6   Histogram of Ordinal Data

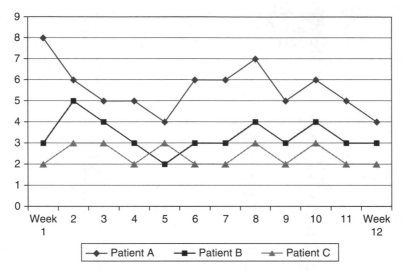

FIGURE 9-7 Frequency Polygon of Continuous Data Related to a 12-Week Weight Loss Program

---

Table 9-7 Practice Descriptive Data Skills

Review collected data: Using the data table and the codebook, answer the following questions.

1. Is there any missing data?

2. Write a statement to summarize the severity of injuries.

3. Write a statement to summarize the location of injuries on property.

Data of Injuries in Three Clinics

Case	Clinic	Number of Injuries in the Last Month	Severity of Injury	Blood Exposure	Description of Injured Person	Location of Injury on Property
1	2	6	1	0	1	3
2	3	4	1	0	1	4
3	1	7	1		1	2
4	2	1	1	1	2	1
5	3	2	2	0	1	4
6	1	1	4	1	3	5
7	2	3	1	0	1	1
8	1	2	1	1	1	3
9	1	5	2	1	2	3
10	3	2	1	0	1	4

Codebook

Variable	Codes
Clinic	1 = Bradbury 2 = Graham 3 = Seffner
Number of Injuries in the Last Month	Numerical value

continues

Table 9-7	Practice Descriptive Data Skills *continued*
Severity of Injury	1 = Basic first aid treatment (e.g., Band-Aid and ointment)
	2 = Medical exam for healthcare provider
	3 = Taken to hospital and released within 23 hours
	4 = Transported by ambulance and admitted to hospital
Blood Exposure	0 = No 1 = Yes
Description of Injured Person	1 = Clinic staff 2 = Patient 3 = Visitor or caregiver
Location of Injury on Property	1 = Parking lot or surrounding landscaped area
	2 = Waiting room
	3 = Back office, file room, break room, exam room
	4 = Lab or procedure room
	5 = Maintenance and grounds building

Answers:

1. In Case 3, the blood exposure data is missing.

2. Of the 10 injuries in the past month, 7 (70%) injuries were treated with basic first aid, 2 (20%) injuries required a medical examination by a healthcare provider, and 1 (10%) injury required the injured individual be transported by ambulance to the hospital for admission.

3. Of the 10 injuries, 2 (20%) injuries occurred in parking lot or surrounding landscaped area; 1 (10%) occurred in the waiting room; 3 (30%) occurred in the back office, file room, break room, or exam room; 3 (30%) occurred in the lab or procedure room; and 1 (10%) occurred in the maintenance and grounds building.

Measures of Central Tendency

Measures of central tendency are used to summarize data and make comparisons between data. Measures of central tendency include the mean, median, and mode.[2]

Mean

The mean is defined as the average score. To find the mean, investigators add all the scores and divide by the total number of scores. Mean scores are used for interval and ratio data, but not for nominal and ordinal data. For example, if investigators asked on a survey "What is your age?" followed by a blank line, the respondents would fill in the blank.

This section presents two ways of calculating a mean. The first example is calculated by hand by merely adding up all the ages and dividing by the number of responses. This method works fine if you have only a small number of responses, such as the 20 in this example.

$$\text{Mean} \quad = \quad 13 + 18 + 14 + 19 + 15 + 14 + 17 + 18 + 13 + 17 + 14 + 16 + 13$$
$$+ 19 + 16 + 14 + 17 + 13 + 19 + 15 = 314, \text{ then divide } 314 \text{ by } 20$$
$$= 15.7 = \text{mean age}$$

The second example is for a larger number of response and utilizes an Excel formula for the calculation. The Excel formula is fx = AVERAGE (A2:A21). See **Figure 9-8**.

On the other hand, suppose investigators asked on a survey "Select your age group," followed by these choices:

1. 13 or less
2. 14–15
3. 16–17
4. 18–19

Investigators would not be able to calculate the mean age, because they are trying to calculate a mean by using nominal data. There are 4 in group 1 (13 or less), 6 in group 2 (14–15), 5 in group 3 (16–17), and 5 in group 4 (18–19).

	A
1	Age
2	13
3	13
4	13
5	13
6	14
7	14
8	14
9	14
10	15
11	15
12	16
13	16
14	17
15	17
16	17
17	18
18	18
19	19
20	19
21	19
22	

FIGURE 9-8 Age Data
Used with permission from Microsoft

Mean score = 1 + 1 + 1 + 1 + 2 + 2 + 2 + 2 + 2 + 3 + 3 + 3 + 3 + 3 + 4 +
4 + 4 + 4 + 4 = 51, then divide 51 by 20 = 2.55

This value shows that the average age is somewhere between 14 and 17, and thus is not accurate, proving the point that means cannot be calculated on nominal or ordinal data. Because the mean is more accurate, it is used for interval and ratio data.

Median

The median is defined as the middle value of the data. When there are an even numbers of scores, the median is calculated by adding the two middle scores together and dividing by two. In **Figure 9-9**, there are 20 age scores, so (15 + 16)/2 = 15.5 is the median. Generally, median is used for ordinal data. The Excel formula is fx = MEDIAN(A2:A21).

	C25		fx	=MODE(A2:A21)	
	A	B	C	D	E
1	Age				
2	13				
3	13				
4	13				
5	13				
6	14				
7	14				
8	14				
9	14				
10	15				
11	15				
12	16				
13	16				
14	17				
15	17				
16	17				
17	18				
18	18				
19	19				
20	19				
21	19				
22					
23		Mean	15.7		
24		Median	15.5		
25		Mode	13		

FIGURE 9-9 Summary of Mean, Median, and Mode
Used with permission from Microsoft

Mode

The mode is defined as the most frequently occurring score. In Figure 9-9, there are two modes because 13 and 14 were both picked the same number of times. When this happens, the data are called bimodal.[2] The mode is used for nominal data. The Excel formula is fx = MODE(A2:A21).

Normal Curve

In this section, several topics related to the normal curve are discussed, including skew, variance, and standard deviation. Let's begin with the normal curve, shown in **Figure 9-10**. If data are evenly distributed, Figure 9-10 shows that mean, median, and mode are the same. In the normal curve, there are equal numbers of variables above and below the mean, median, and mode. For example, if the annual income in one county was evenly distributed, the mean, median, and mode of income remain the same: $43,000 annually. In addition, half the population has an income below $43,000 and half the population has an income above $43,000.

When the mean, median, and mode are not the same number, the curve is lopsided, or skewed. The skew of the curve is positive or negative. In a positive skew, the mean is greater than the median[4] (see **Figure 9-11**).

In Figure 9-11, notice that the mode is not changed by the direction of the skew, because the mode is the most frequent number. In a negative skew, the mean is smaller than the median. For example, if the county has a large proportion of

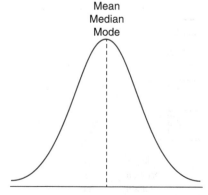

FIGURE 9-10   The Normal Curve

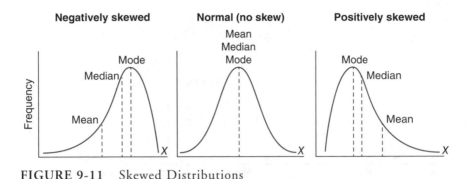

FIGURE 9-11   Skewed Distributions

low-income individuals, the mean is pulled in a negative direction. In a positive skew, the mean is larger than the median. For example, if the county has a large population of wealthy individuals, the mean is pulled in the positive direction.

Lastly, it is often possible to determine the skew by looking at the mean and median instead of constructing a histogram. Let's look at an example of skew. Salaries of personnel in the hospital lab are $280,000, $112,000, $80,000, $78,000, $61,000, $52,000, $39,000, $39,000, and $28,000. The median is $61,000. The mode is $39,000. The mean is $85,444. Without drawing a histogram, it is easy to determine that these data have a positive distribution, because the mean ($85,444) is greater than the median ($61,000).

Standard Deviation and Variance

Standard deviation (Greek symbol sigma, σ) is defined as how much variation or "dispersion" exists from the mean or average. A low standard deviation shows that data are gathered tightly around the mean, whereas high standard deviation shows that data are dispersed or spread out far from the mean. Look at the normal curve in **Figure 9-12**. The vertical line represents the mean score. The area shows one standard deviation from the mean, or 68.26% of the population, with 34.13% above the mean and 34.13% below the mean. The second area represents about 28% (13.59% above the mean and 13.59% below the mean) for a total of two standard deviations, representing about 95.44% of the population. The third area represents about 4% (2.14% above the mean and 2.14% below the mean). By summing, the area of the three standard deviations equals nearly 99% of the population.[3] The remaining 1% is for an infinite number of standard deviations.

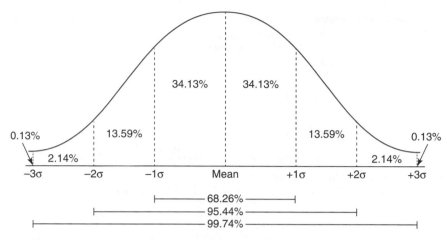

FIGURE 9-12   Standard Deviations Shown on a Normal Curve

Let's begin with an example of exam scores of students from Classes A, B, and C. There were 27 students in each class and 100 points possible on the exam (see **Figure 9-13**). The Excel formulas are *fx* = MEAN(A2:A28); *fx* = STDEV(A2:A28), and *fx* = VAR(A2:A28).

Notice that in Classes A, B, and C, exam scores have a mean of 70.4, but let's suppose that the three instructors decided to assign student grades based on the normal curve. Using **Figure 9-14**, let's calculate how many students are in the first three standard deviations. It is important to notice that exam scores have nothing to do with the number of students in each of the standard deviations.

1st standard deviation: 27 students × 34.13% = 9 students below and
                                       9 students above the mean

2nd standard deviation: 27 students × 13.59% = 4 students below and
                                       4 students above the mean

3rd standard deviation: 27 students × 2.14% = 1 student below and
                                       1 student above the mean

Figure 9-14 shows that as long as the mean score is 70.4 in Classes A, B, and C, the distribution of students remains the same on the normal curve. Regardless of the exam scores, if the instructors used the normal curve to assign grades, 68.26% (1st standard deviation) of students would receive a C, 13.59% (2nd standard deviation) would receive a B if above the mean and a D if below the mean, and 2.14% (3rd standard deviation) would receive an A if above the mean and an F if below the mean.

	A	B	C	D	E	F
1	Class A		Class B		Class C	
2	24		24		63	
3	36		28		64	
4	50		52		65	
5	50		53		67	
6	51		58		67	
7	61		67		67	
8	61		68		67	
9	62		70		68	
10	62		72		68	
11	64		73		70	
12	70		73		70	
13	70		73		70	
14	70		74		70	
15	71		74		71	
16	71		74		71	
17	72		75		71	
18	80		76		72	
19	81		77		72	
20	83		77		72	
21	83		78		72	
22	86		79		72	
23	88		80		73	
24	90		81		74	
25	91		82		74	
26	91		86		76	
27	92		86		77	
28	92		91		79	
29	70.4 Mean		70.4 Mean		70.4 Mean	
30	17.7034 St Dev		15.6236 St Dev		3.816294 St Dev	
31	313.4103 Var		244.0969 Var		14.5641 Var	

FIGURE 9-13   Exam Scores of Classes A, B, and C
Used with permission from Microsoft

Let's try one last comparison using the student grades. Table 9-8 shows that when instructors use the normal curve and the first three standard deviations for distribution of grades, the percentage of students receiving A, B, C, D, and F remain identical. However, the number of points to earn each letter grade changes based on the width of dispersion around the mean. For example, it is much easier to receive an A in Class C, because the exams scored are packed tightly around the mean of 70.4. However, students hoping to receive a C would rejoice about the wide dispersion (high standard deviation) in Class A (see **Table 9-8**).

When investigators present frequency data, they report standard deviations also. This additional information allows the reader to know the spread of the

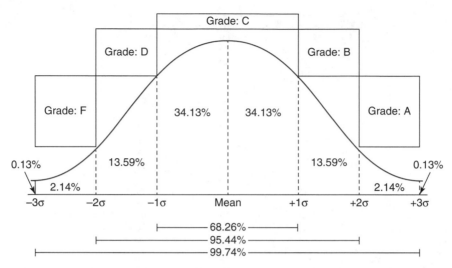

FIGURE 9-14   Distribution of Students on the Normal Curve

data.[4] Using the previous example, if investigators reported only mean scores, it appears that there are no differences among Class A, Class B, and Class C. However, by adding standard deviations, the differences among the classes are apparent.

Table 9-8   Comparison of Usual Grading Scale to Grades Using Normal Curve

	Usual Grading Scale		Grades Using Normal Curve	
	Points	Number of Students (%)	Points	Number of Students (%)
Class A	A 90–100	5 (18.5%)	A 92–100	1 (2.14%)
	B 80–89	6 (22.25%)	B 90–91	4 (13.59%)
	C 70–79	6 (22.25%)	C 61–90	18 (68.26%)
	D 60–69	5 (18.5%)	D 36–60	3 (13.59%)
	F < 60	5 (18.5%)	F < 36	1 (2.14%)
Class B	A 90–100	1 (3.7%)	A 91–100	1 (2.14%)
	B 80–89	5 (18.5%)	B 81–90	4 (13.59%)
	C 70–79	14 (51.85%)	C 58–80	18 (68.26%)
	D 60–69	2 (7.4%)	D 28–57	3 (13.59%)
	F < 60	5 (18.5%)	F < 28	1 (2.14%)
Class C	A 90–100	0 (0%)	A 79–100	1 (2.14%)
	B 80–89	0 (0%)	B 74–78	4 (13.59%)
	C 70–79	18 (66.67%)	C 68–73	18 (68.26%)
	D 60–69	9 (33.33%)	D 64–67	3 (13.59%)
	F < 60	0 (0%)	F < 64	1 (2.14%)

Let's not forget to mention the term *variance*. Variance is defined as the square of the standard deviation.[4] For example, the standard deviation for Class A in Table 9-8 is 17.7034 and the variance is $17.7034 \times 17.7034 = 313.4104$. A further use of variance is beyond the scope of this chapter. In statistics courses, the concept of analysis of variance (ANOVA) is explained in greater detail.

Summary

This chapter began by exploring how data are classified by scales of measurement, including categorical data using nominal and ordinal scales and continuous data using interval and ratio scales. Once the data are collected, it is necessary to organize the data (e.g., frequency distributions and graphic presentations). The chapter ends with a discussion of concepts including measures of central tendency, components of the normal curve, variance, and standard deviation.

Case Study

A national corporation of pharmacy stores hired a research team to determine why some adults chose to receive annual flu vaccines, some adults occasionally receive flu vaccines, and other adults never receive flu vaccines. After a few meetings with the corporate office, the research team members develop the research questions and strategize about the research methods. Researchers hire five graduate students to work 20 hours per week for 15 weeks. A convenience sample is used for survey data collection. Researchers estimate they will need a response rate of approximately 1,000 individuals.

The Health Belief Model is utilized in this research. The main components of the Health Belief Model are perceived benefits, barriers, risks, and severity for performing or not performing the specific health behavior of obtaining an annual flu vaccine.

The research question is:
What are the differences in the perceptions about flu vaccines among adults who receive flu vaccines annually, those who receive them semiregularly, and those who never receive flu vaccines?

continues

CASE STUDY *continued*

For 10 weeks prior to flu season, researchers ask the five graduate students to sit in the waiting area of the local national chain pharmacies with a clipboard. As each person pays for their prescription, clerks invite each customer to participate in the national pharmaceutical chain research related to flu vaccines. If the customer agrees, the clerk introduces the graduate student. A $10 store gift card is offered as an incentive. Prior to conducting the survey, graduate students explain the purpose of the research, obtain consent signatures on the institutional review board–approved consent forms, and keep one copy and give a copy of the consent form to the participating individual. Using clipboards to hold surveys, the graduate student writes responses verbatim for each response.

Survey Questions

1. Have you ever received a flu vaccine?
   Yes
   No
   If Yes, then ask, "Why do you receive flu vaccines each year?"
   If "Yes, but not every year," then ask, "Why not every year?"
   If No, then ask, "What is the reason you do not receive a flu vaccine?"
2. Do your family members receive flu vaccines?
   Yes
   No
   If Yes, then ask, "Why do you think your family members receive flu vaccines each year?"
   If "Yes, but not every year," then ask, "Why do you think they do not receive the flu vaccine every year?"
   If No, then ask, "What is the reason your family members do not receive a flu vaccine?"
3. Do your friends receive flu vaccines?
   Yes
   No
   If Yes, then ask, "Why do you think your friends receive flu vaccines each year?"

continues

CASE STUDY *continued*

> If "Yes, but not every year," then ask, "Why do you think your friends do not receive the flu vaccine every year?"
>
> If No, then ask, "What is the reason your friends do not receive a flu vaccine?"
>
> Now a few questions about you:
>
> 4. What is your age? _____
> 5. What is your employment status? (Check all that apply)
>   Full-time
>   Part-time (less than 30 hours per week)
>   Temporary
>   Seasonal
>   Active-duty military
>   Retired
>
> Because the research is based on a convenience sample, the graduate students conduct as many interviews as possible during their assigned four-hour shifts at the randomly selected national chain stores across various zip codes in their large county. The shifts are randomly assigned as morning, afternoon, and evening hours during weekdays and weekends to ensure responses from a wide variety of customers.
>
> Upon completion of data collection, a spreadsheet is created for entering the data. Graduate students enter the survey data. After checking the data to ensure accuracy, researchers determine the measurements of central tendency and the skew of the curve. Results are presented to the corporate executives of the national pharmaceutical chain. Based on the results, a health education program is developed to increase flu vaccine awareness and compliance. After flu season, research is repeated to determine if the flu vaccine campaign increased flu vaccine compliance.
>
> #### Case Study Discussion Questions
>
> 1. What other survey questions could have been added to the survey to enhance the results?
> 2. What would have been the advantages of using an e-tablet for collecting the data?
> 3. Which measure of central tendency would most likely be used in the data analysis? Why?

Student Activity

Jamestown is a small rural town in the southeastern part of the United States. Historically, the town was mainly a farming community. However, a furniture factory has been the main source of income for most families for the last 50 years. The nearest major city is about 45 minutes away. Recently, the mayor of the town, Mr. Smith, returned from the annual National Conference of Mayors. Among the many topics that were discussed at the meeting was the growing obesity epidemic in the United States. Mr. Smith is very interested in this topic, as he has noticed that more and more people in Jamestown are overweight, including young children. Mayor Smith thought that doing something about the obesity problem in his town would benefit all its citizens. However, before he started working on programs and spending valuable community money and resources, he wanted to make sure that there was indeed a problem with obesity in his community. When he got back from the conference, he went to the local clinic and met with healthcare providers. Also at the meeting was the clerk from the county vital records department. Mayor Smith explained his concerns to them and asked for data that would prove or disprove his suspicions. He asked the healthcare providers how many people at the clinics were overweight (according to the body mass index for their height and weight). He also wanted to know their ages (grouped in 10-year increments) and who among them was diagnosed with an obesity-related illness like type 2 diabetes or chronic heart disease. From the vital records clerk, he wanted to know if obesity-related causes of death had grown over the last decade.

The healthcare providers and the clerk gave Mayor Smith the requested statistics. However, they all came on long lists of paper. Because Mayor Smith is a very busy man, he hired you, a local community college student, to prepare all the data in an easy-to-understand and straightforward fashion that he can present to the city council.

To help you prepare the data, you will need to answer the following questions related to the information sent to you by the doctor's office:

1. What data classification and measurement scale does age represent?
2. What data classification and measurement scale does obesity-related illness represent?
3. If you wanted to show the mayor how many men and women were overweight by age group, what would be the best way to present this?

4. Now suppose you wanted to show the city council which age groups and which gender had the highest numbers of overweight people. What would you do?

5. The clerk gives you the numbers of deaths related to obesity (such as type 2 diabetes and chronic heart disease) for each year over a 10-year period. What would be the best way to show the city council whether obesity is better or worse than it used to be?

After assembling these data for the mayor, he tells you that you are not quite done. He would like you to create some simple descriptive statistics that he can present to the city council. He would like to know the mean, median, and mode of the ages of those individuals who are overweight. Below is a representative sample of 20 people from the data.

25	13	67	7
33	42	11	18
28	31	36	47
52	73	80	15
23	14	44	36

6. What is the mean?
7. What is the median?
8. What is the mode?
9. Based on the information you have, would the distribution curve be normal, positively skewed, or negatively skewed?

Answers

1. Age represents continuous data. Because age has an absolute zero, it is a ratio scale.

2. Obesity-related illness represents categorical data. Like gender, because it has no numerical value, this is a nominal scale.

3. You would present this information to the city council in a simple distribution frequency.

4. The easiest way would be to show this information in a histogram.

5. The best way to show a trend over time using continuous data would be to use a frequency polygon. Even though the types of obesity-related deaths are categorical data, the number of them from year to year

represents continuous data. Because it is continuous data over the last 10 years, we can see whether there is a trend. The trend could be that obesity has gotten worse, has gotten better, or hasn't changed much over the last 10 years.

6. The mean is 34.75, almost 35 years of age.

7. The median age is 29.5.

8. The mode is 36, because there are two people who are 36 years of age.

9. This curve is only slightly positively skewed, because the mean age is slightly larger than the median age.

References

1. The Centers for Disease Control and Prevention. Heart Disease. Available at: http://www.cdc.gov/nchs/fastats/heart.htm. Last updated May 16, 2012. Accessed June 3, 2012.

2. Johnson B, Christensen L. *Educational Research: Quantitative, Qualitative, and Mixed Approaches*, 4th ed. Thousand Oaks, CA: Sage; 2012. http://www.southalabama.edu/coe/bset/johnson/lectures/lec15.htm

3. Kalla S. Measurement of Uncertainty: Standard Deviation. Experiment Resources. Available at: http://www.experiment-resources.com/measurement-of-uncertainty-standard-deviation.html. Accessed on June 3, 2012.

4. Ary D, Jacobs L, Razavieh A, Sorenson C. *Introduction to Research in Education*, 8th ed. Belmont, CA: Wadsworth/Cengage Learning; 2010.

Populations and Samples

Introduction

Researchers conduct studies and evaluators plan, implement, and evaluate programs, but both investigators are discovering information about populations. Because it is often impossible to study the entire population, investigators select a subset or sample of the population. This chapter introduces how probability and inferential statistics are used to make predictions from the random sample selected from the population. The next step involves making decisions that influence the sample size calculation. Once decisions are finalized, the chapter moves on to how to recruit individuals. The recruitment process depends on probability or nonprobability sample designs. Probability sampling involves strict criteria in which every individual in the population has a known chance of getting selected for the sample. Nonprobability sampling is more flexible, inclusive, and not based on chance procedures. With this overview in mind, the chapter begins with a discussion about populations and samples.

Populations and Samples

Let's step back and look closely at the relationship between populations and samples. In statistics, the word *population* is defined as the group or collection of interest for the research. Population does not necessarily indicate only humans. Populations may be soybean crop yields in Iowa, bacteria counts in culture dishes, or cancer clusters in brain tissue. Now let's focus on what a sample is. As previously stated, a sample is a subset of a population. The closer the sample is to representing the whole population, the more accurate the inferences or assumptions that investigators make about the population. If the sample does not represent the population, then the assumptions are less likely to be accurate. As discussed later in this chapter, it is important that the sample is randomly selected from the population to increase the chance that the characteristics match the population.[1]

Probability and Inferential Statistics

Probability is defined as every single event being random. For example, the result of the coin toss at the beginning of a football game is a single and random event. However, if the same coin is tossed 100 times, an approximately equal pattern of heads and tails develops (e.g., 46 heads and 54 tails). If the same coin is tossed 1,000 times, the pattern becomes more accurate (e.g., 480 heads and 520 tails). Probability allows investigators to predict the outcome based on repeating the process, which in this case is tossing a coin.[1]

The word *infer* is defined as to assume or understand. Inferential statistics are mathematical procedures used to assume or understand predictions about the whole population based on data collected from a random sample selected from the population.[2] (These predictions are based on estimates or probability rather than absolute facts.) Investigators use characteristics of the sample (statistics) to estimate the characteristics of the population (parameters). When investigators use inferential statistics, they assume a certain degree of error, because they are never 100% accurate in making assumptions about the population based on the sample. For example, if a pharmaceutical company develops a new beta-blocking drug to reduce hypertension, after completing laboratory and animal studies they *infer* the medication's effectiveness for humans. If they knew the exact human reaction process to the medication, it would be like coin tossing: patients would either improve or get worse after ingesting the new medication. Of course, this simple process does not happen in medical research, so investigators select a random sample from a population of patients diagnosed with hypertension, conduct the study, gather data, and use inferential statistics to estimate the effectiveness of the new medication for the population of adults with hypertension. Because investigators accept a certain degree of error on the effectiveness and possible side effects, the pharmaceutical company states in marketing campaigns that medication effectiveness may vary among patients, and some patients may experience side effects.

Research and Null Hypothesis

Another component of inferential statistics is the development of a hypothesis prior to initiating research. A research hypothesis is a statement of what the investigator expects the relationships to be among the study variables.[2] The four parts of a hypothesis are described by the following questions:[2]

- Is the hypothesis aligned with the current knowledge on the topic?
- What are the expected relationships between the study variables?
- Is the hypothesis able to be tested?
- Is the hypothesis clearly stated?

Let's look at examples of a few research hypothesis statements that answer each of the previously stated questions.

Example 1: Because osteoarthritis improves with moderate exercise, it is hypothesized that adult patients diagnosed with osteoarthritis will achieve greater pain relief when Drug A is taken once per day and 30 minutes prior to moderate exercise.

Example 2: Because obesity is a risk factor for postsurgical wound infections, it is hypothesized that adults diagnosed as obese will experience fewer postsurgical wound infections when their surgical dressings are changed twice per day for the first week after surgery.

In research, the term *null hypothesis* is also used. The null hypothesis states that there is no relationship between the variables.[3] Furthermore, in the null hypothesis, if a relationship is found, it is only by chance. Using the previous example, the null hypothesis would be that for adults diagnosed as obese, there is no relationship between the number of postsurgical wound infections and the number of postsurgical dressings for the first week after surgery. When using the null hypothesis, investigators want their data from the random sample to reject the null hypothesis. They want their data to show that more frequent postsurgical dressing changes are advantageous in decreasing postsurgical wound infections among obese adults.

Investigators must accept or reject the null hypothesis. However, keep in mind that investigators are making this decision based on the sample rather than the population, so their results are always based on incomplete information and are subject to error. If investigators accept the null hypothesis, they are saying that there is a chance of no relationship. Using the previous example, perhaps there is no relationship between wound infections and number of dressing changes. It might be that wound infections have nothing to do with dressing changes but are in fact caused by the mobility or lack of mobility of the obese patients. Nevertheless, researchers accept or reject the null hypothesis, and their decision may be correct or incorrect. Decisions made regarding the null hypothesis have consequences that are labeled type I and type II errors.

Type I errors occur when the null hypothesis is true (there is no relationship between variables) and investigators reject it.[3] From the previous example, investigators report that there is a relationship between postsurgical wound infections and number of dressing changes, thereby rejecting the null hypothesis. The hospital acts on the report and implements an expensive policy of more frequent dressing changes. However, one year later, the hospital observes that the rate of postsurgical wound infections remains the same among obese adult patients. Another team repeats the study and declares that the first study was incorrect because they made a costly type I error (rejection of a true null hypothesis).

Type II error occurs when the null hypothesis is false (there is a real relationship between variables) and investigators accept it.[3] From the previous example, investigators report that there is no relationship between postsurgical wound infections and number of dressing changes, thereby accepting the null hypothesis. Their report states that the investigator found insufficient evidence to increase the number of wound dressings for obese patients. However, one year later, the hospital observes that the rate of postsurgical wound infections remains the same among obese adult patients. Another team repeats the study and declares that the first study was incorrect because they made a type II error (retention of a false null hypothesis). See **Table 10-1**.

Table 10-1   Summary of Type I and Type II Errors

		Truth in Population	
		Null hypothesis is true	Null hypothesis is false
Based on Sample	Rejects null hypothesis	Type I error	Correct
Taken from	Accepts null hypothesis	Correct	Type II error
Population			

From Ary/Jacobs/Cheser/Razavieh/Sorenson. *Introduction to Research in Education*, 8E. © 2010 South-Western, a part of Cengage Learning, Inc. Reproduced by permission. www.cengage.com /permissions

Level of Significance

Before leaving the topic of type I and type II errors, it is necessary to understand the concept of level of significance. Investigators in fear of making type I errors decide to always accept the null hypothesis or always reject the null hypothesis to avoid type II errors. Because neither of these options is feasible, investigators made a decision related to the level of significance. Level of significance is the statistical risk that investigators are willing to accept when making the decision to accept or reject the null hypothesis. If investigators set the level of significance at 0.01, they are willing to accept that 1 out of 100 times, the null hypothesis will be rejected when it is true (type I error). If the level of significance is set at 0.001, the risk of a type I error is 1 in 1,000. Investigators select the level of significance based on the type of investigation and the severity of type I and II errors.[4] In social science, level of significance is typically set at 0.05, because frequently such investigations are based on human behaviors with numerous confounding variables (e.g., age, gender, race/ethnicity, geographical location, environment, education, income, culture). In natural science, level of significance is typically set at 0.01 or 0.001 because research is conducted in controlled environments (e.g., constant temperature, light, humidity, sound, vibration).

Let's recap this complex, but important, section before moving on to determining a sample size. The reader should understand that a sample represents the population, and if the sample does not represent the population, then the assumptions made from that sample are less accurate. Investigators use inferential statistics to estimate the characteristics of the population based on the characteristics of the sample. They assume a certain degree of error because they are making assumptions about the population based on the sample rather than absolute fact. Investigators develop a statement to predict the expected relationship among the study variables; it is called a research hypothesis. The null hypothesis states that there is no relationship among the variables. Based on data gathered from the sample, investigators reject or accept the null hypothesis at the conclusion of their investigation. Investigators make type I errors when the null hypothesis is true and rejected, or type II errors when investigators accept the null hypothesis when it is false. The level of significance allows investigators to set the risk of rejecting a null hypothesis (type I error).

Sample Size Considerations

Why should an investigator be concerned about the number of individuals in the sample for their investigation? Let's look at this question from several viewpoints. As previously stated in this chapter, investigators need to select individuals for the sample who represent the population being studied. For example, if the whole population is 10,000, it does not seem logical for investigators to select 10 individuals for the sample and expect these 10 individuals to represent the population. On the other hand, it does not seem necessary or feasible to select 9,000 individuals for the sample from a population of 10,000. But then investigators ask: If 10 is too few and 9,000 is too many, how many individuals are needed to adequately represent the population? There are no easy answers to this question. The following discussion introduces different aspects of how to determine the appropriate sample size for various types of research or evaluation. However, it is important for readers to realize that the topics presented interact with each other, so determining the ideal sample size is never simple. Let's begin with the topics covered in the discussion. It is not expected that the reader would necessarily be familiar with these topics.

- Margin of error
- Population, sample, and variability
- Confidence level
- Budget and budget justification
- Timeline

Margin of Error

Margin of error is about precision. Generally, investigators do not use a margin of error over 5%. The more precision required, the smaller the acceptable margin of error. For example, if investigators wish to know the level of patient satisfaction, they need to know how many surveys to mail to a random sample of active clinic patients. Investigators want the survey data to represent honest responses related to patient satisfaction from 95% of patients who return the completed surveys. This 5% margin of error is described as plus or minus 2.5%.

In this scenario, investigators are willing to accept that 5% of the patients will not be honest in their survey responses. The best way to think of this concept is to watch the evening news during a national election. Reporters say, "With 36% of the votes counted, we predict that Senator Jones is going to win the election for Colorado." At the bottom of the screen, networks post the margin of error as ±5%, which means that Senator Jones has from 33.5% to 38.5% of the votes based on the accuracy of the exit polls. Networks want to be correct 95% of the time, so they selected a 5% margin of error.[5]

In **Table 10-2**, under margin of error, there are four columns labeled with a percentage. Investigators select the margin of error across the top and population size from the far-left column. For example, if investigators accept a 5% margin of error and the population size is approximately 5,000, the sample size needed is 357. If they wish to increase the level of precision to 2.5% margin of error, the sample size increases to 1,176. Note that decreasing the margin of error by half, from 5% to 2.5%, increased the sample size by more than three times, from 357 to 1,176.

Population, Sample, and Variability

Let's revisit how to use Table 10-2 to determine an adequate sample size. To understand Table 10-2, we begin by defining population size and referring back to the previous discussion on margin of error. Population is defined as the total number of individuals in the group or community from which the sample is drawn. For example, if there are approximately 3,500 clinic patients where the survey data are

Table 10-2   Calculation of Sample Size from Population

Population Size	Margin of Error			
	5.0%	3.5%	2.5%	1.0%
50	44	47	48	50
100	80	89	94	99
500	217	306	377	475
1,000	278	440	606	906
1,500	306	515	759	1,297
2,000	322	563	869	1,655
2,500	333	597	952	1,984
3,500	346	641	1,068	2,565
5,000	357	678	1,176	3,288
10,000	370	727	1,332	4,899
50,000	381	772	1,491	8,056
100,000	383	778	1,513	8,762

Modified from Sample Size Table. Paul Boyd, The Research Advisors. Available at: http://www.research-advisors.com/tools/SampleSize.htm. Reprinted with permission.

collected, the sample size ranges from 346 to 2,565, depending on the margin of error. If the population size is not listed, select the highest number close to the population size. The value in the next column is the sample size based on the margin of error. It is worth noting that for small population sizes, the sample size includes the entire population. Of course, using the population (e.g., 200 or less) as the sample is only possible with availability of adequate funding. For example, if investigators wanted to interview all pediatric transplant nephrologists, they would determine the total number of individuals within this specific medical discipline and then attempt to contact all of them. Lastly, the sample size needs to be large enough so that the data analysis will show a change among the individuals in the sample. For example, investigators are trying to determine if their new Drug A used to treat migraine headaches is better than the current Drug B migraine headache medication. If the sample size is too small, the data analysis would not likely show that Drug A is better, worse, or the same as Drug B.

Variability is another aspect of populations. Variability is defined as the similarities and differences among members of the population. If the population is composed of diverse (heterogeneous) individuals, a larger sample size is required to obtain a higher level of precision. If the individuals are similar (homogeneous) in the population, a smaller sample size is needed to obtain a high level of precision.

Confidence Level

Confidence level is defined as how much certainty investigators have that the sample is a true reflection of the population. In other words, investigators are certain that if other investigators conduct the same study with a different sample from the same population, both studies would yield the same results. In social science, investigators generally use a 95% confidence level, but in natural science, investigators use a 99% level of confidence. Why the difference? Social science investigators are studying behaviors of individuals, communities, and populations, whereas in natural science, experiments are more likely conducted in a controlled (temperature, humidity, light, vibration, etc.) laboratory environment, so results are more precise. For investigators to have a 95% confidence level, it means that 95 out of 100 samples of the same population would obtain the same results. In other words, investigators are willing to accept the risk that 5 times out of 100, the results are different (see **Box 10-1**).

Budget and Budget Justification

When determining sample size, investigators make decisions based on their available funding. Investigators need to consider all costs associated with sample size

BOX 10-1

Case Study: Confidence Level

Investigators wish to study the average height of the population to illustrate a 95% confidence level. They hired five undergraduate students to stand at five different locations in the Newark Airport. After obtaining institutional review board approval, the undergraduate students randomly ask people to participate by simply being measured and receiving a $2 coupon for any food vendor in the airport. Each undergraduate student collected 20 adult height measurements, so the sample size was a total of 100. Investigators analyzed the data and found that one undergraduate student's data showed that 5 out of 20 measurements were much higher than the mean (average) height of the other 95 measurements. When questioned about the data, the student reported that a national basketball team had walked down her assigned terminal and five players volunteered to participate. The basketball players measured over 7 feet in height. Investigators showed the undergraduate students that if the study were conducted 100 times, 95% of the time the mean height would be approximately the same for the true population. Investigators explained that they are willing to accept that 5 times out of 100 (5%), the sample contains a segment of the population with height that is shorter or taller than 95% of the rest of the population.

prior to final decisions. Let's explore how data collection, data entry, and data analysis affect the costs of sample size and selection.

Data Collection

What type of quantitative data will be used? There are two types of quantitative data: primary and secondary data. Primary data is collected by researchers. Secondary data is a set of data that was previously collected.

Investigators gain permission to explore a new research question within the existing data set. Quantitative secondary data include using existing large national data sets that are collected by federal organizations, such as the Centers for Disease Control and Prevention or the National Cancer Institutes.

Investigators also consider the availability of selected individuals. For easier data collection, investigators have a convenient sample of easily assessable individuals. However, in more difficult cases, individuals under study are limited in number or are more difficult to identify.

Data Entry

How will the data be entered for analysis? If the survey data were collected online, there is limited data entry. If the survey data were collected from paper surveys, there are costs associated with data entry.

Quantitative data requires data cleaning, which involves looking at the data spreadsheet and determining what percentage of the data is entered incorrectly or missing from the survey. These errors are corrected by going back to the original survey and correcting the mistakes. Investigators randomly select about 10–15% of the surveys to double-check the data entry for validation. Look at **Table 10-3** for a sample data spreadsheet used in quantitative analysis. Find the data entry errors; there are eight data entry errors total. The answers are located at the end of the chapter.

Table 10-3   Sample Spreadsheet for Quantitative Analysis

Case	v1 Age	v2 Gender 1 = Female 2 = Male	v3 Zip Code	v4 Number of days in Hospital	v5 Satisfaction 1 = Excellent 2 = Very good 3 = Good 4 = Fair 5 = Poor	v6 Recommend 0 = No 1 = Yes
1	45	1	33612	2	5	1
2	62	1	33611	3	5	1
3	57	2	32312	4	4	1
4	33	2	31278	2	4	1
5	47	1	33638	2	3	1
5	68	2	33937	3	4	1
6	71	2	32199	4	5	0
7	73	2	33618	2	3	
8	65	1	33629	1	2	10
9	3	2	32911	1	3	1
10	56	1	32833	3	4	1
11	42	2	33725	4	3	1
12	39	4	33219	38	3	0
13	28	1	34581	1	4	1
14	63	2	33409	3	5	1
15	218	1	33609	3	5	1
16	49	2	32199	3	5	0
17	63	1	33217	2	6	0
18	54	12	33021	1	3	1
19	68	2	93301	2	2	1
20	72	1	33217	3	1	1

Data Analysis

Investigators need to consider the data analysis they will be conducting when selecting the sample size. If descriptive statistics are used (e.g., frequencies and means) then nearly any sample size over 30 is generally sufficient. On the other hand, some complex statistical analyses require a larger sample size (e.g., 200–500). To save time and resources, investigators consult biostatisticians prior to initiating any study to ensure that adequate sampling is achieved for appropriate data analyses. Finally, sample size formulas provide the number of responses needed. However, many investigators add 10–30% to the sample size to compensate for the inability to contact individuals and missing data. Investigators plan for this increase when calculating the research budget.[6]

The cost of data analysis is based on volume of data, the amount of data cleaning needed, complexity of the data analysis performed, and whether there is a need to hire an expert to assist with the analysis (see **Table 10-4**).

Table 10-4 Sample Simple Budget: Quantitative Data

Personnel	Hourly Rate / Number Needed	Hours per Week / Cost per Piece	Weeks	Total
Researcher	$80	20	50	$80,000
Student assistant	$20	25	50	$25,000
Data analysis consultant	$150	10	10	$15,000
Printing				
Recruitment flyers	2,000	0.18		$360
Surveys	1,000	2.15		$2,150
Sample				
Incentives	1,000	10		$10,000
			Total	$132,510

Note: Personnel costs for this simple budget do not include fringe benefits, health insurance, or student tuition.

Budget Justification for Quantitative Data

Personnel:

An investigator will be hired to work 20 hours per week for 50 weeks at $80 per hour, for a total of $80,000.

One student will be hired to work 25 hours per week for 50 weeks at $20 per hour, for a total of $25,000.

A data analysis consultant will be hired to work for 10 hours for the last 10 weeks at $150 per hour, for a total of $15,000.

Sample:

Printing for 2,000 recruitment flyers at $0.18 each will cost $360.

Printing and stapling 1,000 copies of the survey at $2.15 each will cost $2,150.

Incentives for 1,000 participants at $10 each will cost $10,000.

Total: $132,510

Table 10-5　Simple Timeline: Sample 12-Month Timeline for Quantitative Data

Month	Activity	Person Responsible
1st	Establish a funding account for the study; advertise for employ-ment positions	Principal investigator (PI)
2nd	Hire staff	PI
3rd	Develop survey; submit application for institutional review board (IRB) approval for human subjects research	PI
4th	Develop recruitment strategies for participants	PI
5th	Establish a way to provide gift card incentives for participation	PI and student
6th	Quantitative: print surveys or post online	PI and student
7th	Conduct pilot study	PI and student
8th	Revise and submit revisions to the IRB for approval	PI and student
9th	Quantitative: collect survey data	PI and student
10th	Continue to collect data until sample size is achieved	PI and student
11th	Begin to clean data; begin data analysis	PI, student, and data expert
12th	Finalize data analysis	PI, student, and data expert
Wrap-up	Write, edit, and submit final report	PI, student, and data expert

Timeline

In addition to the budget and budget justification, it is important to create a timeline for each study. Although there are multiple types of timelines, each one serves the purpose of keeping the project or study on track (see **Table 10-5**).

Probability and Nonprobability Samples

Let's begin with the basic differences between probability and nonprobability samples. With probability samples, there is no bias in sample selection. The participants are selected based on a strict, objective, and limited criterion such as a random number list. With nonprobability, there is an element of judgment in the selection process. With these two basic differences in mind, let's delve deeper into how probability samples are selected.

Probability Sampling

The first step in probability sampling is to determine the population of interest. Investigators make this decision based on the research questions or evaluation goals and objectives. For example, the population may be based on one or a combination of potential demographic or other specific variables, such as geographical location, gender, age group, ethnicity, religious affiliation, economic status, marital status, type of disease studied, days into remission, and so on.

Once the population is framed, the second step is to determine the different layers within the subset of the population. For example, suppose we have a research question that looks at 10 years of cancer data and asks whether there are different survival rates beyond 12 months for patients with lung cancer based on three things: their stage of disease at diagnosis, type of initial treatment at diagnosis, and age at diagnosis. The first step limits the population of study from *all* types of cancer patients to just lung cancer patients. The second step involves limiting the dataset for patients that survived until at least 12 months after their diagnosis. Then, for the 12-month survivors, the third step would group the survivors by type of initial treatment. Each subsequent step adds another layer until the appropriate groups are formed for further data analyses. This type of probability sampling is systematic and objective. There are no vague decisions, because the sample subject is in one group or the other in the decision tree.[7]

There are several types of probability design, and this discussion includes simple random sampling, quota sampling, and proportionate stratified random sampling.

Simple Random Sampling

Simple random sampling is the most basic way of selecting a group of individuals from a population. The key to simple random sampling is that every individual has an equal chance of being selected from the population. For example, if clinic staff wants to randomly select a group of patients to interview, every active clinic patient must have an equal chance of getting selected. To perform simple random sampling, researchers use a table of random numbers or a computerized random number generator to select the sample of individuals (see **Figure 10-1**).

Simple random sampling has several advantages. It is a straightforward procedure to perform, and investigators may be unable to influence the sample selection (also called bias) because the procedure is controlled by the computer software. Simple random sampling is not feasible for large populations, such as obtaining a list of names of every individual living in a city or county.

Proportionate Stratified Random Sampling

With stratified random sampling, investigators divide the entire population into different subgroups, such as age, gender, and geographical location, which are also called strata. Then the investigators randomly select subjects from each stratum using the same fraction predetermined by investigators. It is important that individuals in each stratum not overlap with other strata. For example, in **Table 10-6**, individuals could not be in both the 70–79 age stratum and the

1. Copy and paste the list of patient names into Column A in Excel.

2. Place the cursor at the top of Column B and type =RAND() into the function toolbar. Hit Enter. In the box of B1, you should see a random number. In this case, it is 0.876972. Now place the cursor on the small black square in the lower right-hand corner of box. With the left-side of the mouse depressed, drag down the B Column.

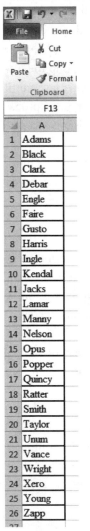

	A
1	Adams
2	Black
3	Clark
4	Debar
5	Engle
6	Faire
7	Gusto
8	Harris
9	Ingle
10	Kendal
11	Jacks
12	Lamar
13	Manny
14	Nelson
15	Opus
16	Popper
17	Quincy
18	Ratter
19	Smith
20	Taylor
21	Unum
22	Vance
23	Wright
24	Xero
25	Young
26	Zapp

	A	B
1	Adams	0.876972
2	Black	0.16729
3	Clark	0.810917
4	Debar	0.836111
5	Engle	0.890288
6	Faire	0.734518
7	Gusto	0.568823
8	Harris	0.16394
9	Ingle	0.449764
10	Kendal	0.135458
11	Jacks	0.215722
12	Lamar	0.786481
13	Manny	0.318046
14	Nelson	0.771621
15	Opus	0.961131
16	Popper	0.985467
17	Quincy	0.734785
18	Ratter	0.987152
19	Smith	0.467334
20	Taylor	0.539435
21	Unum	0.882664
22	Vance	0.040155
23	Wright	0.418034
24	Xero	0.970261
25	Young	0.841087
26	Zapp	0.122716

continues

FIGURE 10-1 Directions for Using Microsoft Excel to Randomize Individuals

3. Highlight Column A and Column B. Click on Sort & Filter in the toolbar. Click on Custom Filter.

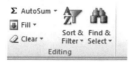

4. Sort by Column B, smallest to largest. Add Level, then sort by Adams.

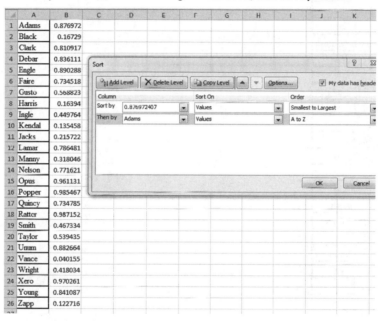

FIGURE 10-1 *continued*

80–89 stratum.[8,9] Individuals may only be in one stratum, so all individuals over age 70 have an equal chance of being randomly selected for study. Stratified random sampling is commonly used for demographic variables, such as age, income, educational attainment, gender, religion, and ethnicity. There are two advantages to using stratified random sampling: (1) investigators obtain representation from subgroups in the given population; and (2) a smaller, but representative, sample size saves investigators' money, time, and effort. For example, if investigators wish to study the elderly population in a retirement community with 1,000 residents, they might use proportionate stratified random sampling. It is essential to

5. Click OK. Keep in mind that each time this procedure is done, the numbers are different and thus the random order of names is different.

	A
1	Adams
2	Gusto
3	Clark
4	Jacks
5	Black
6	Nelson
7	Lamar
8	Ratter
9	Unum
10	Kendal
11	Ingle
12	Taylor
13	Young
14	Harris
15	Zapp
16	Vance
17	Xero
18	Opus
19	Faire
20	Smith
21	Quincy
22	Manny
23	Debar
24	Engle
25	Popper
26	Wright

6. Out of this population of 26 patient names, use the first 20 randomly sorted names from the list. If the population was 1,000 names and the sample size is 200, use the first 200 names of the sorted list.

FIGURE 10-1 *continued*

Table 10-6 Example of Proportionate Stratified Random Sampling

Stratum	Individuals Age 70–79	Individuals Age 80–89	Individuals and over Age 90
Population size	600	280	120
Sampling fraction	1/2	1/2	1/2
Final sample size	300	140	60

remember to use the same sampling fraction across the different population size strata, so that each group is proportionately represented. This sampling ensures no overlap within the sample.

Nonprobability Sampling

Unlike probability sampling, nonprobability sampling does not use random selection. With nonprobability sampling, investigators do not know if the selected sample truly represents the population; therefore, it is less rigorous, less accurate, and less generalizable to the larger population. However, there are situations where investigators desire to select a sample of individuals that represent a specific expertise, demographic characteristic, or condition. This purposeful sampling would not be feasible or practical if investigators used a random sampling design. The following discussion covers several types of nonprobability samples including accidental or convenience sampling, purposive sampling, nonproportional quota sampling, expert sampling, heterogeneity sampling, snowball sampling, and systematic sampling (see **Figure 10-2**).

Accidental or Convenience Sampling

Accidental or convenience sampling is also called intercept sampling or "person on the street" sampling. A few examples of convenience sampling include emailing an online survey to all undergraduate students, asking for personal opinions

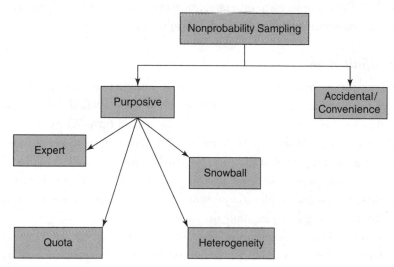

FIGURE 10-2   Nonprobability Sampling

about a specific topic by interviewing students as they walk through the student union (hence, intercept sampling), mailing a paper survey to all pharmacists in a state to gain their opinions about a new state policy on immunizations, and interviewing voters as they exit a polling precinct location. Of course, there are problems with this type of sampling because it is not representative of the population. However, it gives investigators a quick and convenient way to gather data. For example, if investigators want to know the opinions of college students on U.S. healthcare reform, they ask students a few questions as they pass through the student union at a large public university. The sample is not representative of the entire student body, but it is convenient, fast, and relatively inexpensive and provides quick data collection.[2]

Purposive Sampling

With purposive sampling, investigators select individuals with a specific *purpose* in mind. This type of sampling is commonly used by marketing or political advertisement agencies. For example, if marketing researchers want to know the opinions of African American females between the ages of 20 and 40 about a particular presidential candidate, researchers would stand in a busy shopping mall to recruit this specific, purposive sample. After approaching the prospective African American females, they verify their eligibility criteria and then quickly ask a few select questions.[10] In health studies, investigators use purposive sampling to deliberately include individuals who may typically be excluded from the research.[11] For example, purposive sampling would be used if investigators chose to include men with breast cancer in their study.

Quota Sampling

Quota sampling is a technique that uses a small sample that matches characteristics of the target population. For example, suppose the 2010 U.S. Census data states that Bradford County population is composed of 62% White, 18% African American, 12% Hispanic, 6% Asian, and 2% Other racial and ethnic groups and has a gender breakdown that is 51% females and 49% males. Rather than survey the entire population, investigators recruit a sample of individuals who resemble the racial and gender composition of Bradford County. See **Table 10-7** for a quota sampling using a sample size of 500.

According to the information in Table 10-6, once the investigators had 158 white females, they stopped recruiting any additional white females even if more were interested in participating. In this situation, where we have "met the quota," investigators would continue to recruit individuals in the other cells.

Table 10-7 Quota Sampling

	Female (*n* = 255; 51%)	Male (*n* = 245; 49%)
White	158	152
African American	46	44
Hispanic	31	29
Asian	15	15
Other ethnicities	5	5

Nonproportional quota sampling is similar but less restrictive than quota sampling. With nonproportional sampling, investigators specify the minimum number of individuals in each category, but percentage portions are not required to match proportions in the population. Investigators want to ensure that all groups are represented in the study.[10] A 2007 study used nonproportional quota sampling to recruit women at risk for HIV based on their ethnicity and number of sexual partners. Investigators used word of mouth, community organizations, and media sources to recruit equal percentages of White, Black, and Hispanic women, even though equal ethnicity proportions were not representative of the demographics from the women's community. Of the recruited women, 29% were in single-partner relationships and the other 71% were in multipartner relationships. For this study, nonproportional quota sampling allowed adequate representation of women at risk for HIV.[12]

Expert Sampling

Expert sampling is defined as recruiting a group of individuals with known expertise or experience in a specific discipline. This type of sampling is also called a "panel of experts."[10] There are two common reasons for investigators to use expert sampling. First, investigators ask the experts their opinions of the proposed research to gain further insight into solutions or potential pitfalls. Second, investigators ask the experts to support or refute specific topics of interest. This method allows investigators to defend their decisions based on expert opinions rather than merely guessing.[13,14]

Heterogeneity Sampling

Heterogeneity sampling is defined as seeking a wide range of different and diverse opinions. In heterogeneity sampling, investigators are recruiting a diversity of ideas rather than diversity among participating individuals. Investigators are seeking unique and unusual opinions.[10] For example, investigators may use heterogeneity sampling to seek opinions about healthcare reform. They want all opinions rather than seeking how the typical individual voted on the healthcare reform amendment on the ballot, as done with modal instance sampling.

Snowball Sampling

Snowball sampling is defined as when investigators identify one individual who meets the inclusion criteria for the study and then investigators ask the individual if he or she knows someone else who meets the inclusion criteria. With snowball sampling, the sample is not representative, but it can be valuable for specific studies.[10,15] For example, investigators may wish to interview nurses who are retired from the state health department after working there for more than 25 years. However, depending on the research or evaluation topic, snowball sampling poses ethical issues, such as revealing an individual's lifestyle choice or medical condition without consent. For example, if investigators wish to interview medical and nursing students from the lesbian, gay, bisexual, and transgender (LGBT) community, they would talk to medical and nursing students from the LGBT community. After the interviews, the investigators would ask if the students knew other students in the LGBT community who might wish to participate in an interview to increase the sample size. This technique would pose ethical issues if the referred student had not yet made the decision to be identified as a member of the LGBT community. There are numerous other groups of individuals who may not wish to be identified, such as those living HIV/AIDS or other diseases, people diagnosed with mental health challenges, former prisoners, or unemployed or homeless individuals, and many other groups. Investigators need to be aware of such ethical issues when using the snowball sampling technique.

Sampling Bias

When investigators chose a sampling design, they must be aware of potential bias. In research or evaluation, bias is defined as an error caused by systematically selecting one individual or outcome over another.[16] Sampling bias occurs when the selected individuals do not represent the population. When sampling bias occurs, investigators are not able to generalize their findings to the whole population that was supposed to be studied.[2] For example, investigators wanted to study the effectiveness of a hypertension drug on adult patients with diabetes. However, they recruited adult patients with diabetes from a large inner-city Medicaid clinic. This type of sample results in sampling bias, because it is likely that adult patients with diabetes and hypertension receiving Medicaid may have different health issues than adult patients with diabetes and hypertension not receiving Medicaid. Even when investigators select the ideal sampling design, they may encounter bias after the data are collected. After investigators recognize that data are missing, they determine whether the missing data are cause for concern of a nonresponse bias. There are two types of nonresponse bias: item nonresponse and unit nonresponse.[17]

Item Nonresponse Bias

Item nonresponse is best described as individuals leaving several survey questions blank (see **Table 10-8**). When this happens, investigators are faced with making a decision about what to do about the missing responses. In this situation, there are three common ways to handle the missing data, including case deletion, mean replacement, and item deletion.

Case Deletion

With case deletion, investigators determine what percentage of item nonresponse they are willing to tolerate. This percentage changes depending on the type of survey and the sampling design. For example, if an individual completes only 50 out of 100 survey questions, investigators agree that the entire survey is removed from the data collection. However, if an individual leaves 2 out of 100 questions blank, investigators would keep the other 98 responses. Prior to making the final decision on what percentage of blank survey questions are allowed in the data, investigators calculate the overall response rate of survey questions. If the

Table 10-8   Sample of Data Spreadsheet with Missing Data

Case	v1 Age	v2 Gender 1 = Female 2 = Male	v3 Marital Status 1 = Single 2 = Married 3 = Divorced 4 = Widowed	v4 Health Status Today 1 = Excellent 2 = Very good 3 = Fair 4 = Good 5 = Poor	v5 Program Satisfaction 1 = Excellent 2 = Very good 3 = Good 4 = Fair 5 = Poor	v6 Recommend 0 = No 1 = Yes
1	45	1	2	2	5	0
2	62	1	3	3	5	1
3	57		2	4	4	1
4	33	2		2	4	1
5	47	1	4		3	
6	68	2	1	3	4	1

response rate is low, they are less likely to delete an entire survey with a few blank questions, because that would remove the completed responses as well.

Many problems related to item nonresponse are reduced or eliminated by conducting a pilot study. In the pilot study, the exact survey is given to a small sample of individuals to "test" the survey and note any errors. After the pilot study is complete, investigators revise the survey as needed and print the final survey or post it online. Even after conducting several survey pilot testing sessions, it is unlikely but still possible for errors to occur. If the survey is available online for five days, investigators scan through the responses as data become available. Upon review, investigators determine whether individuals complete every question, leave the same questions blank, or leave random questions blank. If many respondents leave the same question blank, then investigators review the specific question to identify problems with inappropriate wording, response choices, or other possible errors. After the problem is identified, investigators decide what they should do about it. If time permits, investigators correct the question and repeat the survey online. If funding permits, paper surveys are reprinted for the remaining data collection sites. Lastly, investigators delete the question from the data analyses.

Mean Replacement

Mean replacement is another way to handle item nonresponse. The word *mean* in statistics is defined as average. The mean is calculated by adding the responses and then dividing the total by the number of responses. In the mean replacement, investigators calculate the mean response for each survey question, then each time individuals leave a survey question blank, investigators fill in the blank with the mean score of how the other individuals responded. For example, 179 out of 200 individuals answered the Likert scale question, "How would you rate your health today? 5 = excellent, 4 = very good, 3 = good, 2 = fair, and 1 = poor." The mean score (average) for the 179 respondents was 3.8 for this question. Investigators would fill in 3.8 on the blank response for the 21 individuals who left this question blank. The same procedure is repeated for each missing response. The disadvantage of this solution is that it causes the survey response to be closer to the mean than it might have been if the individuals actually answered the question. For example, those individuals who left the question blank may have felt poorly and did not wish to complete the survey at all. Their actual responses may have lowered the mean score, but investigators have no way to verify the information.

Item Deletion

Item deletion is defined as deleting only that one question. For example, 87 out of 200 college students answered the Likert scale question, "How many sexual partners have you had in the last 30 days? 7 = six or more sexual partners, 6 = five sexual partners, 5 = four sexual partners, 4 = three sexual partners, 3 = two sexual partners, 2 = one sexual partner, 1 = I did not have any sexual partners in the last 30 days, 0 = I prefer not to respond." If only 87 (43.5%) of college students responded, mean replacement is not appropriate. A better choice is to report that 43.5% responded with a mean score of 2.8 (or between one and two sexual partners) in the last 30 days; however, 56.5% selected "I prefer not to respond."

Unit Nonresponse Bias

In unit nonresponse bias, the word *unit* is defined as if or when a type or group of individuals respond to a survey. The following examples illustrate several types of unit nonresponse bias.

- Unit nonresponse bias occurs when the sampling design, such as quota sampling, is unable to obtain responses from certain segments of the samples. For example, unit nonresponse happens when investigators are seeking 50 individuals in each of four segments—50–59 years of age, 60–69 years of age, 70–79 years of age, and 80–89 years of age—but only 18 of the 50 individuals in the 80–89 years of age category completed the interview. The lack of respondents in one segment causes a bias to occur, because the 32 nonrespondents in the 80–89 years of age segment may have provided responses different from the 18 in that segment who did respond.

- When investigators collect survey data, they keep track of when each survey is returned. When paper copy surveys are returned, investigators label each survey with the date it was received. In addition, each survey is numbered in consecutive order. For online surveys, the survey software assigns a date and time to each survey upon submission. During data analyses, investigators determine if the early responders are different from the late responders. Because late responders are considered to be more like nonresponders, investigators estimate how the nonresponders may have answered. This information provides an estimate of the unit nonresponse bias. For example, let's say that an online survey was emailed to all university employees. Investigators found that administrative assistants responded first without any reminder emails, whereas administrators responded last and only after one or two reminder emails. Investigators use these findings to make further predictions about the profile and reasons why some individuals respond early rather than late.

- Instead of investigators comparing early and late responders, they study the demographic groups or profiles (such as gender, age, ethnicity, and income level) of survey respondents. In the data analysis, investigators compare survey responses of various demographic characteristics. In some studies, investigators compare survey response data to U.S. Census data. If data differ, there may be a nonresponse bias in the study data. For example, survey questions ask for a respondent's zip code, annual household income, and mode of transportation used. If the majority of respondents in the same zip code inflate their annual household income, investigators would note this difference when compared to the U.S. Census. If 90% of respondents in the same zip code say they drive a car as their mode of transportation, investigators could verify the zip and mode of transportation with the U.S. Census. If a bias is noted, investigators would need to question the accuracy of the other survey responses from the same respondents. This type of comparison is called database verification. Investigators compare survey responses with data in a verifiable database, such as U.S. census data. This process allows investigators to verify the accuracy of the data and to determine the accuracy and nonresponse bias. In another example, clinic patients are invited to complete a survey. In the survey, respondents are asked to provide their height and weight. Their responses are verified by the electronic medical record containing the respondents' actual height and weight. With community surveys, database verification is usually not possible.[12]

All of these techniques allow investigators to presume when a bias exists in their data. Discussion of how statisticians adjust the data analysis to account for unit nonresponse bias is beyond the scope of this chapter. However, it is noted that reducing nonresponse bias in the survey development phase saves time and data adjustment in the data analysis phase.[12]

Summary

This chapter began with the definitions of populations and samples. The next section explained the concept of null hypothesis including type I and type II errors and level of significance. With an understanding of null hypothesis, the discussion moved to each component of sample size determination, such as margin of error and confidence levels. The next section explained the difference between probability and nonprobability sampling. The last section presented how sampling bias affects the study results including item nonresponse bias.

Case Study

Nurses from three colleges of nursing in the state of Florida received federal dollars to investigate the history of nursing as a way to facilitate the future of the profession by looking at its past. The research question is, "How does nursing practice in the past influence nursing practice of the future?" For the first two years of funding, the research nursing faculty decided to focus on nurses living in Florida.

For this study, researchers selected a complex sample design. Because this research involves qualitative and quantitative data collection, several different sample designs are used. Researchers decided to begin the research by contacting and interviewing retired nurses residing in Florida. Researchers contacted the Florida Board of Professional Licensure to purchase a list of names and contact information for all registered nurses. However, they were told that because of privacy regulations, the list was not available for purchase, so researchers devised another recruitment strategy.

Phase 1: Prior to the initiation of phase 1, researchers obtained institutional review board approval for this research. For phase 1, snowball sampling was selected to identify a few retired nurses known to the research team. Researchers asked those nurses for the names of other retired nurses living in Florida. The disadvantage with this sampling technique is that the sample is not a representative sample of all retired nurses in Florida, but it remains valuable for the first phase of this research. During this phase, researchers conducted in-depth interviews with retired nurses to gain an overall snapshot of where the profession of nursing was in Florida when they began their nursing careers. Identical questions were asked of each nurse interviewed. Retired nurses were excited to participate in the interviews and gladly shared names of other retired nurses in Florida. Because several of the interviewed nurses lived

continues

CASE STUDY *continued*

in retirement communities, some of the contacts were located down the hall in the same apartment complex. The convenience of snowball sampling outweighed the disadvantages for phase 1 of the project. Upon completion of each digitally recorded interview, transcriptionists were available to transcribe the interviews for immediate review by the nursing researchers. The first snowball sampling yielded interviews mostly from retired white, female nurses. At the time that these nurses began their careers, hospitals in the south remained segregated. Researchers continued to use the snowball sampling to identify retired Black nurses with experience working in segregated Black-only hospitals and, later, integrated hospitals. The general themes of the phase 1 interview paved the way for phase 2.

Phase 2: In Florida, there are approximately 25,500 registered nurses in the workforce. However, every year, more than 16,500 leave nursing for one reason or another, so the net result is approximately 9,000 registered nurses. The required sample size is 370 with a 5% margin of error. However, researchers added 30% to the sample for possible missing data and inability to contact some nurses because of inaccurate contact information. In January 2009, the average age of Florida nurses was 47.7 years, with more than half of the nursing workforce being over age 50. The average age of nurses taking the licensing examination for the first time was 33 years of age.[18]

Because the Florida Board of Professional Regulations Nursing website does not offer data on the gender and ethnicity distribution for Florida nurses, this research uses the ethnic distribution for Florida's population. Because nursing remains a female-dominated field, the sample size reflects female nurses, but researchers recruit male nurses to participate in the study when possible.

Number of Florida Registered Nurses:	9,000
Margin of Error:	5%
Final Sample Size:	370
Additional 30% for missing data:	111
Total:	481

continues

CASE STUDY *continued*

In phase 2, researchers contacted the Florida Nursing Association (FNA) to purchase a list of their member mailing list for registered nurses. Because the FNA is a private association, it is allowed to sell mailing lists of members. Although not all active Florida registered nurses are FNA members, this list serves as an adequate representative sample of all Florida nurses. Because the survey will be mailed to FNA members at their home addresses, they may select to participate by completing and returning the survey or they may decide not to.

Based on the general themes from phase 1, researchers developed survey questions for phase 2. The 80-question survey questions included, but were not limited to, demographic information (e.g., age, ethnicity, marital status, gender, highest education degree), years of nursing employment, location of employment, reasons for staying in nursing, and how nursing has changed during their career. The last question in the survey asked respondents if they would be interested in participating in a 30-minute follow-up telephone interview.

Phase 3: Assuming that the sample size of 481 was achieved in phase 2, researchers utilized random sampling and quota sampling in phase 3. Researchers had funding to conduct 100 30-minute telephone interviews. This process involved dividing the surveys into four piles based on ethnicity of respondents: White, Black, Hispanic, or other ethnicity. The surveys in each pile were assigned consecutive numbers starting with 1. Using a random number generator, survey numbers were pulled until the quota was fulfilled (see **Table 10-9**).[19]

Table 10-9 Quota Sampling Based on Florida Demographics

	White	Black	Hispanic	Other Ethnicities
	57.5%	16.5%	22.9%	3.1%
Final Sample Size: 100	57	17	23	3

Interview questions for phase 3 were generated from survey responses in phase 2. Telephone interviews were conducted to verify if the survey data matched the actual practice and opinions of nurses currently working in nursing.

continues

CASE STUDY *continued*

Case Study Discussion Questions

1. List the various types of sampling techniques combined in this case study.
2. Describe the process of how the researchers will coordinate and conduct 100 30-minute telephone interviews.

Student Activity

Matthew is hired by the March of Dimes Foundation of Nevada to evaluate one of its programs. This educational program has been run in several cities in Nevada to lower the percentage of babies born prematurely and with low birth weight. It invites pregnant women to enroll in a prenatal health class at no charge; it has been in place for 2 years. The class is offered at local women's hospitals and allows women to schedule their prenatal check-ups for the same day that they attend the half-hour class. The class covers many issues, from eating healthy foods and exercising to the importance of stress reduction and social support. The class also offers important prenatal vitamins to the women. Over the last 2 years, 500 women have taken part in the educational classes in different cities. The March of Dimes Foundation of Nevada would like to see if this program is doing as good a job as other groups at lowering rates of premature and low birth weight among women of poor physical and socioeconomic conditions. Matthew decides to conduct a survey. To do this, he must take a sample.

1. What does Matthew need to consider before he starts his research project?
2. What list does he need to have before he can select his sample?
3. What type of sampling method should Matthew use for this study? Why did you choose your answer?
4. What is the appropriate sample size for this study if researchers want to have a 5% margin of error? (Use the following table.)

5. Below is a table that lists one of the strata. Determine the number of individuals that will need to be included in the sample.

Stratum	Did Not Finish High School	Earned High School Diploma/GED	Some College Education	Earned College Diploma
Population size	63	246	74	117
Sampling fraction	50%	50%	50%	50%
Sample size				

6. Suppose one of the clinics had a fire, and some of the patient files were lost. From talking to the prenatal educator, you know that this clinic regularly sees members from a nearby Native American community. You want to make sure that you are including an adequate number of Native Americans. Before completing your sampling frame and starting the research project, you ask a current participant in the program who is a member of this Native American community if she knows of other members who have gone through the program. She gives you the names of 4 other mothers, who then collectively give you an additional 17 names. What type of sampling is this?

Answers

1. Matthew needs to consider how many mothers he will investigate (the sample size).
2. Before he can select his sample, Matthew needs a list of all the women who have attended the program over the last two years. This is called his sampling frame. Matthew will take the sample from the sampling frame.
3. The appropriate sampling method for Matthew to choose is stratified random sampling, because he would like to know more about the physical and socioeconomic conditions of the mothers who have gone through the class in the last two years. Matthew could look at age, race, income, and education level as different strata.
4. The appropriate sample size for this study would be 217 participants.

5.

Stratum	Did Not Finish High School	Earned High School Diploma/GED	Some College Education	Earned College Diploma
Population size	63	246	74	117
Sampling fraction	50%	50%	50%	50%
Sample size	31	123	37	59

6. This is called snowball sampling, where one person who met the criteria you were looking for informed you about others they knew who might also meet that criteria.

References

1. Downing D, Clark J. *Statistics: The Easy Way*, 2nd ed. Hauppauge, NY: Barron's Educational Series, Inc.; 1989.

2. Ary D, Jacobs L, Razavieh A, Sorenson C. *Introduction to Research in Education*, 8th ed. Belmont, CA: Wadsworth / Cengage Learning; 2010.

3. Blair R, Taylor R. *Biostatistics for the Health Sciences*. Upper Saddle River, NJ: Pearson Prentice Hall; 2008.

4. Significance in Statistics and Surveys. Creative Research Systems. Available at: http://www.surveysystem.com/signif.htm. Accessed May 3, 2012.

5. The Research Advisors. Sample Size Table. Available at: http://www.research-advisors .com/tools/SampleSize.htm. Last updated 2006. Accessed May 3, 2012.

6. Israel G. Determining Sample Size. University of Florida, Institute of Food and Agricultural Studies Extension. Available at: http://edis.ifas.ufl.edu/pd006. Accessed May 3, 2012.

7. Doherty M. Probability versus non-probability sampling in sample surveys. *The New Zealand Statistics Review*. 1994;(7):21–28.

8. Castillo J. Stratified Sampling Method. Experiment Resources. Available at: http://www.experiment-resources.com/stratified-sampling.html. Last updated 2009. Accessed May 3, 2012.

9. Stratified Random Sampling. Stat Trek. Available at: http://stattrek.com/survey-research/stratified-sampling.aspx. Accessed May 3, 2012.

10. Trochim W. Nonprobability Sampling. Research Methods Knowledge Base. Available at: http://www.socialresearchmethods.net/kb/sampnon.php. Last updated October 20, 2006. Accessed May 3, 2012.

11. Barbour R. Checklists for improving rigor in qualitative research: A case of the tail wagging the dog? *Brit Med J*. 2001;322:115–117.

12. Morrow K, Vargas S, Rosen R, Christensen A, Salomon L, Shulman L, Barroso C, Fava J. The utility of non-proportional quota sampling for recruiting at-risk women for microbicide research. *AIDS Behav*. 2007;11:586–595.

13. Sampling. Statistics Solutions. Available at: http://www.statisticssolutions.com /academic-solutions/resources/dissertation-resources/sample-size-calculation-and -sample-size-justification/. Accessed September 26, 2013.

14. Stewart D, Strasser G. Expert role assignment and information sampling during collective recall and decision making. *J Pers Soc Psychol.* 1995;69(4):619–628.

15. Browne K. Snowball sampling: Using social networks to research non-heterosexual women. *Int J of Soc Res Meth.* 2005;8(1):47–60.

16. Panzeri S, Magri C, Carraro L. Sampling Bias. Scholarpedia. Available at: http://www.scholarpedia.org/article/Sampling_bias. Last updated 2008. Accessed May 3, 2012.

17. Groves R. Nonresponse rates and nonresponse bias in household surveys. *Public Opin Q.* 2006;70(5):646–675.

18. Kalla S. Measurement of uncertainty: Standard deviation. Experiment Resources. Available at: http://www.experiment-resources.com/measurement-of-uncertainty-standard-deviation.html. Last updated 2009. Accessed May 3, 2012.

19. How to Measure Variability in a Dataset. Stat Trek. Available at: http://stattrek.com/sampling/variance.aspx. Accessed May 3, 2012.

Answers to Table 10-3 Sample Spreadsheet for Quantitative Analysis

Case	v1 Age	v2 Gender 1 = Female 2 = Male	v3 Zip Code	v4 Number of Days in Hospital	v5 Satisfaction 1 = Excellent 2 = Very good 3 = Good 4 = Fair 5 = Poor	v6 Recommend 0 = No 1 = Yes
1	45	1	33612	2	5	1
2	62	1	33611	3	5	1
3	57	2	32312	4	4	1
4	33	2	31278	2	4	1
5	47	1	33638	2	3	1
5	68	2	33937	3	4	1
6	71	2	32199	4	5	0
7	73	2	33618	2	3	No data
8	65	1	33629	1	2	**10**
9	**3**	2	32911	1	3	1
10	56	1	32833	3	4	1
11	42	2	33725	4	3	1
12	39	**4**	33219	**38**	3	0
13	28	1	34581	1	4	1
14	63	2	33409	3	5	1
15	**218**	1	33609	3	5	1
16	49	2	32199	3	5	0
17	63	1	33217	2	**6**	0
18	54	**12**	33021	1	3	1
19	68	2	**93301**	2	2	1
20	72	1	33217	3	1	1

Inferential Statistics

CHAPTER OBJECTIVES

By the end of this chapter, students will be able to:

- Discuss the need for statistics to explain data
- Describe the differences between scientific hypothesis, research questions, null hypothesis, and alternative hypothesis
- Explain the difference between one-tailed and two-tailed inferential statistical tests
- Describe when it is appropriate to use an independent *t*-test and when it is appropriate to use a paired samples *t*-test
- Explain the purpose of correlation coefficients
- Create a scenario to explain the benefits of confidence intervals
- Define type I and type II errors

KEY TERMS

Alternative hypothesis	Null hypothesis
Chi-square	One-tailed tests
Coefficients	*t*-tests
Confidence intervals	Two-tailed tests
Correlations	Type I and type II errors
Inferential statistics	

Introduction

This chapter begins with a discussion of why we need to use statistics to understand data. The first section defines the concepts of scientific hypothesis, research questions, null hypothesis, and alternative hypothesis. After these concepts are understood, the next section explains the difference between one-tailed and two-tailed inferential statistical tests. Building upon this knowledge, various statistical tests are introduced using multiple examples. The chapter concludes with definitions of type I and type II errors. Because it is a common belief among students that learning statistics is difficult, this chapter attempts to present the new terms and definitions as clearly as possible with plenty of applied examples. If at any time a concept is not understood, stop and review the previous section. Using this technique builds a foundation of basic definitions of statistics for future use.

Types of Statistics

Statistics is a branch of mathematics used for data collection, analysis, and interpretation of data.[1] Statistics are used in evaluation and research across most disciplines, including natural science, social science, and business and government. Statistics are used to answer questions related to data. There are two basic types of statistics: descriptive and inferential. Descriptive statistics organize and summarize data without the use of complicated mathematical equations. In this chapter, inferential statistics are defined in detail. For now, think of inferential statistics as the study of drawing associations and conclusions about a population from a random sample of data taken from that population. For example, because it is impossible to study the driving habits of every driver in one county, investigators survey a random sample of drivers and draw conclusions about all drivers in that county based on the sample. Unlike descriptive statistics, inferential statistics use mathematical equations to generate probabilities about a population. These probabilities help researchers, program planners, and evaluators make important decisions about their data. Using Microsoft Excel, this chapter presents a few basic equations or statistical tests as a way to illustrate how inferential statistics are applied to data.

The Need for Statistics

Let's explore why statistics are important to use and understand. For researchers and evaluators, statistics are essential for understanding the data. Without using inferential statistics, it is not possible to determine patterns, make associations, and draw conclusions from the data you have collected. For example, without using inferential statistics, medical researchers would have no way of knowing if one drug was more effective in curing disease than another drug. Researchers could not see patterns in indoor air quality and asthma rates in a community. Evaluators would not know which type of smoking cessation programs was most effective in reducing smoking rates among young adults. Engineers would not know which model of automobile seatbelt was most effective in saving lives. Manufacturers would not know the level of sun protection factor (SPF) needed to provide adequate protection against sun exposure. The list goes on and on, but it is evident that inferential statistics are used to move science forward and thus improve quality of life. Lastly, it is important to note that statistics not only let us know if there are associations and patterns with which to draw conclusions, but also let us know that those associations and conclusions are not due to chance or random error within a particular sample. Though it is part of much more sophisticated statistical techniques than are discussed in this text, higher-level statistics informs researchers not only that a change took place but also, sometimes, how the change took place.

Inferential Statistics

Now let's take the next step in describing inferential statistics in greater detail. As with all investigations, it is necessary to begin with a research question or measurable objectives. Inferential statistics are no different in that each statistical project begins with a question. Think of the question as the roadmap. Travelers begin each trip by determining their destination. Whether traveling by car, train, bus, plane, or ship, travelers plot their journeys by purchasing tickets or programming a GPS device. The same is true with research and evaluation. Investigators do not collect data without first developing a question or roadmap for their study.

For example, suppose you were part of an investigation that wanted to ask, "Do patients with osteoarthritis have greater self-reported pain relief when they use a commonly prescribed drug or a new experimental drug?" As previously stated, it is not feasible to study an entire population, so investigators collect data from a randomly selected sample of the population. As the name implies, investigators use inferential statistics to "infer" or understand how the sample data helps to know the larger population. For example, let's suppose that there are about 20,000 individuals suffering from osteoarthritis in Florida. Because Florida is a large state, it is impossible to recruit all 20,000 individuals to participate in a study related to pain management for osteoarthritis. Instead, investigators recruit 300 individuals with a diagnosis of osteoarthritis from three different clinics. After signing the informed consent documents, they are randomly assigned to one of the two study groups. In the study, 150 patients with osteoarthritis receive the commonly prescribed pain management drug, and the other 150 patients receive the experimental pain management drug.

Prior to the initiation of the actual study, investigators use inferential statistics to determine if the recruited patients have the same characteristics as most other patients with osteoarthritis. For example, investigators want to know if their levels of pain are typical for other patients with osteoarthritis. They want to know what type of health insurance they have, as well as other important characteristics such as age, gender, socioeconomic status, and body mass index (BMI). This type of information allows investigators to know if their study sample is representative of the population of all patients with osteoarthritis. It is important to make sure the sample is representative of the entire population. Investigators want to make sure that if the new experimental pain reliever reduces patients' pain, it is because it really is more effective rather than for some unknown reason related to the particular characteristics of the patients included in the investigation.

After the data are collected, the investigators used inferential statistics to infer whether the experimental pain-relieving drug (1) reduces pain more than the commonly prescribed pain reliever, (2) does not reduce pain as effectively as the commonly prescribed pain reliever, or (3) reduces pain to the same degree as the commonly prescribed pain reliever. This simple example illustrates how investigators move from asking the initial question or objective, to recruiting individuals, to collecting data, to using inferential statistics to determine which drug, if any, is more effective.

Before moving to the next section, let's discuss a little more about statistical tests. Because there are hundreds of statistical tests, evaluators and researchers select the appropriate type of test based on their questions or objectives and the type of data. Using inferential statistics, they draw conclusions related to the data. It is easy for inexperienced researchers and evaluators to use the drop-down menus available in complex statistical computer software programs, but this method does not ensure that the correct statistical test was chosen. Without thoroughly understanding the purpose of various statistical tests, it is easy to receive an incorrect computer-generated result by choosing the wrong test. For this reason, it is important to consult with a statistician to ensure that the correct statistical test is chosen.

In the next section, the discussion turns to scientific hypothesis, research questions, null hypothesis, and alternative hypothesis. All of these terms are useful in understanding inferential statistics.

Scientific Hypothesis

A scientific hypothesis is described as an educated guess based on prior observation, knowledge, or experience that can be supported or refuted through observations or experiments. Scientific hypotheses make predictions that can be duplicated with future research or evaluations. After the same research is repeated multiple times, enough evidence is collected to support or disprove the scientific hypothesis.[2] For example, it took decades of research to gather enough evidence to link tobacco use to lung cancer.

Research Questions

Research questions, like evaluation objectives, provide a clear and concise roadmap on which to focus the study. When creating a research question, it is important to address the issue of what topic or evidence is being supported or refuted in this proposed research. Research questions need to be stated as testable questions that can be specifically studied in an investigation. Let's review a few research questions:

Weak:	What is the relationship between asthma and air quality?
Strong:	For children younger than 10 years of age with asthma, is there a relationship between the day and time of their asthma episodes and the pollen index of their geographical location?
Weak:	Does the application of ice reduce the level of pain after physical therapy?
Strong:	When ice is applied for 20 minutes following a physical therapy treatment session for patients with joint injuries, how do patients report their pain levels 4 hours later?[3]

Null Hypothesis and Alternate Hypothesis

Now that the concepts of scientific hypothesis and research questions are understood, it is time to define the null hypothesis. The word *null* means no difference or no association. The best way to remember the null hypothesis is to understand that the investigator is trying to disprove or refute the statement that there is no difference or no association. In other words, when using inferential statistics, the way that investigators support their hypothesis is to refute the null hypothesis. The null hypothesis refers to the situation in the population. Investigators study a representative sample from the population to find evidence to refute the null hypothesis. You may often hear another term used for the research question, called the alternate hypothesis, when investigators are also discussing the null hypothesis. For example, investigators must assume that their alternate hypothesis is wrong until they find sufficient evidence to the contrary.[4] By using inferential statistics, investigators make a decision to reject or fail to reject the null hypothesis. But what does that mean? Let's look at a few examples so these concepts begin to make sense.

Example 1

Research question:	Do patients with osteoarthritis have greater self-reported pain relief with the commonly prescribed drug or the new experimental drug?
Null hypothesis:	There is no difference between the commonly prescribed drug and the new experimental drug in the self-reported pain experienced by osteoarthritis patients.
Alternate hypothesis:	There is a difference between the commonly prescribed drug and the new experimental drug in the self-reported pain experienced by osteoarthritis patients.

Here is what you need to be thinking when you read this null hypothesis: using inferential statistics to analyze the data collected from the two groups of patients with osteoarthritis, there is enough evidence to reject (or fail to reject) the null hypothesis.

Example 2

Research question:	At the end of 3 months on the Lost-It weight management program, do females working the day shift or females working the night shift lose more weight?
Null hypothesis:	At the end of 3 months on the Lost-It weight management program, there is no difference in weight between females working the day shift and females working the night shift.
Alternate hypothesis:	At the end of 3 months on the Lost-It weight management program, there is a difference in weight between females working the day shift and females working the night shift.

Here is what you need to be thinking when you read this null hypothesis: using inferential statistics to analyze the data collected from the day shift females and night shift females on the Lost-It weight management program, there is enough evidence to reject (or fail to reject) the null hypothesis.

Why can't investigators state that they "accept" or "reject" the null hypothesis? Why is the phrase "fail to reject" used instead of "accept"? It is easier to understand the answer to this question by looking at the previous example. Rejecting the null hypothesis means that the investigation provided evidence to support the notion that there is a difference in weight loss among day shift females and night shift females that is not due to chance alone at the end of 3 months on the Lost-It weight management program. Failing to reject the null hypothesis means that the investigation failed to provide evidence to support the notion that there is no difference in weight loss between day shift females and night shift females at the end of 3 months. Therefore, when the null hypothesis is rejected, the evidence from the data analysis does not support the null hypothesis.[5,6] Investigators should never "accept" the null hypothesis. Doing so would say that they are 100% sure of the null hypothesis in all situations.

Basic Inferential Statistical Tests

One-Tailed and Two-Tailed Statistical Tests

Now that you are starting to understand when to reject or fail to reject the null hypothesis, it is time to introduce the terms *one-tailed* and *two-tailed tests*. Let's begin by stating that investigators determine whether to use a one-tailed or two-tailed test when they state the null hypothesis. The majority of statistical tests allow investigators to select a one-tailed test or a two-tailed test. The discussion begins by defining the one-tailed test.

One-Tailed Test

Investigators use a one-tailed test when their null hypothesis reflects a specific direction. See **Figure 11-1**. The white area shows 95% of all values that, if obtained, fail to reject the null hypothesis. The shaded area shows the 5% of possible values that would reject the null hypothesis, also called the critical area. The critical value shown with an arrow is discussed in detail later in the chapter. One-tailed tests may have the critical value and area on either the far left side or the far right side, depending on the null hypothesis, but only on one side of the normal curve. If investigators select a one-tailed test, the obtained or calculated value might fall in the extreme positive or extreme negative side, depending on what the investigator is studying. It is possible for investigators to falsely reject

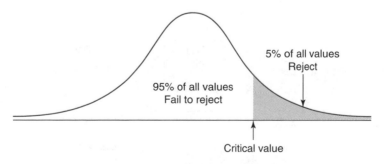

FIGURE 11-1   One-Tailed Statistical Tests

the null hypothesis; thus investigators select a one-tailed test only when they have reason to believe that the difference falls in a specific direction.

Null hypothesis:	When using Drug H, there is no difference in amount of weight gained by patients undergoing chemotherapy.
Alternative hypothesis:	When using Drug H, there is a difference in amount of weight gained by patients undergoing chemotherapy.

Investigators stating this null hypothesis are interested in only the amount of weight gained while taking Drug H. Investigators conducting this study are confident that Drug H improves weight gain among patients undergoing chemotherapy. In this example, investigators must be so confident in the weight gain that they choose to ignore the possibility that some patients taking Drug H may lose weight and thus fall anywhere outside the critical area. Without high confidence based on previous research results, using a one-tailed test results in a serious mistake. Often when patients undergo chemotherapy, they lose weight. Investigators need to be certain that Drug H does not cause weight loss in some patients prior to using a one-tailed test.

Two-Tailed Test

When using a two-tailed test, the normal curve is divided into three sections: the large middle section represents 95% of all possible values, and each of the two side sections represents 2.5% of the possible values. The total of the possible values represented under the normal curve should be 100%. **Figure 11-2** illustrates a two-tailed test, so named because the 5% chance is divided equally (2.5% each) under the two tails of the curve.

Using Excel for Statistics

Now it is time to use Microsoft Excel to learn a few basic statistical calculations. First, it is necessary to add the Excel Analysis ToolPak to your computer

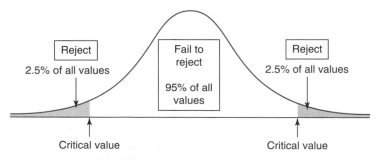

FIGURE 11-2　Two-Tailed Statistical Tests

using the directions in **Figure 11-3**. Once you have added the Analysis ToolPak to your computer, it is easier to follow the examples in the remainder of this chapter. Let's begin by introducing a statistical test called the chi-square test. The symbol χ^2 is used in the literature to refer to this statistical test.

Chi-Square Test

The type of data used for a chi-square test is called nonparametric data because the data does not require normal distribution. Nonparametric data

Step One: Click the File tab, click Options, and then click the Add-Ins category.
Step Two: Select Analysis ToolPak. Click Go and then OK.

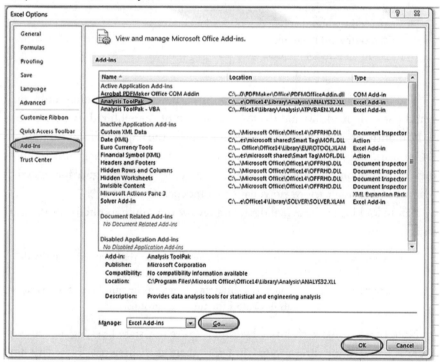

Step Three: Data Analysis appears in the Toolbar under the Data tab.

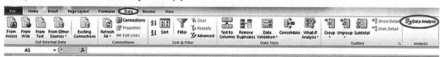

FIGURE 11-3   Installing the Excel Analysis ToolPak
Used with permission from Microsoft

allows investigators to analyze nominal data, such as frequencies.[6] There are several types of chi-square statistical tests. This discussion explains the one-sample chi-square or "goodness-of-fit" test. The one-sample chi-square test requires categorical data for two variables. Each variable has two, three, or four levels. For this example, one variable is dichotomous and offers two responses: yes or no. The second variable is related to age. The categorical data must be independent. Independence is when there is no chance that one responding individual could correctly select more than one response for a single survey question; that is, the responses are mutually exclusive. Review the following survey questions:

At what age did your child complete the required series of immunizations?
   a. 6 months to 12 months
   b. 12 months to 24 months
   c. 24 months or later
Please mark the group that best describes your child's age:
   a. 6 months to 11 months
   b. 12 months to 23 months
   c. 24 months or older

The first example is not mutually exclusive, because a responding individual could correctly mark (a) and (b) for completion of the required immunizations at 12 months or mark (b) and (c) for completion of the required immunizations at 24 months. The violation of independence does not allow investigators to know how many respondents are incorrectly placed in the wrong category for analysis.[6] The second example shows no violation of independence.

Before looking at the actual data, let's review the null hypothesis for this survey question:

Null hypothesis: There is no difference between the numbers of individuals in each of the three age groups.
Alternate hypothesis: There is a difference between the numbers of individuals in each of the three age groups.

Note that the above alternate hypothesis does not state how big a difference there is between the three groups, just that there *is* a difference. Now let's look at some actual data entered into Excel for 60 parents who responded to the survey question (see **Figure 11-4**). The codebook for this survey is as follows: 1 = 6 to 11 months; 2 = 12 to 23 months; and 3 = 24 months or older. **Table 11-1** shows the data in three groups.

Using these data, investigators want to know if the ages of responding individuals are equally distributed, so they conduct a chi-square test to answer this question. Of course, with this example, the reader can merely look at the numbers and see

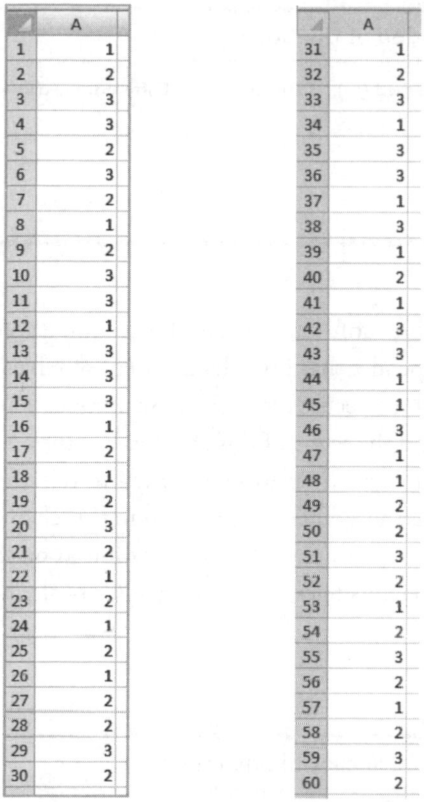

	A
1	1
2	2
3	3
4	3
5	2
6	3
7	2
8	1
9	2
10	3
11	3
12	1
13	3
14	3
15	3
16	1
17	2
18	1
19	2
20	3
21	2
22	1
23	2
24	1
25	2
26	1
27	2
28	2
29	3
30	2

	A
31	1
32	2
33	3
34	1
35	3
36	3
37	1
38	3
39	1
40	2
41	1
42	3
43	3
44	1
45	1
46	3
47	1
48	1
49	2
50	2
51	3
52	2
53	1
54	2
55	3
56	2
57	1
58	2
59	3
60	2

FIGURE 11-4 Actual Data by Age in Years
Used with permission from Microsoft

that the distribution is uneven. However, the purpose of this simple example is to explain the process. When using real datasets, the process is the same, but the datasets are much larger, and it is not as evident if there is a difference. The first column matches the actual or observed data from **Table 11-2**. The second column shows what the investigators expect, or 20 individuals evenly distributed in each category. Conduct the calculations shown in the last column to verify that you understand the equations.

Table 11-1 Actual Data Shown by Age

6–11 months	12–23 months	24 months or older	Total
19	24	17	60

Table 11-2 Calculation of Chi-Square

	Observed (O)	Expected (E)	Difference	$(O - E)^2$	$(O - E)^{2/E}$
6–11 months	19	20	1	1	0.05
12–23 months	24	20	4	16	0.8
24 months or older	17	20	3	9	0.45
Total	60	60			$\chi^2 = 1.30$

The next step is a bit confusing, so read this section carefully. Most statistical textbooks have an appendix that provides a variety of tables called critical value tables that correspond to specific types of statistical tests. How the critical values are calculated is beyond the scope of this chapter, but these values are percentage points used in inferential statistics to reject or fail to reject the null hypothesis.[8] In this text, the critical value tables are provided in this chapter for ease of understanding. Critical value tables may also be easily found on the Internet. For the chi-square test, investigators refer to the Table of Critical Chi-Square Values (see **Table 11-3**).[9]

Table 11-3 Table of Critical Chi-Square Values

Degrees of Freedom (df)	Critical Chi-Square Values	Degrees of Freedom (df)	Critical Chi-Square Values
1	3.8415	21	32.6708
2	5.9915	22	33.9223
3	7.8147	23	35.1703
4	9.4876	24	36.4144
5	11.0706	25	37.6501
6	12.5914	26	38.885
7	14.067	27	40.111
8	15.5073	28	41.3393
9	16.9189	29	42.5564
10	18.3072	30	43.7765
11	19.6746	31	44.9861
12	21.0261	32	46.1949
13	22.363	33	47.3973
14	23.6852	34	48.6062
15	24.9947	35	49.7982
16	26.2967	36	50.9972
17	27.5887	37	52.1894
18	28.8689	38	53.3811
19	30.1427	39	54.5684
20	31.4095	40	55.7596

Table 11-4   Actual Data Shown by Age

18–23 years	24–29 years	30 and over years	Total
34	67	19	120

To use Table 11-3, follow these steps:

1. Determine the degrees of freedom. Degrees of freedom are defined as the number of choices (e.g., 18–23, 24–29, and 30+ years in this example) minus one for the overall category of age. In this example, there are three age group choices and one group called the age variable, so we have 2 degrees of freedom because $3 - 1 = 2$.[10]
2. Look at the far left column and locate 2 degrees of freedom. The critical chi-square value is 5.9915.
3. Decision: Look back at Table 11-2 to find the obtained χ^2 value of 1.30.
4. Compare the obtained χ^2 to the critical χ^2 value of 5.9915. The obtained value (1.30) is less than the critical value. Therefore, investigators fail to reject the null hypothesis. In other words, there is no statistically significant difference between the numbers of individuals in each of the three age groups. In chi-square tests, you want the obtained value to be larger than the critical value.

Let's try another example to confirm your understanding of chi-square tests. The following example asks the same survey question, but yields different responses from the different participating individuals (see **Table 11-4** and **Table 11-5**).

Once again, calculate the degrees of freedom as $3 - 1 = 2$. Look back at Table 11-3 at 2 degrees of freedom and find the critical chi-square value of 5.9915.

Decision: Compare the obtained χ^2 30.14 to the critical χ^2 value of 5.9915. The obtained value (30.14) is greater than the critical value. Therefore, investigators reject the null hypothesis. There is a statistically significant difference in the age group of individuals who answer the survey.

Table 11-5   Calculation of Chi-Square

	Observed	Expected	Difference	$(O - E)^2$	$(O - E)^2 / E$
18–23 years	34	40	6	36	0.9
24–29 years	67	40	27	729	18.23
30+ years	19	40	21	441	11.03
Total	120	120			$\chi^2 = 30.14$

t-Tests

A *t*-test is used to determine if the mean scores between two groups are statistically different. There are two types of *t*-tests: independent and paired samples. Independent *t*-tests look at two groups of individuals (or any other data being measured) examined only once in time. For example, two groups of categorical data (females and males) have blood drawn one time to determine whether there is a difference in the mean scores of their cholesterol levels (continuous data). Paired samples *t*-tests look at one group of individuals tested twice, such as with a pretest and posttest. For example, individuals with diabetes are given a pretest regarding their knowledge of healthy food choices. A pretest mean score is calculated for the group of patients. The individuals attend a diabetes class about healthy food choices. After the class, the same individuals complete a posttest to determine how much information was learned from the class. For a paired samples *t*-test, the pretest mean score is compared to the posttest mean score to determine if there is a statistically significant difference between the two mean scores.

Independent t-Test

Independent *t*-tests determine if there is a statistical difference between the mean scores for two groups examined only one time. For example, let's say that investigators want to know if the Lost-It weight management plan enabled females who work the day shift or females who work the night shift to lose more weight in 12 weeks. As always in inferential statistics, researchers begin by stating the null hypothesis.

Null hypothesis:	There is no difference in weight between day shift females and night shift females at baseline prior to starting the 12-week Lost-It weight management program.
Alternate hypothesis:	There is a difference in weight between day shift females and night shift females at baseline prior to starting the 12-week Lost-It weight management program.

Look at **Figure 11-5** to review the baseline weight for all the participants in the program. In Excel, look at the top line to locate the formula for calculating the baseline mean score for all participants: fx =SUM(C2:C21)/20. After entering the formula, it is necessary to place the cursor where you wish the mean score to appear prior to hitting Enter. Now look at line 22 to see that the mean score for all participants is 188.6 pounds at baseline. Although Figure 11-5 familiarizes the reader with Excel formulas, it does not provide a baseline mean score by day shift and night shift. Note that in Figure 11-5, the codebook denotes column A

	C22		f_x	=SUM(C2:C21)/20	
	A	B	C	D	E
1		Shift	Baseline		
2	1	1	152		
3	2	2	147		
4	3	2	210		
5	4	1	187		
6	5	2	164		
7	6	2	155		
8	7	2	149		
9	8	2	245		
10	9	1	213		
11	10	1	190		
12	11	1	175		
13	12	2	153		
14	13	1	201		
15	14	2	217		
16	15	1	199		
17	16	2	204		
18	17	2	258		
19	18	1	152		
20	19	1	167		
21	20	1	234		
22			188.6		

FIGURE 11-5   Mean Baseline Weight for All Participants
Used with permission from Microsoft

as the case number and column B as their work shift with 1 = day shift females and 2 = night shift females.

To calculate the baseline mean weight by work shift, it is necessary to sort the data. To sort in Excel, go to the toolbar and click on Data, then click on Sort. Highlight columns A, B, and C and then sort by adding levels as seen in **Figure 11-6**. Click OK.

Figure 11-6 shows that the investigators sorted the data, so all the female day shift workers' data are grouped first, followed by the female night shift workers' data. From here, investigators use the formula to calculate the mean score provided in **Figure 11-7**. The female day shift workers' mean baseline weight is 187 pounds, and female night shift workers' mean baseline weight is 190.2 pounds. The female day shift workers had a lower baseline weight than the female night

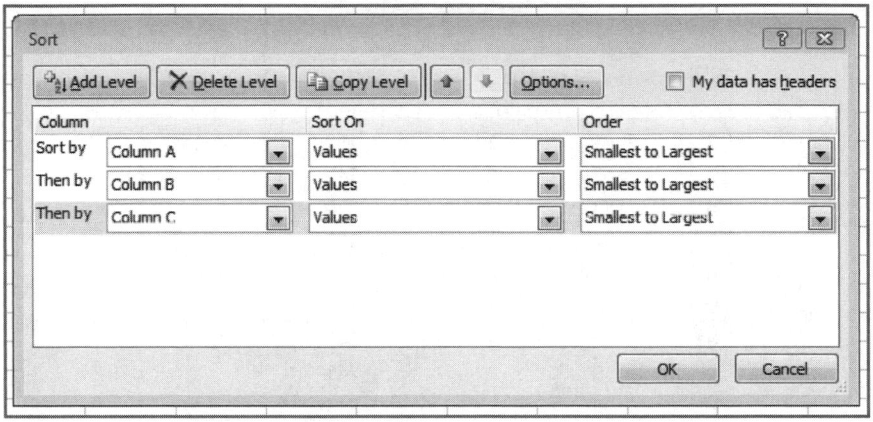

FIGURE 11-6 Sorting Data in Excel
Used with permission from Microsoft

C21 =AVERAGE(B12:B21)

	A	B	C	D	E	F
1	Shift	Baseline	Mean			
2	1	152				
3	1	152				
4	1	167				
5	1	175				
6	1	187				
7	1	190				
8	1	199				
9	1	201				
10	1	213				
11	1	234	187			
12	2	147				
13	2	149				
14	2	153				
15	2	155				
16	2	164				
17	2	204				
18	2	210				
19	2	217				
20	2	245				
21	2	258	190.2			

FIGURE 11-7 Baseline Mean Weight by Female Day Shift and Female Night Shift Workers
Used with permission from Microsoft

shift workers. However, this may be due to simple chance. Investigators want to know if the difference between the baseline weight mean scores is statistically significant, so they conduct an independent *t*-test to reject or fail to reject the null hypothesis.

To calculate the independent *t*-test, go to Formulas on the toolbar, then click on More Functions, then Statistical, then TTEST. The box shown in **Figure 11-8** appears. In the box, enter B2:B11 in Variable 1 Range (day shift workers) and B12:B21 (night shift workers) in Variable Range 2. When you click OK, the results are as shown in **Figure 11-9**.

To understand Figure 11-9, most lines are explained. The lines without explanation are beyond the scope of this chapter.

Line 1: *t*-Test: Two-Sample Assuming Equal Variance.

Line 3: Variable 1 = day shift worker data; Variable 2 = night shift worker data.

Line 4: Mean is the average baseline weight for day shift workers as calculated in Figure 11-7.

Line 5: Variance.

Line 6: Observations: 10 day shift workers and 10 night shift workers.

Line 7: Pooled Variance.

Line 8: Hypothesized Mean Difference.

Line 9: df (degrees of freedom) is 20 (10 day shift workers + 10 night shift workers) observations – 2 groups (day shift workers and night shift workers) = 18.

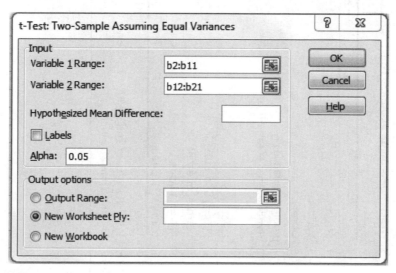

FIGURE 11-8 Using Excel to Calculate an Independent *t*-Test
Used with permission from Microsoft

	A	B	C
1	t-Test: Two-Sample Assuming Equal Variances		
2			
3		*Variable 1*	*Variable 2*
4	Mean	187	190.2
5	Variance	692	1752.622222
6	Observations	10	10
7	Pooled Variance	1222.311111	
8	Hypothesized Mean Differen	0	
9	df	18	
10	t Stat	-0.204665245	
11	P(T<=t) one-tail	0.420065063	
12	t Critical one-tail	1.734063607	
13	P(T<=t) two-tail	0.840130126	
14	t Critical two-tail	2.10092204	

FIGURE 11-9 Results of Independent *t*-Test
Used with permission from Microsoft

Line 10: *t*-Stat is −0.2046 and is called the obtained *t*-value. It is calculated by Excel using a formula. (Note: It is possible to calculate a *t*-test by hand, but the formula is beyond the scope of this introductory chapter, so the Excel formula is illustrated.)

Line 11: *p*-value (one tail)

Line 12: *t*-critical (one tail)

Line 13: *p*-value (two tail): Calculated by Excel; probability of *t*-value happening by chance is 0.84013.

Line 14: *t*-critical (two tail): Look at **Table 11-6**.

Note: Before proceeding to making a decision about the null hypothesis, it is important to become familiar with Table 11-6. As previously mentioned, there are critical value tables for most types of inferential statistic calculations.

Now let's follow the steps to make a decision regarding the null hypothesis for the *t*-test:

1. The first step in reading Table 11-6 is to determine the number of cases. In this example, there are 20 cases or participants. As previously stated,

Table 11-6   Table of Critical *t*-Values

Degrees of Freedom (df)	One-tailed 0.05	Two-tailed 0.05 (0.025 in each tail)	Degrees of Freedom (df)	One-tailed 0.05	Two-tailed 0.05 (0.025 in each tail)
1	6.3138	12.707	21	1.721	2.08
2	2.9200	4.3026	22	1.717	2.074
3	2.3534	3.1824	23	1.714	2.069
4	2.1319	2.7764	24	1.711	2.064
5	2.0150	2.5706	25	1.708	2.06
6	1.9432	2.4469	26	1.706	2.056
7	1.8946	2.3646	27	1.704	2.052
8	1.8595	2.3060	28	1.701	2.049
9	1.8331	2.2621	29	1.699	2.045
10	1.8124	2.2282	30	1.698	2.043
11	1.7959	2.2010	35	1.69	2.03
12	1.7823	2.1788	40	1.684	2.021
13	1.7709	2.1604	45	1.68	2.014
14	1.7613	2.1448	50	1.676	2.009
15	1.7530	2.1314	55	1.673	2.004
16	1.7459	2.1199	60	1.671	2.001
17	1.7396	2.1098	65	1.669	1.997
18	1.7341	2.1009	70	1.667	1.995
19	1.7291	2.0930	75	1.666	1.992
20	1.7247	2.0860	80	1.664	1.99

Adapted with permission from https://www.statstodo.com/TTest_Tab.php.

the statistical term *degrees of freedom (df)* for the *t*-test is calculated by subtracting 1 for each group from the total number of groups. In this example, there are two groups (day and night shift workers), so 20 − 2 = 18 degrees of freedom.

2. Locate 18 degrees of freedom on Table 11-6. The critical *t*-test value is 2.1009 for a two-tailed test.

3. Look back at Figure 11-9 to find the calculated or obtained *t*-value of −0.2046.

4. Compare the obtained *t*-value of −0.2046 to the critical *t*-value of 2.1009.

5. If the obtained *t*-value does not exceed the critical value, the investigators fail to reject the null hypothesis. Investigators report that the null hypothesis is the best explanation and there is no difference in weight between females and males at baseline prior to starting the 12-week Lost-It weight management program. In other words, the decision is that there is no significant difference between the baseline weight of day and night shift workers.

The mean is 187 pounds for day shift workers and 190.2 pounds for night shift workers. Because the obtained *t*-test value of −0.2046 is between −2.1009 and +2.1009, investigators *fail to reject* the null hypothesis. There is no statistically significant difference between the baseline weight of the female day shift and female night shift workers.

Now let's return to the example, using **Figure 11-10**. An alternative way to determine whether the null hypothesis is rejected or failed to reject is to look at

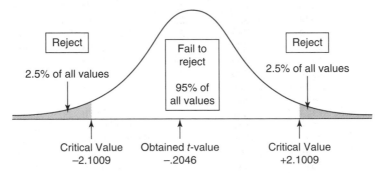

FIGURE 11-10 Illustration of Failing to Reject the Null Hypothesis Using a Two-Tailed Test
Adapted from One and Two-Tailed Tests from Cliffs Notes. Available at: http://www.cliffsnotes.com/study_guide/One-and-Two-Tailed-Tests .topicArticleId-267532,articleId-267495.html. Reprinted by permission of Houghton Mifflin Harcourt.

line 13 in Figure 11-9, p(T<=t) two-tail = 0.8401. The "p" stands for probability value. To determine whether to reject or fail to reject the null hypothesis, the p-value must be less than 5%, or 0.05. In this example, $p = 0.8401$; it is larger than 0.05, and therefore researchers fail to reject the null hypothesis due to lack of evidence to reject the null hypothesis.

This second example of an independent t-test uses the same null hypothesis with a different dataset.

Null hypothesis:	There is no difference in weight between female day and night shift workers at baseline prior to starting the 12-week Lost-It weight management program.
Alternate hypothesis:	There is a difference between female day and night shift workers at baseline prior to starting the 12-week Lost-It weight management program.

Figure 11-11 shows the data. The baseline mean score for 20 female day shift workers is 149.6 pounds, and the baseline mean score for 20 female night shift workers is 200.8 pounds.

As with the first example, in Excel, select the t-Test: Two-Sample Assuming Equal Variance (see **Figure 11-12**). When you click OK, the results are as shown in **Figure 11-13**.

To understand Figure 11-13, each line of interest is explained here:

Line 1: t-Test: Two-Sample Assuming Equal Variance was selected by the investigator.

Line 3: Variable 1 – female day shift worker data; Variable 2 = female night shift worker data.

Line 4: Mean is the average baseline weight for day shift females (149.6 pounds) and night shift females (200.75 pounds).

Line 6: Observations: 20 female day shift workers and 20 female night shift workers.

Line 8: Hypothesized Mean Difference.

Line 9: df (degrees of freedom) is 40 observations (20 day shift female workers + 20 night shift female workers) – 2 groups had their weight measured one time (female day shift workers and female night shift workers) = 38.

Line 10: t-Stat is –4.636, calculated by Excel, and is called the obtained t-value.

Line 11: p-value (one tail).

Line 12: t-critical (one-tail).

Line 13: p-value (two-tail): Calculated by Excel is 0.000004113 and is the probability of the t-value happening by chance. (Hint: In Excel, E-05 equals placing five zeros in front of first number.)

	A	B	C	D
1	1	97		
2	1	109		
3	1	117		
4	1	118		
5	1	118		
6	1	123		
7	1	124		
8	1	139		
9	1	145		
10	1	145		
11	1	149		
12	1	156		
13	1	157		
14	1	158		
15	1	163		
16	1	189		
17	1	193		
18	1	194		
19	1	197		
20	1	201	Mean	149.6
21	2	156		
22	2	158		
23	2	165		
24	2	168		
25	2	172		
26	2	173		
27	2	173		
28	2	180		
29	2	184		
30	2	190		
31	2	194		
32	2	195		
33	2	201		
34	2	210		
35	2	212		
36	2	231		
37	2	252		
38	2	260		
39	2	261		
40	2	280	Mean	200.8

FIGURE 11-11 Mean Baseline Weight for Female Day and Night Shift Workers
Used with permission from Microsoft

Line 14: *t*-critical (two-tail): Look at Table 11-6. The critical *t*-value is 2.024. Note: Table 11-6 illustrates a condensed Table of Critical *t*-Values. It shows the crtical *t*-value for 35 degrees of freedom as 2.03 and for 40 degrees of freedom as 2.021. In a comprehensive version of a Table of Critical *t*-Values, the actual critical *t*-value for 38 degrees of freedom is 2.024.

FIGURE 11-12 *t*-Test: Two-Sample Assuming Equal Variance
Used with permission from Microsoft

Compare the obtained *t*-value of −4.636 to the critical *t*-value of 2.024. If the obtained *t*-value is more extreme than the critical *t*-value, the investigators reject the null hypothesis. Investigators report that there is a significant difference in weight between female day shift workers and female night shift workers at baseline prior to starting the 12-week Lost-It weight management program. In other words, investigators can say that the difference is not due to chance.

	A	B	C
1	t-Test: Two-Sample Assuming Equal Variances		
2			
3		*Variable 1*	*Variable 2*
4	Mean	149.6	200.75
5	Variance	1033.410526	1401.460526
6	Observations	20	20
7	Pooled Variance	1217.435526	
8	Hypothesized Mean Difference	0	
9	df	38	
10	t Stat	-4.63577824	
11	P(T<=t) one-tail	2.05658E-05	
12	t Critical one-tail	1.68595446	
13	P(T<=t) two-tail	4.11315E-05	
14	t Critical two-tail	2.024394164	
15			

FIGURE 11-13 Results of Example Two for Independent *t*-Test
Used with permission from Microsoft

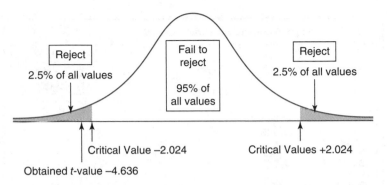

FIGURE 11-14 Illustration of Rejecting the Null Hypothesis

The mean is 149.6 pounds for female day shift workers and 200.75 pounds for female night shift workers. Because the *t*-test value of −4.636 is outside the range between −2.02439 and +2.02439, investigators reject the null hypothesis (see **Figure 11-14**). Because the *t*-value is in the shaded critical area, investigators have enough evidence to *reject* the null hypothesis. There is a statistically significant difference between the baseline weight of the female day shift workers and the female night shift workers.[6]

Paired Samples t-Test

Paired samples *t*-tests compare the mean scores of one group tested twice. For example, let's say that investigators want to know if the Lost-It weight management program was effective in helping day shift females (column A) lose weight

	A	B	C
1	1	152	142
2	1	152	140
3	1	167	160
4	1	175	158
5	1	187	180
6	1	190	173
7	1	199	187
8	1	201	189
9	1	213	201
10	1	234	209

FIGURE 11-15 Comparison of Baseline Data and 12th Week Data for Day Shift Workers
Used with permission from Microsoft

between their initial weigh-in (column B) and the end of the program after 12 weeks (column C). See **Figure 11-15**.

Null hypothesis:	There is no difference between the baseline weight and the 12th week weight for female day shift workers participating in the Lost-It weight management program.
Alternate hypothesis:	There is a difference between the baseline weight and the 12th week weight for female day shift workers participating in the Lost-It weight management program.

To understand **Figure 11-16**, each line of interest is explained here:

Line 1: *t*-Test: Paired Two Sample for Means was selected by the investigator.

Line 3: Variable 1 = female pre-weight data; Variable 2 = female post-weight data.

Line 4: Mean is the average pre-weight for female day shift workers (187 pounds) and post-weight (173.9 pounds).

Line 6: Observations: 10.

Line 8: Hypothesized Mean Difference.

Line 9: df (degrees of freedom) is 10 observations (one group of female day shift workers with their weight measured twice) − 1 group of female day shift workers had their weight measured two times (pretest and posttest weights) = 9.

Line 10: *t*-Stat is 7.6904, calculated by Excel, and is called the obtained *t*-value.

Line 11: *p*-value (one tail).

Line 12: *t*-critical (one tail).

Line 13: *p*-value (two tail): Calculated by Excel as 0.00000301 and is the probability of the *t*-value happening by chance. (Hint: In Excel, E-05 equals placing five zeros in front of the first number.)

Line 14: *t*-critical (two tail): Look at Table 11-6. The critical *t*-value is 2.2621.

	A	B	C
1	t-Test: Paired Two Sample for Means		
2			
3		Variable 1	Variable 2
4	Mean	187	173.9
5	Variance	692	557.4333333
6	Observations	10	10
7	Pearson Correlation	0.98251345	
8	Hypothesized Mean Difference	0	
9	df	9	
10	t Stat	7.694058975	
11	P(T<=t) one-tail	1.50919E-05	
12	t Critical one-tail	1.833112933	
13	P(T<=t) two-tail	3.01838E-05	
14	t Critical two-tail	2.262157163	

FIGURE 11-16   Results of Paired Samples *t*-Test
Used with permission from Microsoft

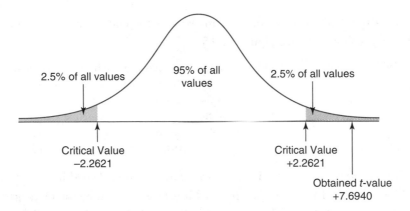

FIGURE 11-17 Illustration of Paired Samples *t*-Test

Adapted from One and Two-Tailed Tests from Cliffs Notes. Available at: http://www.cliffsnotes.com/study_guide/One-and-Two-Tailed-Tests.topicArticleId -267532,articleId-267495.html. Reprinted by permission of Houghton Mifflin Harcourt.

For females, the average baseline weight is 187 pounds and the average weight at the 12th week is 173.9 pounds. The paired samples *t*-test yields a *t*-value of 7.6940. With 9 degrees of freedom, the critical *t*-value is 2.2621. Look at **Figure 11-17** to determine the decision. Because the obtained *t*-value is in the shaded critical area, investigators reject the null hypothesis. In other words, there is a statistically significant difference between the pre-weight and post-weight for day shift workers who participated in the Lost-It weight management program.[6]

Lastly, let's determine whether to reject or fail to reject the null hypothesis based on the *p*-value. Look at Figure 11-13 and see that the two-tailed *p*-value is 0.000003018. Knowing that the *p*-value must be less than 0.05, researchers decided to reject the null hypothesis.

Correlation Coefficients

Statistical tests help tell investigators if there are relationships or associations between two variables that are measured. For example, does a new drug affect pain reduction among patients? Is there a relationship between the type of work that a person does and their ability to lose weight in a weight reduction program? Though very important, statistical tests can only tell us if there is or is not a relationship. They cannot give us any more information about those relationships, such as how strong it is or whether it has a positive or negative effect on the variables. That is where correlation coefficients come in.

Correlation coefficients define a numerical relationship between two continuous variables (also called a Pearson product-moment correlation). There are other types of correlations, but this chapter introduces bivariate correlations that show the relationship between two continuous variables. Let's begin this discussion by providing a simple example of how correlations are used in everyday life. When parents take their child to the pediatrician, the child is weighed and measured. These data are plotted on the child's growth chart in their medical records. The pediatrician is interested in knowing if the child is proportional for his age for height and weight. This would help tell the pediatrician if the child is growing normally as compared to other children of the same age group. If the plot on the growth chart shows the child in the 90th percentile for height and the 40th percentile for weight, the pediatrician recommends healthy choices of food in order to add calories to child's diet because he is somewhat underweight. If, on the other hand, the percentiles were reversed, the pediatrician recommends a reduction in calories because the child's weight exceeds the recommended weight for the child's height. At each visit, the pediatrician plots the height and weight trends for each child. Pediatricians are more concerned about the child following a consistent pattern over time (e.g., 40th percentile for height and weight or 90th percentile for height and weight). Pediatricians become concerned when children's growth patterns are inconsistent. Keep in mind that growth charts are one of several criteria used by pediatricians to determine the overall health of a child (see **Figure 11-18**).[11]

The numerical value of a correlation is called a correlation coefficient and depicts two concepts: direction and strength. Direction is described as positive or negative. Positive direction occurs when variables on the *x*-axis increase as variables on *y*-axis increase. For example, pediatric growth charts show height and weight, both of which are continuous data. Negative direction occurs when variables on the *x*-axis increase as variables on *y*-axis decrease. For example, data shows that as duration of exercise increases, weight decreases. Strength is described as how dispersed the dots are on the scatter plot. Wide dispersion means less strength and narrow dispersion shows greater strength. Scatter plots describe the direction and strength of the correlations shown on a graph (see **Figure 11-19**). If the scatter plot dots are closer together, the strength is strong (−1.00 to +1.00), which means that for every unit of increase on the *x*-axis, there is an equal increase in every unit on the *y*-axis. The reverse is also true for negative correlations. As the scatter plot dots become more widely dispersed, the strength weakens to close to 0. For example, in Figure 11-19A, the dots line up in a straight line perfectly. The direction is positive and the strength is +1.00. Now turn to **Box 11-1**.

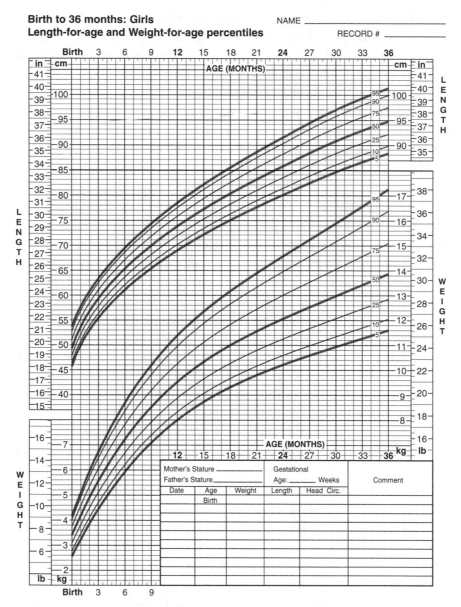

FIGURE 11-18 Birth to 36 Months Growth Chart for Girls

Reproduced from the Centers for Disease Control and Prevention. Growth Charts. Available at: http://www.cdc.gov/growthcharts. Accessed on June 3, 2012.

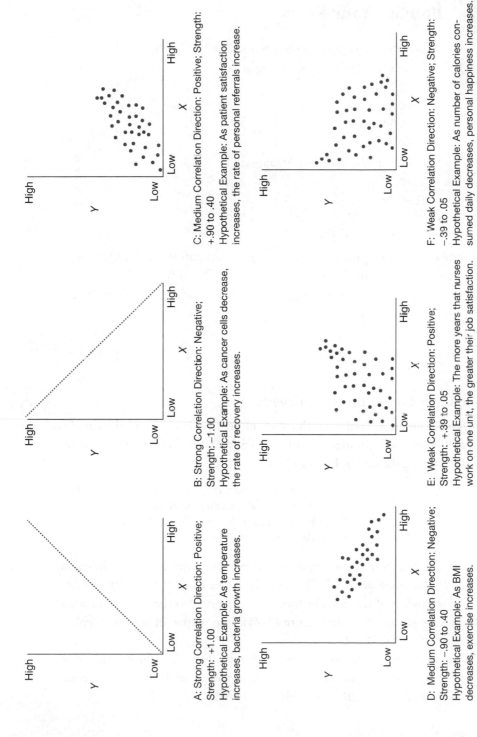

FIGURE 11-19 Six Scatter Plots of Continuous Data Showing Strength and Direction of Correlations

BOX 11-1

Practice Your Skills

Answer the following questions by looking back at Figure 11-19.

1. Which correlation is the strongest?
   a. –0.75
   b. +0.48
   c. –0.20
   d. +0.65

2. Which correlation is the strongest?
   a. +0.18
   b. +0.20
   c. –0.30
   d. –0.18

Answers: 1. (a), –0.75, is the strongest correlation of the choices. See Figure 11-19, Example D.

2. (c), −0.30 is the strongest correlation of the choices. See Figure 11-19, Example E.

Computing Correlation Coefficients

When determining a correlation, the result of the calculation is called a correlation coefficient and is reported in statistical writing as "r". Let's begin with a null hypothesis using the data in **Figure 11-20**.

Null hypothesis: There is no correlation ($r = 0$) between height and weight for female day and night shift workers.

Alternate hypothesis: There is a correlation between height and weight for female day and night shift workers.

Next, enter the formula to calculate a correlation coefficient in the function (fx) toolbar in Microsoft Excel. The formula on the left is the correlation coefficient for height and weight. The formula on the right is the correlation coefficient for weight and BMI (see **Figure 11-21**). Information on how to calculate BMI can be found in Box **11-2**.

When the CORREL formula is entered into the fx toolbar, the box shown in **Figure 11-22** appears. Enter Array 1 for height and Array 2 for weight. Repeat the same process for CORREL for weight and BMI.

	A	B	C
1	Height	Weight	BMI
2	72	230	29.5
3	61	210	39.7
4	64	170	29.2
5	67	154	24.1
6	71	189	26.4
7	68	149	22.7
8	66	156	25.2
9	59	114	23
10	73	256	35.7
11	61	108	20.4
12	71	224	31.2
13	78	305	35.2
14	64	142	24.4
15	65	126	21
16	67	136	21.3
17	62	118	21.6
18	70	208	29.8
19	67	129	20.2
20	58	97	20.3

FIGURE 11-20   Data for Height, Weight, and BMI for Female Day and Night Shift Workers
Used with permission from Microsoft

B21			f_x	=CORREL(A2:A20,B2:B20)	
	A	B	C	D	E	F
1	Height	Weight	BMI			
2	72	230	29.5			
3	61	210	39.7			
4	64	170	29.2			
5	67	154	24.1			
6	71	189	26.4			
7	68	149	22.7			
8	66	156	25.2			
9	59	114	23			
10	73	256	35.7			
11	61	108	20.4			
12	71	224	31.2			
13	78	305	35.2			
14	64	142	24.4			
15	65	126	21			
16	67	136	21.3			
17	62	118	21.6			
18	70	208	29.8			
19	67	129	20.2			
20	58	97	20.3			
21		0.830357				

FIGURE 11-21   Formulas to Calculate Correlation Coefficient
Used with permission from Microsoft

BOX 11-2

BMI Calculator and Information

The National Heart, Lung, and Blood Institute (http://nhlbisupport.com/bmi/bminojs.htm)[14] provides a free BMI calculator, if you wish to calculate your own BMI. Body mass index is the correlation of body fat based on height and weight.

BMI categories:

- Normal weight = 18.5–24.9
- Overweight = 25–29.9
- Obesity = BMI of 30 or greater

National Heart, Lung and Blood Institute; National Institutes of Health; U.S. Department of Health and Human Services.

Let's explore Figure 11-22 further.

1. Look at **Table 11-7**.[16]
2. The degrees of freedom is calculated: 19 (number of individuals in the data) – 2 (number of variables: height and weight) = 17.
3. Using 17 degrees of freedom, locate the critical value of 0.4555.

From Figure 11-22, the formula result (obtained r value) is +0.8303. The obtained value is more extreme than the critical value and therefore falls in the critical area for rejecting the null hypothesis (see **Figure 11-23**). Investigators

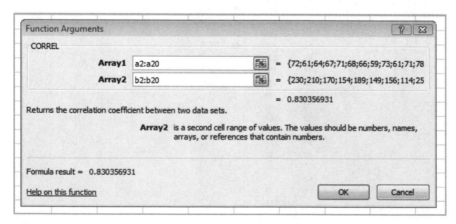

FIGURE 11-22 Correlation Formula Results
Used with permission from Microsoft

Table 11-7   Critical Values for Correlation Coefficients

Degrees of Freedom (df)	One-tailed 0.05	Two-tailed 0.05 (0.025 in each tail)	Degrees of Freedom (df)	One-tailed 0.05	Two-tailed 0.05 (0.025 in each tail)
1	0.9877	0.9969	11	0.4762	0.5529
2	0.9000	0.9500	12	0.4575	0.5324
3	0.8054	0.8783	13	0.4409	0.5139
4	0.7293	0.8114	14	0.4259	0.4973
5	0.6694	0.7545	15	0.4120	0.4821
6	0.6215	0.7067	16	0.4000	0.4683
7	0.5822	0.6664	17	0.3887	0.4555
8	0.5494	0.6319	18	0.3783	0.4438
9	0.5214	0.6021	19	0.3687	0.4329
10	0.4973	0.5760	20	0.3598	0.4227

Data from Quantitative Psychology at Middle Tennesee State University. Available at: http://capone.mtsu.edu/dkfuller/tables/correlationtable.pdf

reject the null hypothesis. There is a statistically significant correlation between height and weight for adult females and males.

It is essential to remember that with correlations, one variable does not mean that it *causes* another variable to change; it simply means that two things are numerically related or associated. For example, gaining weight never means the individual will grow taller. In another example, more people drown when the temperature is over 90 degrees. In this case, the high temperature has nothing to do with drowning, but rather means more people swim in warm weather. In reverse, just because more people are swimming does not make the temperature rise.

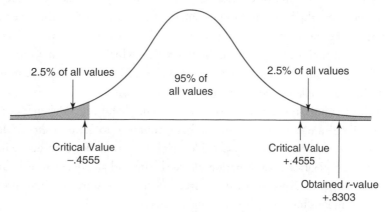

2.5% of all values

95% of all values

2.5% of all values

Critical Value −.4555

Critical Value +.4555

Obtained *r*-value +.8303

FIGURE 11-23   Illustration of Correlation Coefficient for Rejecting the Null Hypothesis

Confidence Intervals

Now that you have been introduced to the concept of rejecting and failing to reject the null hypothesis with chi-square tests, t-tests, and correlation coefficients, it is time to present the topic of confidence intervals. The confidence interval provides more information than simply rejecting or failing to reject the null hypothesis. By using the null hypothesis, investigators know that there is a statistically significant difference between the mean scores, whereas the confidence interval calculates an estimate of the magnitude of the difference.

Let's explore this definition in greater detail for improved understanding. Remember at the beginning of this chapter, you learned that in inferential statistics, investigators were unable to gather data from the whole population, so they select a representative sample of individuals to participate in their study. Investigators collect and analyze their data. If they use a t-test in the analysis, they would calculate a mean score. This mean score is derived from the sample, not of the whole population. Because investigators cannot study the whole population, they are always left wondering how well the mean score for the sample estimates the actual mean score for the whole population. To ease their speculation, they calculate a confidence interval. Confidence intervals provide a range, including a lower and upper limit, of where the mean score of the population is likely to be contained.[15] Because investigators only have data from the sample, they estimate the confidence interval range from the data collected from the sample representing the population.[16]

So how do the investigators decide their level of certainty in the calculated confidence interval? Good question. First, investigators set the desired level of their "confidence," and this value is represented by a percentage. In most cases, investigators set the level of confidence at 95%, so they can state that they are 95% certain that the lower and upper ranges of the calculated confidence interval capture the mean score of the population. In other words, the 95% confidence interval indicates the range of values within which the mean score would fall 95% of the time if investigators repeated the study with an infinite number of sample size samples taken from the same population.[17]

For this example, the data from the second example for the independent t-test (Figure 11-13) are used to present the basic equation to introduce confidence intervals. Because Excel does not provide a simple formula for confidence intervals, this example uses a combination of Excel data and an equation that can be calculated by hand. (Note: Most specialized statistical software programs provide drop-down menus for ease of calculating confidence intervals.)

The following steps explain the equation used to calculate a confidence interval.

1. To calculate a confidence interval, you need to use Excel formulas to determine the values for mean scores, standard deviation, sample size, degrees of freedom, and the critical *t*-value.

   Mean scores: Day shift females: 149.6 pounds

   Excel: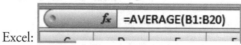

   Night shift females: 200.75 pounds.

   Excel: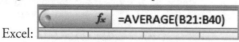

   Standard deviation: Day shift females: 32.14

   Excel: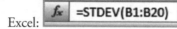

   Night shift females: 37.43

   Excel: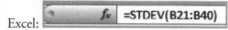

   Sample size: Day shift workers: 20 and night shift workers: 20
   Degrees of freedom: 40 − 2 = 38
   Critical *t*-value: 2.0243

2. To understand the confidence interval formula, it is necessary to know the meaning of each symbol.

   $\bar{X}_1$ = Mean score 1 (day shift workers: 149.6 pounds)
   $\bar{X}_2$ = Mean score 2 (night shift workers: 200.75 pounds)
   s_1^2 = Standard deviation of day shift workers (32.14) squared = 1,033
   s_2^2 = Standard deviation of night shift workers (37.43) squared = 1,401
   n_1 = Number of day shift workers = 20
   n_2 = Number of night shift workers = 20

Decision: Investigators are 95% confident that the mean difference between day shift worker baseline weight and night shift worker baseline weight is between −73.48 pounds and −28.81 pounds (see **Figure 11-24**). Why are these numbers negative? The answer is because the female day shift workers start the Lost-It

$$(\bar{X}_1 - \bar{X}_2) - \begin{matrix}\text{Critical}\\ t\text{-Value}\end{matrix} \times \sqrt{\frac{S_1^2}{n_1} + \frac{S_2^2}{n_2}}$$

Lower Limit:

$$(149.6 - 200.75) - 2.024 \times 11.03 = -73.4865$$

Upper Limit:

$$(\bar{X}_1 - \bar{X}_2) + \begin{matrix}\text{Critical}\\ t\text{-Value}\end{matrix} \times \sqrt{\frac{S_1^2}{n_1} + \frac{S_2^2}{n_2}}$$

$$(149.6 - 200.75) + 2.024 \times 11.03 = -28.8133$$

FIGURE 11-24 Confidence Interval Upper and Lower Limits

weight management programs weighing between 28.81 and 73.48 pounds less than the female night shift workers.[18]

If evaluators were aware of this weight difference, they may plan, implement, and evaluate a program with a specific focus on the weight loss challenges faced by the female night shift workers that are different from the female day shift workers.

Now let's compare the limited information received by conducting an independent *t*-test (Figure 11-9) and the expanded information received by adding the confidence interval (Figures 11-21 and 11-22). As shown in **Figure 11-25**, investigators have enough evidence to *reject* the null hypothesis and to state that

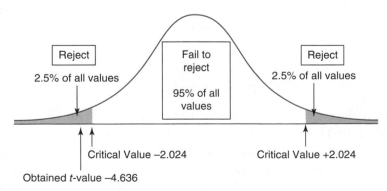

FIGURE 11-25 Rejecting the Null Hypothesis

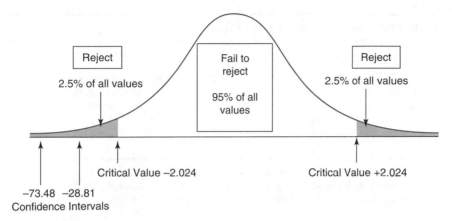

FIGURE 11-26   Rejecting the Null Hypothesis with Confidence Intervals

there is a statistically significant difference between the baseline weights of the day shift and night shift workers.[6]

However, **Figure 11-26** gives us the same information plus added information about the magnitude of the difference between the female day shift workers' baseline weight and the female night shift workers' baseline weight with the inclusion of the confidence intervals. Now investigators have enough evidence to reject the null hypothesis and to state with 95% confidence that the mean weight difference between day shift and night shift workers for the population is between 21.81 pounds and 73.48 pounds.

There are last important concepts about confidence intervals. First, if the lower and upper values include 0, the investigators fail to reject the hypothesis. For example, if the lower value is −1.89 and the upper value is +3.73, the spread includes 0, so the "fail to reject" is correct. Second, when the confidence interval is extremely wide (e.g., −6.79 to −218.09), the sample size is too small and needs to be increased for a more accurate representation of the population.

Type I and Type II Errors

Type I and type II errors build on the concept of the statistical significance level and rejecting the null hypothesis. Investigators make a type I error when they falsely reject the null hypothesis when looking at differences between the intervention group and the study group in what they are studying. For example, if

Table 11-8 Summary of Type I and Type II errors

Researcher's Decision		Actual Situation	
		Null hypothesis is really true.	Null hypothesis is really false.
	Reject the null hypothesis.	Type I error	Correct
	Fail to reject the null hypothesis.	Correct	Type II

Adapted from Ary D, Jacobs LC, Razavieh A. *Introduction to Research in Education*, 6th ed. Belmont, CA: Wadsworth/Thompson Learning; 2002; and Salkind NJ. 2010. *Statistics for People Who Think They Hate Statistics*, 2nd ed. Thousand Oaks, CA: Sage; 2010.

the null hypothesis is "For patients with diabetes, there is no difference between Drug A and Drug B for treating their chronic hypertension," investigators commit a type I error when they report that Drug A and Drug B are different, when in fact there is no difference.[6,19]

It is helpful to think of type II errors as the opposite of type I errors. Type II errors occur when investigators *fail to reject* the null hypothesis when there is a difference between the control and study groups. For example, investigators commit a type II error when they report that there is no difference between Drug A and Drug B on the outcome variables being studied. This is a serious error because healthcare providers prescribe Drug A and Drug B assuming that both drugs are the same, when in fact the drugs are different.[6,19] Type II errors are also defined as failing to reject a false null hypothesis. See **Table 11-8** for a summary of these definitions.[20] Practice your skills with **Box 11-3**. See **Box 11-4** for more resources.

BOX 11-3

Type I and Type II Errors Practice Problems

Practice with a few more examples.
Example 1
Null hypothesis: There is no difference between the Medical College Admissions Test (MCAT) scores of 1st-year medical school students and 4th-year medical school students at a highly ranked state university.

continues

BOX 11-3

Type I and Type II Errors
Practice Problems *continued*

Data report: The MCAT scores of the 1st-year medical school
students are higher than the MCAT scores of the
4th-year medical school students.

Researcher decision: Reject the null hypothesis, because the null
hypothesis is false.

a. Correct decision

b. Type I error

c. Type II error

Example 2

Null hypothesis: There is no difference between the blood glucose levels
of patients with diabetes before and after they attend a
diabetes education course.

Data report: The hemoglobin A1C levels of patients are lower after they
attend the diabetes education course.

Researcher decision: The researcher fails to reject the null hypothesis.

a. Correct decision

b. Type I error

c. Type II error

Example 3

Null hypothesis: There is no difference in job satisfaction between
the night shift nursing staff and the day shift
nursing staff.

Data report: The job satisfaction is the same between night shift and
day shift nurses.

Researcher decision: Researchers reject the null hypothesis, when the
null hypothesis is really true.

a. Correct decision

b. Type I error

c. Type II error

Answers: 1 = a, 2 = c, 3 = b

BOX 11-4

Websites That Provide Free Confidence Interval and Sample Size Calculators

http://www.surveysystem.com/sscalc.htm
http://www.dssresearch.com/KnowledgeCenter/toolkitcalculators
/samplesizecalculators.aspx
http://www.raosoft.com/samplesize.html
http://www.nss.gov.au/nss/home.nsf/NSS/0A4A642C712719DCCA2571
AB00243DC6?opendocument
http://www.gifted.uconn.edu/siegle/research/samples
/samplecalculator.htm
http://www.macorr.com/sample-size-calculator.htm
http://www.custominsight.com/articles/random-sample-calculator.asp

Summary

This chapter introduces inferential statistics, then defines scientific hypothesis, research questions, null hypothesis, and alternative hypothesis. How to conduct basic inferential statistical tests using Excel was introduced using chi-square tests and *t*-tests as examples. After defining correlation coefficients, the chapter concluded with a discussion of confidence intervals and type I and type II errors. The purpose of this chapter is to provide a brief introduction of using this technique and build a foundation of basic definitions of statistics for future use.

Case Study

At the Glendale Hospital Rehabilitation Center, the nurses wanted to initiate a pilot study in which dog owners and their certified trained pet therapy dogs are allowed to visit patients in the rehabilitation unit. The pets provide companionship for the patients, and the pet owners also provide a source of conversation for the patients. The nurses wrote a proposal for the new program and presented it to the hospital board.

continues

CASE STUDY *continued*

Because the pet owners and their certified trained dogs volunteer in hospitals and rehabilitation units, there is no cost to the institution to initiate a volunteer pet therapy program. The only budget item was to utilize the services of a program evaluator, so the board members approved the pet therapy proposal after limited discussion. Immediately, the nurses hired Thad Davis to assist as an evaluator with this project. Thad, a senior at a nearby university, was a volunteer in the rehab center and was familiar with the patients' needs.

The nurses placed an advertisement in the local newspaper to recruit local dog owners and their certified trained dogs to participate in the new pet therapy program. The advertisement listed specific guidelines: dog owners and certified and trained dogs with documentation of current vaccinations. After 18 families volunteered, the dogs were "interviewed" and 12 certified trained dogs were selected. The dogs were categorized by size: small (≤ 15 pounds), medium (16–50 pounds), and large (51+ pounds).

Thad created a patient survey to determine which patients were interested in participating in pet therapy. In the current group of patients, he found that 28 of the 40 patients were interested. As new patients were admitted, they were invited to participate if desired. **Figure 11-27** shows the patient survey data after the first month of the pilot pet therapy program.

Codebook

Gender:	1 = female; 2 = male
Dog at home:	0 = no; 1 = yes
Satisfaction with pet therapy:	1 = poor, 2 = fair, 3 = good,
	4 = very good, 5 = excellent
Dog size:	1 = small, 2 = medium,
	3 = large

Thad wanted to make sure he had enough knowledge and skills to determine if the program was successful, so he met with his faculty advisor at the university. After meeting with his professor, Thad was thrilled to learn that his basic statistics skills were sufficient to analyze the data.

continues

CASE STUDY *continued*

	A	B	C	D	E	F	G
1	Gender	Age	Days in Unit	Dog at Home	# of Pet Visits	Satisfaction	Dog Size
2	1	72	12	1	1	5	1
3	2	78	32	1	2	5	1
4	2	72	7	1	3	5	1
5	1	68	14	1	2	5	2
6	2	70	26	1	2	5	2
7	1	83	21	0	3	5	3
8	2	84	18	0	2	5	2
9	2	71	16	1	3	4	3
10	1	76	12	1	2	4	1
11	1	83	7	1	3	5	2
12	1	91	20	1	1	4	3
13	1	79	19	1	2	5	2
14	2	84	17	1	3	4	1
15	1	83	13	1	2	3	3
16	1	67	5	0	2	5	2
17	1	79	17	1	3	3	1
18	2	62	13	0	3	4	3
19	1	67	20	1	3	5	3
20	2	64	18	0	2	5	3
21	2	65	9	1	3	5	2
22	1	67	10	1	2	3	1
23	1	71	11	1	1	2	3
24	1	78	21	0	3	5	2
25	2	74	8	1	3	5	1
26	1	89	14	1	3	4	3
27	1	83	16	0	2	5	2
28	2	81	19	0	1	4	3
29	1	75	20	1	3	5	3

FIGURE 11-27 Patient Pet Therapy Survey
Used with permission from Microsoft

Case Study Discussion Questions

Here are the research questions that Thad answered:

1. What are the mean scores for age, days in rehab unit, number of pet visits, satisfaction with pet therapy, and dog size?
2. Is there a statistically significant difference between having a dog at home and the age of patients in the rehab unit?

continues

CASE STUDY *continued*

3. Is there a statistically significant difference between having a dog at home and satisfaction with the pet therapy?
4. What is the correlation coefficient between number of pet visits and satisfaction with pet therapy, and between dog size and satisfaction with pet therapy?

Use the data to practice your Excel skills to answer the research questions.

In addition, Thad created another survey for staff members (nurses, occupational therapists, physical therapists, and patients technicians) participating in the pilot study of pet therapy. Most of the staff ($n = 26$) participated in the pilot pet therapy program, though a few declined due to pet allergies or other undisclosed personnel reasons. **Figure 11-28** shows the data collected from the rehab unit staff.

	A	B	C	D	E
1	Staff Job	Staff Satisfaction	Unit Disruption	Perceived Patient Satisfaction	Continue Program
2	1	3	1	5	1
3	1	2	1	5	1
4	1	3	1	5	1
5	2	1	2	4	1
6	1	2	1	5	1
7	2	3	2	3	1
8	1	4	2	5	0
9	1	5	3	5	1
10	1	3	2	4	1
11	2	3	2	5	1
12	1	2	2	3	0
13	1	2	1	5	0
14	1	2	1	3	1
15	1	3	1	2	1
16	1	3	1	4	1
17	1	4	2	5	1
18	2	4	3	4	0
19	1	2	1	5	1
20	1	2	2	3	1
21	2	1	1	5	0
22	2	1	1	4	1
23	1	3	1	5	1
24	2	2	3	3	1
25	1	3	1	5	0
26	1	4	1	5	1
27	1	5	1	4	1
28					

FIGURE 11-28   Staff Member Satisfaction Survey
Used with permission from Microsoft

continues

CASE STUDY *continued*

Codebook

Staff job:	1 = nursing/patient care,
	2 = therapist
Staff satisfaction of pet therapy:	1 = low, 2 = medium, 3 = high
Unit disruption:	1 = low, 2 = medium, 3 = high
Perceived patient satisfaction:	1 = poor, 2 = fair, 3 = good,
	4 = very good, 5 = excellent
Continue pet therapy:	0 = no, 1 = yes

Here are the research questions that Thad answered related to the staff survey:

1. Is there a statistically significant difference between staff position and staff satisfaction?
2. What percentage of the staff wish the pet therapy program to continue?

Answers

General Research Questions

1. Mean scores for age (75.57), days in rehab unit (15.54), number of pet visits (2.32), satisfaction with pet therapy (4.43), and dog size (2.11).
2. There is no statistically significant difference between having a dog at home and age of patients.
3. There is no statistically significant difference between having a dog at home and satisfaction with the pet therapy.
4. There is no statistically significant correlation between number of pet visits and satisfaction with pet therapy. There is no statistically significant correlation between dog size and satisfaction with pet therapy.

Staff Survey Research Questions

1. There is no statistically significant difference between staff position and staff satisfaction.
2. Of the responding staff, 76.9% wish the pet therapy program to continue.

Student Activities

Below are some practice questions to help familiarize yourself with the concepts you have learned in this chapter.

Turn the following problem statements into an appropriate research question, a null hypothesis, and an alternate hypothesis.

1. Leila is a community organizer in a low-income urban center. She believes that there are a lot fewer grocery stores that offer fresh fruits and vegetables in her neighborhood than in other, wealthier neighborhoods in the same city. If this is true, she would like to try to encourage local grocers to carry more fruits and vegetables.
   Research question:

   Null hypothesis:

   Alternate hypothesis:

2. Carl is a nursing administrator in the emergency room of a busy hospital. He thinks that patients have better satisfaction with their care and that nurses make fewer mistakes when they are allowed to take a nap when they are on the night shift. If this is true, he would like to allow nurses to take naps on long breaks.
   Research question:

   Null hypothesis:

   Alternate hypothesis:

3. Samuel works for the local YMCA. He believes that retired adults who participate in group exercises at the YMCA have lower blood pressure than those who participate in exercise on their own. He thinks that not

only does the exercise help them physically, but socializing with others helps lower their stress. If this is so, he would like to institute more group classes especially for retirees.

Research question:

Null hypothesis:

Alternate hypothesis:

Based on the following alternate hypotheses, should the researcher use a one- or two-tailed statistical test?

4. Alternate hypothesis: There are fewer grocery stores that provide fresh fruit and vegetables in District A than in District B.

5. Alternate hypothesis: There is a significant difference in patient satisfaction when nurses are allowed to take a nap while on night shift.

6. Alternate hypothesis: Retired adults who participate in exercise on their own at the YMCA have higher blood pressure than those who participate in group exercise.

After running the appropriate statistical tests for several research questions, decide which null hypothesis to reject, fail to reject, and accept.

7. After running a chi-square statistical test, you find that the obtained chi-square value is 6.0123 and the critical chi-square value is 5.9915. What is your judgment?

8. After running a two-tailed t-test, you obtain a p-value of 0.035. What is your judgment?

9. Based on a visual inspection of the normal curve in **Figure 11-29**, what is your judgment?

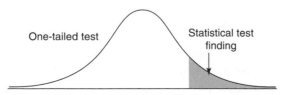

FIGURE 11-29

10. Researchers have run a confidence interval. Their upper limit was 0.75 and their lower limit was −1.03. What is your judgment?

Answers

1. Research question: Are there significantly fewer grocery stores that offer fresh fruits and vegetables in Leila's neighborhood than in other, wealthier neighborhoods within the city?
   Null hypothesis: There is no difference in the number of grocery stores that offer fresh fruits and vegetables.
   Alternate hypothesis: There is a significant difference in the number of grocery stores that offer fresh fruits and vegetables.

2. Research question: Do nurses provide better care to emergency room patients if they are allowed to take a nap on night shift?
   Null hypothesis: There is no difference in patient satisfaction and number of mistakes when nurses are allowed to take a nap while on night shift.
   Alternate hypothesis: There is a significant difference in patient satisfaction and the number of mistakes when nurses are allowed to take a nap while on night shift.

3. Research question: Do retired adults participating in group exercise classes at the YMCA have lower blood pressure than those retired adults who only participate in solo exercise at the YMCA?
   Null hypothesis: There is no difference in blood pressure between retired adults who participate in group exercise and those who do their exercises on their own.
   Alternate hypothesis: There is a difference in blood pressure between retired adults who participate in group exercise and those who do their exercises on their own.

4. One-tailed statistical test. This is because we are asking if there is directionality in the difference (i.e., that there are fewer stores in District A than in District B).

5. Two-tailed statistical test. This is because we are not assuming that there are better or worse patient satisfaction outcomes, only that there are different outcomes. Therefore, we would expect that any extreme differences could be on either end of the normal curve.

6. One-tailed statistical test. This is because we are asking if there is directionality in the difference (i.e., that solo exercisers have higher blood pressure than those who participate in group exercise).

7. Reject the null hypothesis. The obtained chi-square value is larger than the critical chi-square value.

8. Fail to reject the null hypothesis. Normally, if you were running a one-tailed t-test, a 0.035 would be statistically significant if you had an alpha level of 0.05. However, because we split the alpha level in two (for each side of the normal curve) in a two-tailed t-test, a significant significance would be a p-value of less than 0.025. Because 0.035 is greater than 0.025, we fail to reject the null hypothesis.

9. Reject the null hypothesis. Because the obtained statistical test is in the critical area of the normal curve, we would reject the null hypothesis.

10. Fail to reject the null hypothesis. Because the confidence interval includes 0, we must fail to reject the null hypothesis.

References

1. Lincoln LM. *Think and Explain with Statistics.* Boston, MA: Addison-Wesley Publications; 1986.

2. Zimmerman KA. What Is a Scientific Hypothesis? Live Science. Available at: http://www.livescience.com/21490-what-is-a-scientific-hypothesis-definition-of-hypothesis.html. Published July 10, 2012. Accessed November 3, 2012.

3. George Mason University Writing Center. How to Write a Research Question. Available at: http://writingcenter.gmu.edu/?p=307. Published March 8, 2012. Accessed November 3, 2012.

4. Lane DM. HyperStat Online. Rice University. Available at: http://davidmlane.com /hyperstat/A29337.html. Last Updated March 1, 2008. Accessed November 3, 2012.

5. Cliffs Notes. Stating a Hypothesis. Available at: http://www.cliffsnotes.com/study _guide/Stating-Hypotheses.topicArticleId-267532,articleId-267491.html. Accessed November 3, 2012.

6. Salkind NJ. *Statistics for People Who Think They Hate Statistics*, 2nd ed. Thousand Oaks, CA: Sage Publications, Inc.; 2010.

7. Cliffs Notes. One and Two-Tailed Tests. Available at: http://www.cliffsnotes.com /study_guide/One-and-Two-Tailed-Tests.topicArticleId-267532,articleId-267495 .html. Accessed November 3, 2012.

8. Statistics Mentor. The T-Table Critical Values. Available at: http://www.statisticsmentor .com/tables/table_t.htm. Accessed November 3, 2012.

9. StatsToDo. T Test Tables. Available at: http://www.statstodo.com/TTest_Tab.php. Accessed on September 27, 2013.

10. Dallal GE. *The Little Handbook of Statistical Practice.* Seattle, WA: Amazon Digital Services, Inc.; 2012.

11. Centers for Disease Control and Prevention. Growth Charts. Available at: http://www .cdc.gov/growthcharts. Accessed on June 3, 2012.

12. Rice University. Online Statistics Homepage. Values of Pearson Correlation. Available at: http://onlinestatbook.com/chapter4/pearson.html. Accessed November 3, 2012.

13. Fuller DK. Middle Tennessee State University. Critical Values for Pearson's Correlation Coefficient. Available at: http://capone.mtsu.edu/dkfuller/tables/correlationtable.pdf. Accessed November 3, 2012.

14. The National Heart, Lung, and Blood Institute. Calculate Your Body Mass Index. Available at: http://nhlbisupport.com/bmi/bminojs.htm. Accessed November 3, 2012.

15. National Institute of Standards and Technology. What are Confidence Intervals? Available at: http://www.itl.nist.gov/div898/handbook/prc/section1/prc14.htm. Last Updated April 1, 2012. Accessed November 3, 2012.

16. Yale University. Confidence Intervals. Available at: http://www.stat.yale.edu/Courses/1997-98/101/confint.htm. Accessed November 3, 2012.

17. Utah Office of Public Health Assessment. Confidence Intervals in Public Health. Available at: http://health.utah.gov/opha/IBIShelp/ConfInts.pdf. Accessed November 3, 2012.

18. Statistics Lectures. Confidence Intervals for Independent Samples t-Test. Available at: http://www.statisticslectures.com/topics/ciindependentsamplest/. Accessed November 3, 2012.

19. Campbell RB. University of Northern Iowa. Type I and II Error. Available at: http://www.cs.uni.edu/~campbell/stat/inf5.html#TI. Accessed November 3, 2012.

20. Ary D, Jacobs LC, Razavieh A. *Introduction to Research in Education*, 6th ed. Belmont, CA: Wadsworth/Thompson Learning; 2002.

Budgets and Cost Analyses

Introduction

This chapter begins with different types of budgets including personal budgets, evaluation and research budgets, and budget summaries. Once the basic components of budgets are understood, the next section links the budget concepts to the various types of cost analyses. Evaluators and researchers use cost analysis techniques to determine the most effective and efficient health procedures, treatments, and programs.

Budgets

This section describes different types of budgets. We begin with personal budgets. If a student does not understand his or her own budget, it can be difficult to develop budgets for other purposes. Our first example of a budget utilizes the concept of the federal poverty level in the United States. Why do evaluators and researchers need to be concerned about the income of participants? If investigators use income as a variable in their study, they should take the concept of poverty level into consideration when interpreting the final results or making recommendations to stakeholders. Next, a sample budget for research or evaluation is examined along with a budget justification. Lastly, profit and loss statements for a small company are shown. For this chapter, Microsoft Excel is used to show examples of various types of budgets.

Personal Budgets

Let's begin with developing a simple budget for an individual who recently graduated from a four-year university with an undergraduate degree and is now working full-time. This exercise introduces the basics of using an Excel spreadsheet for budgets. When using Excel, it is essential to use the function (*fx*) toolbar located in the toolbar ribbon. For example, in **Figure 12-1**, the required federal taxes are 7.65% and income taxes are about 10%, so the taxes that are subtracted from the gross income every paycheck is 17.65%. Note that cell G3 is the recent graduate's pay before taxes and G4 is the taxes (see the function [*fx*] toolbar). The equation for the graduate's take-home pay in cell H4 is cell G4 subtracted from cell G3 (G3 − G4= $1,841). You should also remember that months are calculated as 4.3 weeks, as shown in E3. This individual has a monthly excess of $6. Note that the annual income is $21,196 and the annual expenses are $21,114.

To practice Excel skills, try creating your own monthly budget in an Excel spreadsheet. Using the function (*fx*) toolbar will help save you time. For example, you can calculate numerous separate equations without using the *fx* toolbar. If it is necessary to change one number to balance the budget, you need to recalculate every item. However, if the *fx* toolbar is used, numerous items change instantly without any additional steps. Note that the sample budget in Figure 12-1 does not include any credit card bills or other expenses. If you use a credit card to pay for items, subtract the amount from your checking account so you have enough money to pay off the credit card statement each month. This technique saves having to pay interest on the debt incurred. Also remember to save for vacations and emergencies, so you have a cushion of money in reserve for planned and unplanned expenses. Vacations are more enjoyable when you are not incurring debt while having fun.

	G4		▼	f_x	=G3*F4				
	A	B	C	D	E	F	G	H	I
1								Monthly	Annual
2	Income		Hours	Pay/Hour	Weeks				
3		Job	40	$ 13	4.3		$ 2,236		
4		Income Tax				17.65%	$ 395	$ 1,841	
5		Health Insurance					$ 75	$ 1,766	$ 21,196
6									
7	Expenses								
8		Rent					$ 475		
9		Utilities					$ 120		
10		Internet/Phone					$ 120		
11		Food		$ 75	4.3		$ 323		
12		Public Transportation		$ 25	4.3		$ 108		
13		Hair/Clothes/Shoes		$ 35	4.3		$ 151		
14		Entertainment		$ 30	4.3		$ 129		
15		Medical/Dental					$ 60		
16		College Loan					$ 150		
17		Vacation Savings					$ 50		
18		Personal Savings					$ 75		
19								$ 1,760	$ 21,114
20									
21								Extra	$ 82
22									

FIGURE 12-1   Sample Budget
Used with permission from Microsoft

The next type of budget to investigate might belong to a member of the 15% of the population (46.2 million people) who lived in poverty in the United States in 2011.[1] Why does an investigator need to think about this type of budget? The reason is that investigators work with many types of people, including individuals and families living in poverty. For example, during a medical treatment evaluation, if participants are required to make return visits to the clinic for follow-up care or medication, the investigation team needs to be aware of transportation options and costs. If a study is taking place at a community clinic in a neighborhood with lower socioeconomic status, it is likely that participants are at or below the poverty level. Therefore, proximity of public transportation is of consideration if investigators expect individuals to comply with return visits. Another consideration would be the need to have accommodating clinic appointment times for participants with shift-work employment and limited flexibility. Lastly, investigators should not jump to the conclusion that individuals who fail to keep appointments are forgetful, disorganized, or not interested in their health; rather, investigators should remain mindful of exploring the barriers that keep individuals in poverty from seeking appropriate healthcare services (e.g., employment schedules, lack of transportation, low literacy, lack of health literacy). **Figure 12-2** shows a sample budget for a single person living at the federal poverty level. The U.S. federal poverty guidelines are $11,170 for one person and $23,050 for a family of four.[2] Keep in mind that the federal minimum wage is $7.25 per hour, but many states have increased their minimum wage levels.[3]

Evaluation and Research Project Budgets

All evaluations and research projects have budgets. Whether a study is a multimillion-dollar grant funded by the National Institutes of Health or a $1,000 evaluation in a small community agency, the principal investigator is in charge of tracking the funding and verifying that the money is spent appropriately. Even if the institution has a finance department to track grant funding, it is ultimately the responsibility of the individual conducting the evaluation or research to provide the appropriate oversight.

It should also be noted when investigators apply for grant funding, the budget is a critical component to the grant application. Whether the funding comes from the federal government, a private organization, or a community agency, the funding is highly regulated and frequently audited to prevent fraud and waste. For example, investigators must calculate grant budgets accurately for each budget category. There are many rules and regulations regarding grant budgets in order to protect against waste, misuse, and fraud. It is not possible for investigators to move money from one category to another (e.g., salaries to travel expenses) without written permission from the funding agency. Furthermore,

	H13		f_x	=SUM(G6:G12)				
	A	B	C	D	E	F	G	H	I
1	Income		Hours	Pay/Hour	Weeks			Monthly	Annual
2		Job	25	$ 7.25	4.3		$ 779		
3						17.65%	$ 138	$ 917	$ 11,003
4									
5	Expenses								
6		Rent		$ 95	4.3		$ 409		
7		Food		$ 62	4.3		$ 267		
8		Public Transportation		$ 20	4.3		$ 86		
9		Mobile Phone		$ 10	4.3		$ 43		
10		Clothes		$ 15	4.3		$ 65		
11		Drug Store		$ 4	4.3		$ 17		
12		Savings		$ 7	4.3		$ 30		
13								$ 916	$ 10,991
14									
15								Extra	$ 12
16									

FIGURE 12-2   Budget for a Single Individual Living at the U.S. Poverty Level of $11,170
Used with permission from Microsoft

it is not possible to alter the number or salary rate of personnel on the grant budget. There are also specific regulations guarding against purchasing equipment and food. For instance, an investigator may not purchase a new laptop without a specific need to use the laptop for data collection in the community. Lastly, most large institutions and universities have contracts with certain vendors that guarantee the lowest price (e.g., rental car companies, print goods suppliers, airlines). Investigators are required to use only these vendors, even if there is some inconvenience involved, such as longer layovers or less direct routes. It is important to know the regulations and specific rules for your institution related to budget spending. In all situations and circumstances, it is up to the investigator to abide by the budget regulations at their institutions or else risk censure, fines, and even criminal investigation. When it doubt, find out the policy prior to making the purchase or changing any line of an approved budget.

Now let's expand this discussion by examining a budget for an evaluation or research project. These budgets include an Excel spreadsheet, but also a budget justification. When a budget is created for a project, it is not simply turning in a total projected amount of money required to successfully complete the evaluation or study. It is necessary to justify why the amount of money is required. The budget justification is a written description that explains the specific expenditures of the proposed budget. Budget justifications allow the institution or organization funding the proposed project to determine if the planned costs are reasonable. **Figure 12-3** shows a sample budget for an evaluation project, and **Box 12-1** shows the budget justification.

In the budget justification in Box 12-1, you will notice that there is an item called indirect costs. Indirect costs are a percentage of the total expenses for the evaluation or research project that are collected by the institution or agency hosting the project. For example, universities charge investigators a variable rate for funded research. This amount provides funding to the university to pay expenses used by the project staff but not listed on the research budget (e.g., building utilities and maintenance, office furniture, and the cost of general administrative and personnel work).

Budget Summaries: Profit and Loss Statements

As already noted, budgets serve multiple purposes for investigators, such as tracking available resources, costs, and payments. Budgets also summarize information. A budget summary is called a profit and loss statement. These statements

	A	B	C	D	E	F	G
1	Personnel	Salary	FTE	Subtotal	Percent	Benefits	Total
2	Principal Investigator	$ 100,000	0.20	$ 20,000	0.28	$ 5,600	$ 25,600
3	Director	$ 80,000	1.0	$ 80,000	0.28	$ 22,400	$ 102,400
4	Team Leader	$ 65,000	1.0	$ 65,000	0.28	$ 18,200	$ 83,200
5	Adm Assistant	$ 45,000	1.0	$ 45,000	0.28	$ 12,600	$ 57,600
6	Data Collector	$ 40,000	0.25	$ 10,000	0.28	$ 2,800	$ 12,800
7	Data Entry Clerk	$ 40,000	0.25	$ 10,000	0.28	$ 2,800	$ 12,800
8							
9	Biostatistician	$ 175	50				$ 8,750
10							
11	Incentives	$ 25	200				$ 5,000
12							
13	Mileage	$ 0.49	200	12			$ 1,176
14							
15	Printer	$ 600					$ 600
16	Computers	$ 3,000					$ 3,000
17	Office Supplies	$ 300		12			$ 3,600
18	Paper	$ 200		12			$ 2,400
19	Printer Cartiridge	$ 75		12			$ 900
20	Postage	$ 30		12			$ 360
21	Space Lease	$ 1,800		12			$ 21,600
22	Telephone/Internet	$ 300		12			$ 3,600
23	Utilities	$ 200		12			$ 2,400
24						Subtotal	$ 347,786
25					Indirect	$ 0.15	$ 52,168
26						TOTAL	$ 399,954

FIGURE 12-3   Sample Budget for an Evaluation Project
Used with permission from Microsoft

Sample Budget Justification

BOX 12-1

Personnel

Ima Wright, PhD, serves as principal investigator with 0.20 full-time equivalent (FTE) commitment for $20,000 salary and $5,600 benefits, for a total of $25,600.

Alison Richards, PhD, serves as director with 1.00 FTE commitment for $80,000 salary and $22,400 benefits, for a total of $102,400.

Barbara Villiotti, MA, serves as team leader with 1.00 FTE commitment for $65,000 salary and $18,200 benefits, for a total of $83,200.

Erica Patterson, BS, serves as administrative assistant with 1.00 FTE for $45,000 salary and $12,600 benefits, for a total of $57,600.

continues

BOX 12-1

Sample Budget Justification *continued*

Daniel Kohler, BSPH, serves as data collector with 0.25 FTE for $10,000 salary and $2,800 benefits, for a total of $12,800.

Marie Gomez, BSPH, serves as data entry clerk with 0.25 FTE for $10,000 and $2,800 benefits, for a total of $12,800.

Consultant

R. C. Blair, PhD, serves as biostatistician consultant with a salary of $175 per hour for 50 hours, for a total fee of $8,750.

Incentives

Each of the 200 participants will receive a $25 gift card upon completion of the online survey, for a total for $5,000.

Mileage

Mileage of 200 miles per month for 12 months at $0.49 per mile for a total of $1,176.

Office

One printer used for office printing needs is $600.

Two computers at $1,500 each totals $3,000.

Miscellaneous office supplies at $300 per month for 12 months totals $3,600.

Copy paper and stationary at $200 per month for 12 months is $2,400.

One printer cartridge at $75 per month for 12 months is $900.

Postage at $30 per month for 12 months is $360.

Office space lease at $1,800 per month for 12 months is $21,600.

Telephone and Internet charges at $300 per month for 12 months total $3,600.

Utilities at $200 per month for 12 months are $2,400.

Subtotal of expenses: $347,786

Indirect costs are calculated at 15%: $52,168

Total expenses: $399,954.00

allow individuals, departments, or large companies to determine at a glance if they are gaining or losing money and in which areas (see **Table 12-1**).

Cost Analysis

Now that the budgets have been introduced, it is time to understand the concept of cost analysis. Simply stated, cost analysis combines the budgets and costs; in this discussion, these will be related to healthcare costs. Although most

Table 12-1 Sample Profit and Loss Statement

Complete Hospital Linen Services

January 1, 2014, to December 31, 2014

GROSS INCOME
Gross sales	$1,100,000
Other income	$300,000
TOTAL GROSS INCOME	$1,400,000

NET INCOME
Income before taxes	$1,400,000
Personal income taxes	$448,000
TOTAL NET INCOME	$952,000

EXPENSES
Cost of goods sold	$400,000
Accounting and legal fees	$12,000
Advertising	$58,000
Insurance	$59,000
Maintenance and repairs	$18,000
Supplies	$6,000
Payroll expenses	$24,000
Postage	$2,000
Rent	$65,000
Licenses	$6,000
Taxes	$75,000
Telephone/internet	$8,000
Travel/transportation/gas	$48,000
Utilities	$19,000
Other	$1,500
TOTAL EXPENSES	$801,500
Subtract Expenses from Net Income **NET GAIN**	**$150,500**

investigators are not expected to know the complexities of financial analysis and how they relate to their work, it is important to have a basic understanding of the various types of cost analyses. From the viewpoint of evaluation, some cost analyses are performed to determine if the program is effective or if the project is providing the "biggest bang for the buck." Cost analysis information is useful when presenting results to various stakeholders. This discussion of cost analysis includes cost benefits, cost effectiveness, cost utility, and cost feasibility, each providing answers to different questions. Let's begin with brief definitions prior to exploring each type of cost analysis in detail (see **Table 12-2**).

Cost-Benefit Analysis

Cost-benefit analysis compares monetary costs among several similar products, programs, or procedures. Cost-benefit analysis is typically used for making

Table 12-2   Summary of Type of Cost Analysis

Type of Cost Analysis	Definition
Cost benefit	Comparison of the monetary costs across several similar programs
Cost effectiveness	Comparison of total costs to total benefits
Cost utility	A type of cost-effectiveness analysis; comparison of benefits gained from different health outcomes (e.g., quality of life)
Cost feasibility	Comparison of project's cost as compared to the attained value and benefits

short-term decisions. Given limited resources, cost-benefit analysis is used to allocate sparse resources in community organizations (e.g., hospitals, school districts, and police and fire departments). For example, if a brand-name medication offers similar benefits as a generic brand medication, the cost-benefit analysis reveals the advantage of purchasing the generic brand. In other words, investigators identify costs and benefits associated with products, programs, and procedures.

Examples of benefits include reduction of postsurgical infection rates, time savings, reduction in personnel costs, improved patient satisfaction, and reduction in disposable waste products. Values are expressed monetarily and are stated as a ratio. For example, if Surgical Gauze X costs $1,000 per carton of 50 packages ($20 per pack) and is proven to be more absorbent than Surgical Gauze Y, which costs $500 per carton of 50 packages ($10 per pack), the initial monetary ratio is 1:2, or half the cost for 50 packages. However, upon closer examination, the cost-benefit analysis shows that during an actual surgical procedure, so many surgical gauze packs are used that surgical nurses do not report that they noticed the greater absorbency of the more expensive gauze. Because the nurses report that the expensive Surgical Gauze X packs are harder to open, they frequently open several packs prior to surgery to save time during the procedure. This time-saving techniques causes greater expense in the long run if the open packs are not used and are discarded. Therefore, after all factors are considered, the ratio may increase to 1:4, making Surgical Gauze Y much less expensive because there is less waste.

Cost-benefit analyses do not include consideration of the program effectiveness, which is how well the program performs. Although the advantage of cost-benefit analysis is the ability to determine a broad comparison of overall costs across programs, there are several disadvantages. First, it is difficult to determine all of the actual costs and benefits of a program. For example, should safety be measured by less crime, fewer reports of bullying in schools, less family violence, and/or fewer police reports or emergency department admissions from violence? Second, benefits associated with costs may not be seen for years. For example, the positive benefits of the human papillomavirus (HPV) vaccine may not be noted in HPV-related cancer rate reductions for more than a decade. Third, the program costs spent this year do not have the same monetary value as when the benefits are realized. In other words, the clinic immunization supplies that cost $20,000 in 2010 might cost $40,000 in 2020. It is difficult to make an accurate cost comparison because of inflation.[4]

Also, cost benefits are expressed in terms of the common unit of money. Evaluators may explore the positive and negative effects of adding county health clinic hours on Saturday and extending the hours, changing them from 9:00 a.m. to 5:00 p.m. to 8:00 a.m. to 8:00 p.m. This change would deter county health clinic patients from using the community hospital emergency department for routine clinic services. The evaluators would use the current clinic expenses and income to calculate the costs per patient over one month and then calculate the budget if the hours of operation were extended. **Figure 12-4** shows a hypothetical budget.

	A	B	C	D	E	F	G
1	EXPENSES			INCOME			
2	Building				Billable Patient Visits		
3		Utilities				Initial	
4		Maintenance				Intermediate	
5		Security				Extended	
6		Parking			Patient Procedures		
7	Personnel					Laboratory	
8		Physicians				Office	
9		Pharmacists			Pharmacy		
10		Nurse Practitioners				Medications	
11		Nurses			Clinic Subsidy		
12		Support Technicians				Federal	
13		Clerks				State	
14	Supplies						
15		Office Supplies					
16		Medical Supplies					
17		Dispoable Supplies					
18	Legal, Accounting, Computer Support						
19			TOTAL				TOTAL
20							
21	Current Budget						
22		Total per month/number of patients			Total per month/number of patients		
23		$500,000 / 500 patients = $1000 per patient			$400,000 / 500 patients = $800 per patient		
24					Clinic Subsidy = $200 per patient		
25		Total	$1000 per patient		Total	$1000 per patient	
26							
27	Extended Hour Budget Projection						
28		Total per month/number of patients			Total per month/number of patients		
29		$800,000 / 900 patients=$888 per patient			$900,000 / 900 patients = $1000 per patient		
30					Clinic Subsidy = $200 per patient		
31		Total	$888 per patient		Total	$1200 per patient	
32					Net Gain: $312 per patient		

FIGURE 12-4   Summary of Monthly Expenses and Income for Community Clinic
Used with permission from Microsoft

In this sample, the clinic expenses for the current hours of operation equal the clinic income. In other words, the clinic "breaks even" on its budget, but does not provide extra money for improvement or expansion. If the hours of operation are extended, the clinic's income will likely exceed the clinic's expenses. This occurs because some expenses, such as building and parking maintenance, legal and accounting fees, and computer support, remain the same regardless of hours of operation, as they are flat-rate expenses. The net gain of $312 per patient × 900 patients provides an additional $280,800 of income per month. This additional new revenue could be used to upgrade laboratory equipment, install electronic medical record computer software, and provide salary increases for the clinic personnel. This example illustrates that a cost-benefit analysis allows the county health department to not only increase its bottom line, but also find ways to better serve the community. The community clinic is open longer hours, making it convenient for families and individuals who work during the day to make appointments after 5:00 p.m. Because they can make appointments after 5:00 p.m., they are less likely to utilize expensive emergency department services unnecessarily. This change increases revenue and allows the clinic to invest in better equipment and training that will ultimately benefit patients.

Another term used for making decisions, such as changing clinic hours in our example, is called *return on investment (ROI)*. For example, the county commissioners ask how many months it will take before the clinic sees the projected extra revenue generated (i.e., their ROI) from hiring and training the extra clinic personnel to staff the extended hours of operation. One last note: keep in mind that the sample budget (see Figure 12-4) does not calculate the cost savings to the community by reducing the unnecessary overuse of the emergency department at the local county hospital. This earned money would be part of the ROI.[5]

This discussion includes some of the challenges associated with cost-benefit analysis. First, the most difficult part of cost-benefit analysis in health is calculating equivalencies between two products.[6] For example, when searching for an apartment, individuals evaluate location, distance to work and school, the nearest public transportation, availability of parking, amenities, price per square foot, cost of utilities, and overall satisfaction with floor plan and neighborhood. When selecting a healthcare service, decisions are based on subjective (personality of healthcare provider and communication style) as well as objective (convenience of location, type of insurance accepted, type of medical specialist required) criteria. Although all healthcare providers are required to have state licensure or board certifications, it is often difficult to determine expertise and skill. Therefore, individuals often rely on word-of-mouth when choosing healthcare providers—thus making equivalencies, or how a product is measured by different criteria, challenging.

An example of trade-offs would be an individual selecting an apartment with less living space at a higher cost for an ideal, convenient location. However, in health care, trade-offs are not limited to selecting one healthcare provider over another. For individuals on a limited budget, examples of trade-offs could be choosing between an annual mammogram, a dental appointment, or an ophthalmology appointment. Even at the national level, paying for preventive health care is always difficult to acquire funding for because only trends from data over several years or decades allow decision makers to determine how preventive services affect health in the future.

Another challenge in healthcare cost-benefit analysis is related to ethics. Because cost-benefit analysis deals with monetary trade-offs rather than effectiveness, ethical dilemmas enter into decisions. For example, if an individual has enough income to pay $1,000 per month for an apartment, then the apartment search is limited to that budget. If the apartment price exceeds the income, then after a few months, the individual could default on the rent, resulting in eviction or not paying for other important bills or services. This scenario is not the same in health care. If an individual arrives at the emergency department in need of life-saving surgery, the surgery is performed and somehow the cost is paid. If the injured individual does not have health insurance or income to pay the hospital bill, it is written off as bad debt by the hospital. When this scenario occurs over and over in numerous hospitals, the healthcare system begins to question who should and should not receive medical care. For example, ponder the following possible ethical questions:

1. Should preterm infants weighing less than one pound be resuscitated at birth?
2. Should individuals over the age of 70 years be eligible for organ transplants?
3. Should morbidly obese patients who develop diabetes be eligible for long-term dialysis treatment when their kidneys no longer function?
4. Should individuals with a 20-year or more history of tobacco use be eligible to receive treatment for lung cancer?
5. Should individuals over 90 years of age be given any type of treatment after a cancer diagnosis?

As can be seen in these questions, it is impossible to put a value on human life or to fund every research project that might improve or save a human life. It is less controversial to think in terms of reducing the risk of acquiring a disease or dying.[6]

Third, the healthcare industry explores the cost benefit of safety for employees. So why do evaluators need to know about occupational safety? The simple response is that healthcare facilities are required by federal law through the Occupational Safety and Health Administration (OSHA) to protect their employees, patients, and visitors. Evaluators with specialized training in the field of environmental and occupational health are qualified to conduct OSHA evaluations in a variety of settings including clinics, hospitals, assisted living facilities, retirement communities, and day care centers. OSHA establishes a hierarchy of protection used to remove or reduce risk and increase safety measures.[7] For example, OSHA requires specific items such as the installation of reflective skid-resistant strips on stairwell steps to avoid a fall. In addition, OSHA becomes involved in administrative controls including written procedures, training, limited exposure, audits, and inspections. For example, hospital transport workers need to receive adequate training on how to lift and move patients without sustaining a back injury. Lastly, OSHA regulates the use of personal protective equipment such as safety glasses, clothing, gloves, respirators, and barriers. For example, a healthcare worker must use gloves and protective face shields to guard against blood-borne pathogen exposure. Even in the best scenario, employees still sustain injuries. These injuries are expensive because the employer pays the healthcare costs, the injured worker is paid their salary while recuperating, and temporary workers must be hired to replace the injured worker during convalescence. Additional hidden costs involve possible legal fees, increased insurance liability rates, and the time required to complete OSHA forms and further investigations.[8] Some clinics find it less expensive to hire an external OSHA evaluator to investigate the potential risks within the facility rather than experience an incident and have to pay increased liability insurance rates. Such external evaluators assess the severity and likelihood of risk (see **Table 12-3**).

Of course, healthcare organizations are always striving to reduce safety risks and minimize injuries involving employees, staff, and visitors. Even if the clinic complies with every OSHA requirement, it is likely that individuals will incur injuries. In the final report, the external evaluators summarize all the injuries, in order of severity, that occurred inside and outside the clinic over the past year, including those of employees, patients, and visitors. In addition, the external evaluators provide recommendations to the healthcare facility related to the costs and benefits of making specific changes. For example, suppose a report of injuries states that several employees slipped on the tile floor when using the side entrance of the clinic. No one was seriously hurt, but one nurse sprained her wrist and the lab technician bruised her shoulder. Upon further investigation,

---

Table 12-3 Simple Job Hazard Analysis

		Severity	
		Low	High
Likelihood	Low	A	B
	High	C	D

Box A: Low severity and low likelihood
A clerk gets a paper cut while retrieving some documents from the printer.

Box B: High severity and low likelihood
The patient fails to disclose his HIV status prior to receiving services at a small walk-in clinic for a severe laceration on his leg. While injecting Novocain (numbing medicine) around the wound prior to stitching, the healthcare provider is accidently stuck with the needle.

Box C: Low severity and high likelihood
The hospital cafeteria is known for its delicious homemade pizza. It is also well-known among the hospital staff that the pizza needs to time to cool prior to eating it. Many workers have sustained mild burns on the roofs of their mouths because they were too anxious to eat the hot pizza before the cheese had a chance to cool a little.

Box D: High severity and high likelihood
A nurse works in the emergency department. He is hit in the face by a combative patient while attempting to restrain the patient. The nurse sustains a severe injury because his arm became entangled in the bedrail as he fell to the floor after losing his balance from the force of the facial hit.

---

the external evaluators found that the side entrance sidewalk is not sloped and usually wet because of poor drainage and no awnings over the door. Because both injuries happened when it was raining, the external evaluators provide two recommendations, including the cost and benefits: (1) low cost and modest benefit: when it rains, the janitor places laminated carpet mats inside the side entrance; (2) high cost and high benefit: fix the poor drainage problem by reconstructing the sidewalk with a proper slope and install an awning over the side entrance, so the side entrance remains dry even when it rains. The clinic administration examines the recommendations and selects the best option.[9]

Cost-Effectiveness Analysis

Cost-effectiveness analysis is a comparison of costs among programs, procedures, or interventions designed to accomplish similar outcomes. However, unlike cost-benefit ratios, cost effectiveness is not expressed in monetary terms. For example, if the outcome is the same, cost-effectiveness analysis compares the cost of treating patients infected with a common virus to the cost of immunizing the population. As the name implies, cost effectiveness compares similar interventions in terms of usefulness or effectiveness, such as a bottle of antibiotics containing 5 pills with instructions to ingest 1 pill per day for 5 days versus a bottle of antibiotics containing 20 pills with instructions to ingest 1 pill in the morning and 1 pill in the evening for 10 days. Although both antibiotics show the same results in the laboratory, the 5-pill antibiotic has higher effectiveness. Why? Because it is more likely that a patient will take 1 pill per day for 5 days than 2 pills per day for 10 days. Once individuals begin to feel better, they are less likely to complete the full 10-day supply of pills.[10]

As another example, a pharmaceutical manufacturer makes Vaccine A and Vaccine B to prevent sexually transmitted infections (STIs). Vaccine A requires one injection, is 100 times more effective in preventing STIs, provides up to 4 years of proven effective protection, and costs $150. Vaccine B requires three injections spaced 30 days apart, provides adequate protection for 12 months, and costs $10 per injection. However, Vaccine B shows little effectiveness in preventing sexually transmitted infections if only one or two injections are received. Healthcare providers are faced with a dilemma. The following list illustrates a few of the many questions that need to be considered by healthcare providers and their patients:

1. Is the expensive one-time cost of Vaccine A enough to deter individuals from receiving it?
2. Is it better to recommend the low-cost Vaccine B and hope for maximum compliance with receiving the three required injections?
3. What are the risks of acquiring sexually transmitted infections if only one injection of Vaccine B is received?
4. Do insurance companies cover the cost of either vaccine?
5. Is the copay the same for both vaccines?

Investigators and healthcare providers explore the advantages and disadvantages for each comparison. See **Figure 12-5** for a summary of cost-effectiveness comparison.

As seen with the example of Vaccine A and Vaccine B, there are challenges in cost-effectiveness analysis. First, cost effectiveness starts with a common unit (e.g., a specific disease or disability). However, over time individuals may mature, gain knowledge, and adopt specific preventive behaviors, such as increased condom use to prevent sexually transmitted diseases, that influence the common

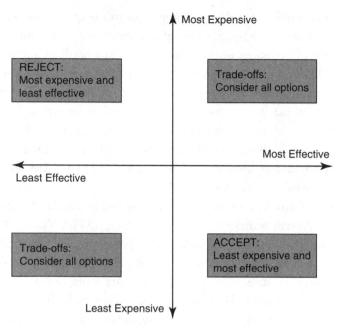

FIGURE 12-5   Summary of Cost-Effectiveness Comparison

outcomes. Because the preventive behaviors change the outcomes, evaluators make adjustments in the analysis because the outcomes are no longer identical. Second, cost-effectiveness decisions are not as simple Figure 12-5 might imply. As in the example, there is no box for selecting Vaccine A, because it is the most effective and most expensive. In most situations, evaluators need to consider all the options. Usually evaluators provide recommendations with scenarios and ideal choices. For example, evaluators may recommend to legislatures that the state subsidize Vaccine A for all adolescents, regardless of ability to pay, because the vaccine is so effective in preventing STIs. Because Vaccine B is less effective and requires three injections, it is unlikely that adolescents would comply with follow-up appointments. Therefore, evaluators would recommend that Vaccine B be removed from the list of vaccines available for the adolescent population.

Cost-Utility Analysis

Cost-utility analysis is a type of cost-effectiveness analysis that compares quality of life gained by dollars spent used to gain it.[11] To understand cost-utility analysis, it is necessary to understand the terms *quality-adjusted life years (QALY)* and *disability-adjusted life years (DALY)*. As expected, cost-utility analysis is controversial, because it attempts to place value on the health status of human individuals and society. Unlike cost effectiveness, which compares similar benefits or outcomes, cost-utility analysis compares health interventions or procedures with different benefits.

Quality-Adjusted Life Years

Quality-adjusted life years is a calculation combining quantity and quality of health to quantify outcomes based on treatment or other activities that influence health. Investigators measure QALY by using secondary data from large epidemiological studies as well as medical records across similar medical conditions to compare and predict life expectancies. QALY measures the cost of producing one year of quality living. Quality living data is collected and defined in several ways, including self-report of individuals, medical chart reviews, and caregiver assessment. For example, one 24-year-old person with spinal cord paralysis is involved in paraplegic sporting events and ranks QALY as good, whereas another 24-year-old person with spinal cord paralysis becomes socially isolated because of depression and ranks QALY as poor. Life circumstances vary as to how individuals view their quality of life. From the researchers' viewpoint, QALY is a single unit that measures the state of health on a ranked scale from 0 (immediate death) to 100 (perfect health). It is possible for the calculation to yield a negative number when an individual is living indefinitely with poor quality of life.[12]

Cost-utility analysis calculates QALY in years.[13] If it costs $100,000 to gain one year of life for an individual with a specific illness, the cost utility is $100,000 per year. With limited healthcare resources, cost-utility analysis compares maximum benefits gained from different health treatments to produce health outcomes. In other words, cost-utility analysis influences whether an individual should or should not be treated for a specific disease.[14] In general, health interventions that yield low QALYs are given fewer scarce resources. Although this type of calculation is appealing to decision makers, cost-utility analysis raises several questions. How is quality of life defined among individuals? Are the calculations valid, and do they measure what is intended to be measured? Are the calculations reliable or repeatable across populations? Is one population adversely affected by the calculation more so than another? For example, is one ethnicity more likely to suffer from a specific disease than another ethnic group? Lastly, what ethical issues are involved in each of the cost-utility calculations?[15]

Disability-Adjusted Life Years

Another type of cost-utility analysis is disability-adjusted life years. DALY measures the years one lives with a disability and years of life lost because of premature death from that disability.[16] When individuals experience a disease or disability caused by environmental exposure, natural disaster, or health behavior risks, the term *disability-adjusted life year* is used. One DALY is defined as one lost year of "healthy" life. Across a population, the total DALYs measure the gap between no disease and disability. The World Health Organization developed DALY to measure a population's health by comparing nonfatal and fatal outcomes when prioritizing health resources.[16] DALYs are used to calculate the magnitude of disease and health risks globally,[17-19] nationally, and at local levels. DALY estimates are also used to measure the effectiveness of prevention programs for specific diseases[20] when recommending funding priorities.[21] Although DALY calculations are not always agreed upon by global experts, they provide a standardized cost-effectiveness analysis of public health interventions in low- and middle-income countries.[22,23]

Even with the limitations, DALYs use standardized disability definitions to compare the health impact of a wide range of medical conditions.[24] If DALYs are the only calculation used, it is possible that factors causing disabilities receive less funding than if several measurements are used. As with any social determinant of health, it is necessary to investigate all aspects of the disability including the functional limitations, physical activities, and social interactions.[25] See **Box 12-2** for an example of cost-utility analysis in general.

Cost-Feasibility Analysis

Cost-feasibility analysis is defined as a comparison of the cost required for the project compared to the overall projected value of the project.[26,27] For example, a medical treatment is proven valuable for a common but non-life-threatening illness; however, the cost is prohibitive for the general population. Evaluators use a SWOT (strengths [advantages], weaknesses [disadvantages], opportunities [prospects for growth], and threats [awareness of internal or external warnings]) analysis to conduct a cost-feasibility study. Gathering data to support each component of the SWOT analysis allows evaluators to report comprehensive findings to the stakeholders and decision makers.[28] SWOT analyses are also used to evaluate current program objectives or to determine future objectives based on results of previous SWOT analyses.

For a cost-feasibility study, evaluators conduct a SWOT analysis to explore the viability of a current or future project. For example, if the hospital administrative board is considering expanding the cardiac care unit, it conducts a cost-feasibility study to explore all aspects of the return on investment. Keep in mind that the costs are not only monetary but are also related to patient satisfaction, the community need for more cardiac care patient beds, the

BOX 12-2

Example of Cost-Utility Analysis

In 2006, researchers used cost-utility analysis to demonstrate cost effectiveness in medical interventions. They reviewed the published literature to compare which of three treatments was most effective in preventing coronary heart disease (CHD) in men. The three daily treatments included taking aspirin only, statin medication only, or a combination of aspirin and statin medications. Their findings suggested that a combination of aspirin and statin medications is the most effective method of preventing coronary heart disease in men. The authors used cost-utility analysis because they compared the lifetime effects of 10 years of either aspirin therapy, or statin therapy, or a combination aspirin and statin therapy, or no therapy in middle-aged men with a 7.5% risk of CHD. Their findings suggested that aspirin therapy was less costly than no therapy for men having a CHD risk of 7.5% and greater. The addition of statin therapy increased the cost-utility ratio but proved to be more cost-effective only for the men who had a greater than 10% risk of CHD.[29]

Data from Pignone M, Earnshaw S, Tice JA, Pletcher MJ. Aspirin, statins, or both drugs for the primary prevention of heart disease events in men: A cost-utility analysis. *Ann Intern Med.* 2006;144(5):326–336.

availability of highly trained nursing staff, expanding the size of the hospital, and the loss of valuable space used for parking.

Another way to think about cost feasibility is to answer this question: Is the problem worth solving at a reasonable cost? For this aspect of cost feasibility, evaluators explore four different aspects of feasibility: technical, economic, operational, and organizational. Technical feasibility investigates whether it is possible to solve the problem with existing technology. For example, does the hospital have the current electronic medical records technology needed to analyze patient records to address research questions rather than only billing and finance questions? Economic feasibility compares the costs of solving the problem versus the benefits of solving the problem. If the costs are excessive, the benefits are not obtainable. Operational feasibility investigates whether the program implementation is compatible with the environment (e.g., physical, political, economic, or administrative). Take, for example, the operational feasibility of implementing an art and music therapy program in the hospital if the hospital board members strongly believe that these types of complementary medical therapies are not valuable in the healing and recovery process. Lastly, organizational feasibility relates to the strategic plan of the organization. If the proposed project is not in alignment with the long-term goals of the organization, then there is no point in moving forward with the funding and implementation of the project.

Summary

This chapter began with a detailed description of types of budgets, including personal, research financial plans, and profit and loss statements. This discussion was followed by an introduction to the various types of cost analysis. Evaluators and researchers use cost analysis techniques to determine the most effective and efficient health procedures, treatments, and programs.

Case Study

For the last 10 years, Ellen Ferguson has owned and directed Caring for Women, Inc., a small women's health clinic in Iowa. The clinic provides well-women care, such as contraceptive services, preconception through menopause counseling, annual physical examinations, and routine medical services for minor healthcare needs such as urinary tract infections, sexually transmitted infections, and upper respiratory infections. Because the clinic is located near a local high school and a university, female students, staff, and faculty receive health care at the clinic. There are five employees: the director, the office manager, two nurse practitioners, and one medical assistant. Because the clinic is run by nurse practitioners, Dr. Ferguson pays a medical director a monthly stipend to serve as the medical backup for the nurse practitioners treating women in the clinic. After years of struggling to keep the clinic open, Dr. Ferguson decides to conduct a cost analysis to decide whether to close the clinic. She gets out her textbooks and reviews the various types of cost analysis techniques. She decides that cost-benefit analysis is inappropriate, because she is not interested in comparing her clinic with other clinics in the area and she is not allocating limited resources to

continues

CASE STUDY *continued*

different programs. She also determines that cost-utility analysis does not pertain to her clinic, because cost-utility analysis involves expected quantity and quality of life among her patients. The remaining two techniques are cost-effectiveness and cost-feasibility analyses. Dr. Ferguson decides to explore both techniques because she wants to ensure that all aspects are considered. After completing the cost-effectiveness summary, she realizes that the clinic must find a way to increase the number of patients coming through the door without increasing overhead costs, in other words, the most effective but least expensive solution (see **Figure 12-6**).[10]

Dr. Ferguson holds a team meeting to brainstorm possible ideas for increasing revenue to keep the clinic open. Because the clinic staff is dedicated to keeping the clinic open, they decide that they could begin to offer various cosmetic treatments as well as medical health care. After reviewing the clinic schedule, they realize that there are often gaps in the

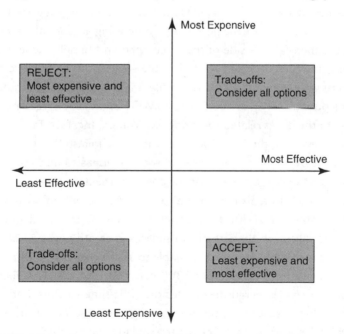

FIGURE 12-6   Summary of Cost-Effectiveness Comparison

continues

CASE STUDY *continued*

appointments. These appointment gaps are expensive, because the nurse practitioners are being paid even though they are not seeing patients and thus not generating revenue for the clinic. It is suggested that the clinic could offer massage therapy and esthetician services (e.g., facials, microdermabrasion, waxing). They decide to hire an esthetician for three days per week (Monday, Wednesday, and Friday) and a massage therapist for three days per week (Tuesday, Thursday, and Saturday) on a consultation basis. The esthetician and massage therapist will split their fees with the clinic. For example, if the massage therapist receives $100 per hour, the clinic receives $50. The advantages for the esthetician and massage therapist include the following: (1) no overhead costs (e.g., space rental, utility payments, telephone/internet costs), (2) a permanent address for advertising purposes, (3) steady exposure to the clinic patients, (4) a location to store a massage table and supplies, (5) and free parking. The clinic staff decides to convert the third exam room into the esthetician service and massage therapy room. The suggested ideas are at no cost and have the potential of generating additional revenue to keep the medical care side of the clinic open and fiscally viable. Before making any final decisions related to the suggestions from clinic staff, Dr. Ferguson conducts a cost-feasibility analysis with the assistance of her accountant. They decide to use a SWOT analysis for greater clarification of the issues related to Caring for Women, Inc. (see **Table 12-4**).

After reviewing the SWOT analysis with the clinic staff, Dr. Ferguson makes the decision to move forward with the ideas to add esthetician services and massage therapy. At the advice of the accountant, the decision is limited to a six-month trial period. At the end of six months, Dr. Ferguson meets with the accountant to review the fiscal status of the clinic. Although the esthetician services generate about $1,500 per month, the massage therapist is unable to secure a steady stream of clients and thus only adds about $300 per month to the clinic income. Unfortunately, Dr. Ferguson decides that it is time to close Caring for Women, Inc., because she can no longer generate sufficient income to pay the salaries of her staff. She is interested in selling Caring for Women, Inc., but soon realizes that it is difficult to sell a medical practice. Besides

continues

CASE STUDY *continued*

> ### Table 12-4   SWOT Analysis for Caring for Women, Inc.
>
> | STRENGTHS | WEAKNESSES |
> |---|---|
> | Personalized care for women | Not enough patients to generate needed income |
> | Accepts all types of health insurance | |
> | Ease of scheduling appointments | Does not offer obstetrical/prenatal care |
> | Dedicated clinic staff and medical director | Gaps between appointments |
> | Easy-to-find location | |
> | Convenient free parking | |
>
> | THREATS | OPPORTUNITIES |
> |---|---|
> | Large women's health clinic based at nearby university | Offer esthetician services and massage therapy |
> | Inability to qualify for large employer health insurance contracts | Advertise more for new services |

the equipment and office furniture and supplies, there is little to sell. She is closely connected to the local Planned Parenthood clinic, so she contacts them. They are willing to purchase the Caring for Women, Inc., patient files and computer database in hopes of increasing their own patient population seeking personalized medical care. The purchase price is negotiated for $30,000. In addition, Planned Parenthood hires the office manager and medical assistant. The nurse practitioners are hired by the university-based women's health clinic, and Dr. Ferguson becomes a women's health researcher at the university. For continuity of care, Planned Parenthood contacts the Caring for Women, Inc., patients via postcard immediately after the sale is final. They are pleased to report that their clinic has seen an increase in revenue from the purchase of Caring for Women, Inc., after only 6 months.

Case Study Discussion Questions

1. Create one profit and loss statement showing a 15% profit and one profit and loss statement showing a 15% loss.
2. Discuss other options that the staff could have tried to attract more income.

Student Activity

The following is an example of a personal budget. Study the budget and then answer the questions about it.

Brad is 26 years old and works in a small marketing firm in a medium-sized city. This budget reflects his income and expenses for a typical month (see **Table 12-5**).

1. How much money does Brad earn (before taxes) in a:
    Week:
    Month:
    Year:
2. How much money in state and federal taxes is withheld from Brad's pay-check every two weeks?
3. Calculate Brad's take-home pay for one month.

Table 12-5   Brad's Budget

Category	
Income	
Salary $23.00 per hour	40 hours per week
Expenses	
Federal income tax	22%
State income tax	3%
Social Security/Medicare	6.2%
Medical insurance	$64.00 per month
Life insurance	$15.00 per month
401(k) contribution	4%
Savings	?
Rent	$750 per month
Auto payment	$230 per month
Auto insurance	$160 per month
Water	$24 per month
Gas	$60 per month
Electricity	$75 per month
Cable/internet	$140 per month
Phone/cell phone	$93 per month
Other utilities	$34 per month

4. How much discretionary money does Brad have after paying his living expenses from his take-home income?

5. Suppose Brad wants to start saving more money. He considers several amounts. How much money would he need to save each month if he saved 5%, 10%, and 15% of his discretionary money?
5%:
10%:
15%:

6. Suppose Brad wants to save the maximum amount of 15% of his discretionary money each month. How much money does Brad then have left over to use each week for going out, paying for gas for his car, and entertainment?

Answers

1. How much money does Brad earn (before taxes) in a:
Week: $920
Month: $3,956
Year: $44,160

2. How much money in state and federal taxes is withheld from Brad's paycheck every two weeks? $574.08

3. Calculate Brad's take-home pay for one month. $2,606.24

4. How much discretionary money does Brad have after paying his living expenses from his take-home income? $1,040.24

5. Suppose Brad wants to start saving more money. He considers several amounts. How much money would he need to save each month if he saved 5%, 10%, and 15% of his discretionary money?
5%: $52.01
10%: $104.02
15%: $156.04

6. Suppose Brad wants to save the maximum amount of money each month. How much money does Brad then have left over to use each week for going out, paying for gas for his car, and entertainment? $221.05

References

1. De Navas-Walt C, Proctor BD, Smith JC. U.S. Census Bureau. Current Population Reports, P60-243. *Income, Poverty and Health Insurance Coverage in the United States: 2011.* Washington, DC: U.S. Government Printing Office; 2012.

2. Families USA. 2012 Federal Poverty Guidelines. Available at: http://www.familiesusa.org/resources/tools-for-advocates/guides/federal-poverty-guidelines.html. Accessed November 3, 2012.

3. United States Department of Labor. Minimum Wage Laws in the States. Available at: http://www.dol.gov/whd/minwage/america.htm. Accessed February 3, 2013.

4. The Organisation for Economic Co-operation and Development (OECD). OECD Health Data 2012: How Does the United States Compare. Available at: http://78.41.128.130/dataoecd/46/2/38980580.pdf. Accessed November 3, 2012.

5. Rochester Institute of Technology, Department of Outreach Education and Training. Cost Benefit Analysis. Available at: https://www.rit.edu/~w-outrea/training/Module5/M5_CostBenefitAnalysis.pdf. Accessed November 3, 2012.

6. Watkins T. San Jose State University Department of Economics. An Introduction to Cost Benefit Analysis. Available at: http://www.sjsu.edu/faculty/watkins/cba.htm. Accessed November 3, 2012.

7. Occupational Safety and Health Administration. OSHA Laws and Regulations. Available at: http://www.osha.gov/law-regs.html. Accessed November 3, 2012.

8. Occupational Safety and Health Administration. Safety and Health Management Systems eTool. Available at: http://www.osha.gov/SLTC/etools/safetyhealth/. Accessed November 3, 2012.

9. Dixon I, Lundeen A. *Cost Effective Analysis: An Employer Decision Support Tool.* Washington, DC: National Business Group on Health Center for Prevention and Health Services; 2004.

10. Musgrove P, Fox-Rushley J. Cost-effectiveness analysis for priority setting. In: Jamison DT, Breman JG, Measham AR, Alleyne G, Claeson M, Evans DB, Jha P, Mills A, Musgrove P, eds. *Disease Control Priorities in Developing Countries.* Washington, DC: The World Bank; 2006.

11. The World Health Organization. Cost-utility analysis. In: *Introduction to Drug Utilization Research.* Oslo, Norway: The World Health Organization; 2003. Available at: http://apps.who.int/medicinedocs/en/d/Js4876e/5.4.html. Accessed November 3, 2012.

12. Bandolier. QALY. Available at: http://www.medicine.ox.ac.uk/bandolier/booth/glossary/QALY.html. Accessed November 3, 2012.

13. Pettinger T. Cost Utility and Cost Effectiveness Analysis. http://www.economicshelp.org/blog/93/economics/cost-utility-and-cost-effectiveness-analysis/. Published December 4, 2007. Accessed September 23, 2013.

14. Vanhook P. Cost-utility analysis: A method of quantifying the value of registered nurses. *Online J Issues Nurs.* 2007;12(3).

15. McGregor M. Cost–utility analysis: Use QALYs only with great caution. *CMAJ.* 2003;168(4):433–434.

16. The World Health Organization. Health Statistics and Health Information Systems. Metrics: Disability-Adjusted Life Year. Available at: http://www.who.int/healthinfo/global_burden_disease/metrics_daly/en/. Accessed November 3, 2012.

17. Murray CJ, Acharya AK. Understanding DALYs (disability-adjusted life years). *J Health Econ.* 1997;16(6):703–730.

18. Murray CJL, Lopez AD, eds. *The Global Burden of Disease: A Comprehensive Assessment of Mortality and Disability from Diseases, Injuries, and Risk Factors in 1990 and Projected to 2020.* Cambridge, MA: Harvard University Press; 1996.

19. Lopez AD, Mathers CD, Ezzati M, Jamison DT, Murray CJL, eds. *Global Burden of Disease and Risk Factors.* Washington, DC: World Bank; 2006.

20. Lopez AD, Mathers CD, Ezzati M, Jamison DT, Murray CJ. Global and regional burden of disease and risk factors, 2001: Systematic analysis of population health data. *Lancet.* 2006;367:1747–1757.

21. Cadilhac DA, Carter RC, Thrift AG, Dewey HM. Why invest in a national public health program for stroke? An example using Australian data to estimate the potential benefits and cost implications. *Health Policy.* 2007;83(2–3):287–294.

22. Gross CP, Anderson GF, Powe NR. The relation between funding by the National Institutes of Health and the burden of disease. *N Engl J Med.* 1999;340(24):1881–1887.

23. Schackman BR, Neukermans CP, Fontain SN, Nolte C, Joseph P, Pape JW, Fitzgerald DW. Cost-effectiveness of rapid syphilis screening in prenatal HIV testing programs in Haiti. *PLos Med.* 2007;4(5):e183.

24. Thacker SB, Stroup DF, Carande-Kulis V, Marks JS, Roy, Gerberding JL. Measuring the public's health. *Public Health Rep.* 2006;121(1):14–22.

25. Grosse SD, Lollar DJ, Campbell VA, Chamie M. Disability-adjusted life years: Not the same. *Public Health Rep.* 2009;124(2):197–202.

26. Young GIM. Feasibility studies. *Appraisal Journal.* 1970;38(3):376–383.

27. Jyoth BN, Babu GR, Krishna IVM. Object oriented and multi-scale image analysis: Strengths, weaknesses, opportunities and threats—A review. *J Computer Science.* 2008;4(9):706–712.

28. Hofstrand D. Iowa State University Extension and Outreach. How to Do and How to Use a Feasibility Study. Available at: http://www.extension.iastate.edu/agdm/wholefarm/html/c5-64.html. Accessed November 3, 2013.

29. Pignone M, Earnshaw S, Tice JA, Pletcher MJ. Aspirin, statins, or both drugs for the primary prevention of heart disease events in men: A cost-utility analysis. *Ann Intern Med.* 2006;144(5):326–336.

Reports and Presentations

Introduction

After investigators spend endless hours conducting their studies, it is time to present their findings. This chapter provides details on how to create effective written reports, oral presentations, panel discussions, lectures, and poster presentations related to research and evaluation results. First, types of written reports are discussed and the development of each element is defined, including reference styles and overcoming writer's block. Second, effective ways to communicate are reviewed, including oral presentations, ways to prepare useful slide presentations, and powerful rehearsal strategies. Lastly, the chapter concludes with techniques to create winning poster presentations with key bullet points.

Types of Written Reports

It is not unusual for students to experience a feeling of dread when given an assignment to write a report. However, because writing is an essential skill throughout your academic studies as well as in your future professional careers, it is important to learn some basic components of report writing. Prior to discussing types of reports, we divide this section into manageable components to make composing the whole report less daunting.

Let's begin with the discussion of three types of reports: research, evaluation, and technical. Keep in mind that even though each type of report is unique, every report should be written clearly and concisely. Research reports focus on results of the research. They also compare the current results with previous results, if known. Research reports are published in peer-reviewed journals and contribute to the overall body of knowledge related to the specific topic. Research reports are written for a generalized audience within a wide field of study (e.g., medicine, nursing, public health, pharmacy). Evaluation reports present the findings of an evaluation, including best practices, processes, program impact, and long-term outcomes. Like research reports, evaluation reports may be published in peer-reviewed journals. However, there are evaluation firms that conduct high-quality evaluations, but their reports are not published in peer-reviewed journals. Their evaluation findings are available on the Internet as technical reports or governmental documents, such as final reports produced for the U.S. Government Accountability Office. Both research and evaluation reports provide the reader with recommendations for future investigations. Technical reports aim to state how the problem was solved or to propose solutions. Technical reports are generally not published in peer-reviewed journals and are written for a specific audience (e.g., stakeholders, board members, nonprofit organizations, funding agencies). Technical reports are written using specialized language for an audience of experts, such as computer science software programmers.

After determining the type of report that is appropriate, the next step is to answer a few questions about the purpose of the report.

Who is the audience?

- If the audience is a professor, then it is likely that the professor explained the purpose of the writing assignment in class or in the syllabus. If students have questions, they should ask for greater clarification from the professor before starting the assignment.

- If the audience members are also stakeholders (e.g., funding agency members, community members, board of directors), then the report should address their concerns.
- If the audience is a funding agency, then the report answers the questions or objectives related to the original reason for conducting the evaluation or research.

In all situations, reports should be well organized and written in clear, understandable language. For example, if the report targets computer science engineers implementing an update of a hospital's electronic medical records software, the report does not need to define the technical terms understood by the computer science engineers. However, if the same report is written for the hospital administrators, the technical language is replaced with easy-to-understand terms.

How will the report be used?

- If the report is for a course assignment, the report will be used for a grade. Therefore, the report is written to match the grading rubric provided by the professor.
- If the report is used for seeking additional funding for a community report, the report emphasizes current results as well as recommendations and future needs.
- If the report is used to obtain buy-in from stakeholders, then the report focuses on the positive effects of the current activities.

Once the audience and purpose of the report are identified, the writer thinks about these questions:

- What are the specific elements of the report (e.g., number of pages, font, font size, margins, placement of tables and figures, reference style)?
- What is the explicit message or aim of the report?
- What are the key points you wish to communicate?
- What information is needed to make your findings understandable that should be collected prior to writing the report (e.g., maps, data, graphs, tables, figures)?

After these questions are addressed, it necessary to outline the report. Begin the outline with basic information. Even the simplest of outlines helps to start the writing process (see **Table 13-1**). More details are added to each segment of this

Table 13-1 Simple Report Outline

Introduction
Background
Key Points
  1.
  2.
  3.
  4.
Recommendations
Conclusion
References

outline later in this chapter. However, it is best to start with a basic outline rather than add all the details in the beginning.

As you create the outline, it is useful to think about the readers. The report provides information to meet the needs of the audience. Review **Table 13-2**. In sample 1, the audience is interested in the overall strengths, weaknesses, opportunities, and threats of the clinic. Sample 2 directs the audience to specific areas within the clinic. Both outlines could be either appropriate or inappropriate based on the designated needs of the audience.[1]

Elements of the Report

Now that the simple outline is complete, let's begin to delve into the specific elements of the report. For this discussion, the elements expand the basic outline and provide greater detail for the reader. Although most reports have similar

Table 13-2 Example of Two Basic Report Outlines

Sample 1: Basic Report Outline		Sample 2: Basic Report Outline	
Strengths	Patient Services and Staffing	Patient Services and	Strengths
	Accounting and Finance	Staffing	Weaknesses
	Plant Maintenance and Grounds		Opportunities
Weaknesses	Patient Services and Staffing		Threats
	Accounting and Finance	Accounting	Strengths
	Plant Maintenance and Grounds	and Finance	Weaknesses
Opportunities	Patient Services and Staffing		Opportunities
	Accounting and Finance		Threats
	Plant Maintenance and Grounds	Plant Maintenance	Strengths
Threats	Patient Services and Staffing	and Grounds	Weaknesses
	Accounting and Finance		Opportunities
	Plant Maintenance and Grounds		Threats

Table 13-3   Sample Author Guidelines

Taylor & Francis Group	http://www.tandf.co.uk/journals/ifa.asp
Springer Publishing	http://www.springerpub.com/content/downloads /Springer_Publishing_Manuscript_Guidelines.pdf
American Psychological Association	http://www.apa.org/pubs/authors/instructions.aspx
American Dental Association	http://www.ada.org/995.aspx
New England Journal of Medicine	http://www.nejm.org/page/author-center/manuscript- submission

sections, if you are writing for a specific journal, you should verify its author guidelines. Author guidelines describe the required components of manuscript and reference style desired by the agency or publisher requesting the report (see **Table 13-3**).

Now let's explore each element of the report. Under each section, a more detailed outline or description is provided in the discussion.

Title Page

The title page includes the title, author(s), and date of submission. In some situations, the name of the funding agency or report recipient is listed on the title page. The title of the report should describe the scope of the report in a few words. Here are a few examples of titles.

Incomplete description:
   Forms of Violence Directed at Women

Complete description:
   Forms of Violence Directed at Women: Online Education Modules to Educate Registered Nurses About Recognizing Relationship Violence Among Their Pregnant Patients

Incomplete description:
   Disparities Among Breast Cancer Screening Rates

Complete description:
   Disparities Among Breast Cancer Screening Rates: A Secondary Analysis of Data from the 2000–2010 Behavioral Risk Factor Surveillance System

Incomplete description:
   Emergency Contraception: The Role of the Pharmacist

Complete description:
   Emergency Contraception: Assessing the Knowledge, Attitudes, and Dispensing Practices Among Pharmacists Practicing in Texas

Table of Contents

The table of contents provides the reader with a list of the major and minor segments of the report. Because page numbers are provided, it allows the reader to turn to the section that is of most interest. It indicates how the information is organized. All tables and figures are included in the table of contents.

Abstract or Executive Summary

Although abstracts or executive summaries are shown first, they are written last. The abstract is a summary of the entire report. Abstracts are provided at the beginning of scientific or academic reporting. They provide a concise summary of complex research. This allows a reader to ascertain the purpose and main findings of the research and decide whether they want to continue reading. Abstracts are usually written after all other parts of the manuscript, so that the findings and recommendations are not erroneously reported. Always double-check the guidelines, as abstracts and executive summaries often have length limits. Abstracts may range from 50 to 400 words in length. Within the word limit, the writer tells the whole story: what the problem was, how the problem was researched, what the data analysis methods were, what the results were, and what the recommendations are. In a similar fashion, executive summaries are usually 2 to 3 pages and also tell the overall summary of the report findings.[2] In the report, the abstract or executive summary is placed on a separate page is and written as a single paragraph without any indentation. Keep in mind that an abstract or executive summary may be the only portion of the report read by a general audience. Therefore, it is important that these sections include the most important findings or key points, are clearly written, and are logically organized.

Introduction

An introduction is not a rewritten version of the abstract; rather, the introduction sets the tone of the report (see **Box 13-1**). The introduction is divided into three sections:

1. The statement of the problem provides a brief review of the issues and states the accomplishments completed to date.
2. The purpose of the study briefly describes how this study builds on or adds to the current knowledge.
3. The scope of the study explains the methods used in this research or evaluation.

BOX 13-1

Outline of an Introduction Section

Introduction
    Statement of the problem
    Purpose of the study
    Scope of the study

The extent of specific details in the introduction depends on the audience. For example, a technical report for colleagues needs fewer details and explanation than a quarterly report for a funding agency, such as the National Institutes of Health.

Literature Review or Background

A literature or background section provides the current knowledge regarding a given topic area, including substantive, theoretical, and methodological findings (see **Box 13-2**). The literature review starts with a broad focus and ends narrowly. Depending on the scope of the topic, the literature review is either comprehensive or selective. The decision between comprehensive or selective is based on the purpose of the report and possible length restrictions. If there is no length restriction as in a thesis or dissertation, a comprehensive review of the literature is used—for example, the historical overview of healthcare provider responses to HIV/AIDS in the United States since the 1980s. A selective review

BOX 13-2

Outline of a Literature Review Section

Literature review or background
    State the limitations of the review
        Broad topic: historical background or specific limitations
        Focus of topic
        Narrow focus of topic
        Gap in knowledge for the topic
    Transition from review to purpose of reported research

of literature is typical for journal articles. The selective literature review begins with a broad overview of the historical side of the topic and ends with specific targeted literature related to the need for the research. Developing a detailed outline ensures maximum clarity and explains the need for the research. The outline shows the connection between the known body of knowledge on the topic and its relationship to the proposed research. A selective literature review is limited and clearly states those limits for the reader. For example, "This review of the literature is focused on research conducted after 2010 on the topic of best practices in health education programs for adults diagnosed with type 2 diabetes." Because literature reviews summarize knowledge, direct quotes are sometimes included in this section. Lastly, a literature review ends with a brief summary that serves as a transition to the next component of the report.

Methods

The methods section of a written report shows how a researcher went about answering the research questions or how an evaluator addressed the goals and objectives of an evaluation (see **Box 13-3**). The methods section is often used to judge the validity of the research or evaluation. The best way to organize the methods section is to think of a recipe. For example, cookies taste awful if the recipe fails to include the key ingredient of sugar. In the same respect, if this section fails to include enough detail, readers are unable to judge the validity of the findings and duplicate the study. Researchers duplicate studies to defend or refute the results. This section, like other sections, must be organized in a logical sequence: what was investigated, what was found, what interpretations were made, and what judgments were made. Use short, informative headings

---

BOX 13-3

Outline of a Methods Section

Methods
  Institutional review board approval process
  Study design
  Sampling
  Setting
  Pilot test
  Data collection

and subheadings. An easy way to remember the components of this section are: who, what, when, where, why, and how.

Study design:
Describe whether a theory provided the foundation for the study. If so, which theory, and why was it selected? If no theory was used, explain why that decision was made.
Was the study a randomized control trial with both control and experimental groups of participants?
Identify the design, and describe why it was selected. Did the design include a pretest and a posttest?

Sampling:
Describe the inclusion and exclusion criteria for participants.
Identify why the inclusion and exclusion criteria were used.
Describe how the participants were recruited.
How many participants were needed for the study? How many participants actually participated in the study? Describe why the number of participants was not reached.
How many participants were lost to follow-up in the study? Why?

Setting:
Where did the study take place?
Why was this setting selected for the study?
What made the chosen site ideal or unique for this study?
If there were multiple sites, how and why were the sites chosen?

Data collection:
Quantitative data collection
What surveys, questionnaires, or instruments were used to collect data?
How were instruments collected: via mail, in person, or online?
How were data entered for analysis?
Were some surveys tested with double entry to verify accuracy?
Were any tests conducted to verify reliability and validity?
Qualitative data collection
What types of data were collected: interviews, focus groups, or existing documents?
Describe the interview/focus group guidelines.

Prior to describing the methods used, researchers and evaluators must acknowledge that institutional review board approval was obtained prior to conducting any portion of the investigation.

Results

The section describes the findings of the research study or evaluation (see **Box 13-4**). Results are presented concisely. Results tell us the statistics found

BOX 13-4

Outline of a Results Section

Data analysis
   Statistical methods
   Qualitative methods
Response to research question(s)
   Description of analysis output
   Tables, graphs, and figures

by quantitative statistical analysis or themes found through qualitative analysis. Generally, if collected, the demographics are presented first, so readers learn about the studied population prior to reviewing the results. Although a few demographics are typically discussed briefly in the narrative, all demographics are shown in a table format (see **Table 13-4**).

Keep in mind that tables and figures are labeled sequentially throughout the document (e.g., Table 1, Table 2, Figure 1, Table 3, and Figure 2). If the report is divided into chapters, the tables and figures are numbered within each chapter. For example, for Chapter 1 there is Table 1.1 and Table 1.2, for Chapter 2 there is Table 2.1, Table 2.2, Figure 2.1, and Figure 2.2, and so on.

After the demographics, the data used to address the research questions or objectives are presented. For example, if a paired samples *t*-test was used to

---

Table 13-4   Sample of Demographic Data Presented in a Results Section

Description of Demographic Data

For demographics, 224 (86%) of the clinic staff responded to the survey. For gender, there were 107 (48%) females and 117 (52%) males. For age, there were 78 (35%) clinic workers in the 20–29 age group, 83 (37%) in the 30–39 age group, 43 (20%) in the 40–49 age group, and 20 (8%) in the 50+ age group. As for education, there were 6 (3%) of the clinic staff reporting less than a high school degree, 17 (7%) with a high school diploma, 19 (8%) with some college credits, 153 (68%) with a college degree, and 29 (14%) with a graduate degree.

Table A. Demographic Data (*n* = 224)

Variable	Number	Percentage
Gender	Females	107 (48%)
	Males	117 (52%)
Age	20–29 years	78 (35%)
	30–39 years	83 (37%)
	40–49 years	43 (20%)
	50+ years	20 (8%)
Education	< High school	6 (3%)
	High school	17 (7%)
	Some college	19 (8%)
	College degree	153 (68%)
	Graduate degree	29 (14%)

determine the difference between pretest surveys and posttest surveys, those results are presented. For example, "Of the 224 clinic staff who responded, there was a pretest mean score of 64 and posttest mean score of 97, with a t-test showing a statistically significant difference ($t = 7.08$; $p = 0.03$)." For each research question, the same process is followed throughout the results section. Keep in mind that investigators do not merely cut and paste the statistical results from the statistical software package into the results section of the report. Investigators also do not add any statistics outside those that are meant to address the research question.

For example, investigators notice an interesting correlation in the data analysis while they are conducting the statistics. This interesting correlation is not added to the results section merely because it is a unique finding. If this new finding is indeed unique, it is advised that the investigators explore it further and perhaps report it in the discussion or in another manuscript.

Discussion, Conclusion, Recommendations, and Future Research

The purpose of the discussion section is to compare the results of the current study to the results of similar studies published in the literature (see **Box 13-5**). The results of the current study may defend or refute the results of previous studies, with researchers adding what is different about their samples or methods that may have contributed to the differences in the findings. When findings vary from study to study, you cannot assume researcher error or study weakness; but the differences could be based on study participants, geographical location, age, culture, income, or education. For example, the participants of the previous study lived in

BOX 13-5

Outline of Discussion, Conclusion, Recommendations, and Future Research Sections

Discussion
    Defend or refute literature
        Limitations
Conclusion
Recommendations
Future research

an urban area, whereas the participants of the current study live in a remote rural area. This geographical difference could have contributed to the difference in findings. Another example may show that results for one age group of participants are different from the results for another age group for the same intervention.

Limitations are the weaknesses of your research or evaluation and are reported in the discussion section. Because all investigations have limitations, it is advised that the final report should reflect any recognized weaknesses. For example, if the results show that only 16% of the participants completed the posttest survey, it should be noted as a weakness. This weakness may be the result of an issue with the study design, how the survey was administered, or the survey questions themselves. Putting this information in the limitations section allows investigators to improve future studies by addressing these issues at the beginning. However, it would be up to the investigators to state what methods were utilized to try to improve the response rate, such as reminder postcards and phone messages. On the other hand, a weakness may not have been noticed until late in the research and could not be corrected. For example, an error on the survey was not noticed until after 700 participants had completed the survey and data entry began. This error might be the following:

Survey question (incorrect):	Correct version would be:
Please select the category that includes your age:	
a. 20–30 years	a. 20–29 years
b. 30–40 years	b. 30–39 years
c. 40–50 years	c. 40–49 years
d. 50–60 years	d. 50–59 years
e. 60+ years	e. 60+ years

Participants who are 30, 40, 50, or 60 years of age would not be able to select only one choice. This overlap would cause a serious error in inferring any results related to the age variable. At this point, the survey would be not resubmitted for completion, but rather the error would be mentioned as a limitation.

In the limitations section, it is also important to pay attention to the language of the discussion. Even if the project had numerous major limitations, it is critical not to assign blame or make excuses for any aspect or weakness of the study. Focus on presenting possible solutions to establish trust rather than doubt in the report. The information presented in the report remains neutral and without commendation.

Conclusions are a final, brief interpretation of the results. Most conclusions are written in a few sentences or paragraphs. Keep in mind that the abstract or executive summary and the conclusion are the most frequently read segments of reports. The information in the conclusion should be presented in order of importance. The conclusion does not include any speculation, but rather only the evidence supported by the results of the current study. Recommendations follow the conclusion and present direct suggestions or action items for the decision makers reading the report. If an evaluation team has a list of suggestions, the recommendations may be presented in bullet points (see **Box 13-6**).

Future research is the final section of the narrative portion of the report. This section states specifically what further studies the researchers recommend. For example, if two published studies had similar results and the current study refuted those results, researchers suggest conducting a similar study to confirm the newly found information. For example, if researchers in Asia, France, and the United States detect one viral strain of the flu, but each researcher noted different onset symptoms, then a report would likely suggest further research related to the onset symptoms.

BOX 13-6

Sample Recommendations

Based on the results of this evaluation, the following recommendations are proposed:

- Change the clinic's hours of operation from 9:00 a.m. to 5:00 p.m. to 8:00 a.m. to 6:00 p.m. to improve clinic access to working individuals.
- Use flexible scheduling for staff to cover the additional hours of operations without increasing staff salary expenses.
- Move the children's play area from the current location to the north side of the waiting room to keep the children away from the path of patients entering through the side doorway of the clinic.
- Switch the current staff break room and the last exam room in the same hallway; this switch would allow the staff more privacy instead of having the break room next to the waiting room.
- Repair the crack in the slope of the sidewalk near the front entrance to ease access for patients with disabilities.
- Trim the large shrubbery near the exit driveway of the parking lot to improve safety for staff and patients entering and leaving the clinic.

BOX 13-7

Outline of References and Appendices

References

Appendices

References and Appendices

There are numerous reference styles (see **Box 13-7**). It is important to follow the style indicated in your journal author guidelines. If there are no author guidelines, as in a technical report, then investigators may select one of the commonly used recognized styles. However, whichever style is chosen, it is important to use it consistently throughout the report. This attention to detail is important for the quality of the overall report. See **Box 13-8** for a list of referencing styles.

Appendices appear at the end of the report. The information placed in an appendix is usually not essential to explaining your findings, but it still supports your analysis. The appendices are placed in order of reference in the narrative and labeled with letters. For example, the narrative may refer to Appendix A when discussing a specific document that is too long for placement in the actual report. The appendices are listed as Appendix A, Appendix B, and so on. The

BOX 13-8

Useful Websites for Referencing Styles

APA is most commonly used to cite sources in the social sciences.
http://owl.english.purdue.edu/owl/resource/560/01
MLA is most commonly used to write papers and cite sources in the liberal arts and humanities.
http://owl.english.purdue.edu/owl/resource/747/01
The Chicago Manual of Style covers a variety of topics from manuscript preparation and publication to grammar, usage, and documentation and is most commonly used in literature, history, and the arts.
http://owl.english.purdue.edu/owl/resource/717/01
AMA is most commonly used to cite sources in medicine.
http://medlib.bu.edu/facts/faq2.cfm/content/citationsama.cfm

page numbering that started with the title page continues through to the end of the appendices.

Sometimes writers experience a condition where they cannot produce any new or creative material. This is called writer's block. Often this happens when you have been working on the same project for a long period of time, or you are writing something that has some element of technical difficulty. Every writer has experienced this phenomenon. However, every writer has tips and tricks that help them deal with it. (see **Table 13-5**).[3]

Table 13-5   Writer's Block Problems and Solutions

Problem	Solution
If you do not know enough about the topic, you can't write about it.	Go research and read what other people have written about the topic.
You feel that you need to start at the beginning.	Start with an area that you know. For example, if you understand three key points, then begin writing at that point.
The blank screen looks intimidating and scary.	Write something; write anything—just begin writing. Nothing is written perfectly on the first try.
Your schedule does not allow you to dedicate 2 hours of time to writing.	Resolve to only write one paragraph each day. It is necessary to fit writing into your life rather than trying to dedicate a specific time.
You lose interest in writing about one topic area.	Leave the unfinished topic and move on to something that is interesting.
You do not think of yourself as a good writer.	The way to get better at writing is to write more. Just like in sports, you need to practice the skill to improve.
You have an outline, but it is not helping.	Spend a little time adding details to the outline. You may recognize that some topics need to be rearranged for greater clarity.
You do not think that what you have written makes sense.	Read that section aloud. The spoken word helps to identify possible flaws in written materials.
You keep thinking that other people will not like what you write.	Find a trusted friend or writing coach to critique your work. Be prepared for honest comments. You would not expect to learn how to play golf without a coach. Writing is the same.
You get stuck on one word.	Don't waste time fretting over one word or phrase. Simply type XXX and come back to it later. Type one word and then click on the thesaurus to search for a synonym that might fit.
You are hopelessly stuck.	Take a short break (e.g., go for a walk, get something to drink, make a phone call). If a short break does not solve the problem, save your document and come back to the task in a few hours or the next day.
Your deadline is close and you are about to panic.	This situation is a fatal flaw. No one writes well under stress. Pace yourself. Know your deadline and determine how much of the report needs to be completed each week to make the deadline. This detailed plan allows for planned and unplanned life events. Best of all, a slow, steady writing pace allows you to sleep at night and not panic.

Adapted from Charlie Jane Anders. The 10 Types of Writer's Block (and How to Overcome Them). Available at: http://io9.com/5844988/the-10-types-of-writers-block-and-how-to-overcome-them. Published October 6, 2011. Accessed November 3, 2012.

Presentation of Results

Now that the report is written, it is time to decide how to present the information. There are two basic formats: oral presentations and written presentations. Let's begin with oral presentations.

Oral Presentations

There are numerous situations in which investigators are asked to present their findings in front of an audience. Here are a few examples of oral presentations:

- The funding agency asks the evaluator to come to a board meeting.
- The researchers present the results at a local, state, or national conference.
- The investigators offer to discuss the evaluation process as a guest lecture in an academic course.

After the type of presentation is determined, the investigator decides how he or she wishes to prepare the presentation. There are several questions to answer:

- Who is the audience?
- What is the size of the audience?
- Where is the presentation (e.g., conference room, classroom, auditorium)?
- What is the proposed length of the presentation?
- What type of design is appropriate?
  - Will PowerPoint be used?
  - If so, is the computer equipment and screen available?

Let's discuss a few examples related to types of presentations.

Example 1

Ms. Irene Williams completes an evaluation for the local hospital related to the loss of revenue at the hospital's gift shop. She is asked to present her findings to the auxiliary board so they can agree on whether the gift shop should remain open 7 days per week. Ms. Williams is told that 10–12 individuals will attend the meeting. The auxiliary board meets in the hospital's conference room equipped with a laptop, projector, and screen. Because her presentation will be during the regular monthly meeting, it will be one of several items on the agenda. She will have 15 minutes to present the results of the 6-month evaluation project.

Ms. Williams decides to create five PowerPoint slides that include a title slide, the purpose of the evaluation, her methods, results, and recommendations. Her PowerPoint slides follow the 5 × 5 rule, which is to have a maximum of five bullet points on each slide and no more than five words per line of each bullet point. She rehearses her presentation a few times to make sure it stays within 10 minutes so that the audience can have 5 minutes to ask questions. She also prepares a one-page handout that summarizes the key points of her presentation.

On the day of the presentation, Ms. Williams dresses in a dark business suit and arrives 45 minutes early. She brings two different electronic modes of her presentation in case one is not compatible with the hospital's equipment. She does not want to be rushed in traffic and wants to have plenty of time to park, find the conference room, and set up the computer prior to individuals entering the room. Because she is well prepared, but not over-rehearsed and tense, her presentation sounds more like a conversation than a script. The audience is comfortable asking a few questions, and Ms. Williams leaves 5 minutes of the allotted agenda time to clarify her recommendations. Her presentation is a well-prepared success.

Example 2

Mr. James Sutton receives an email stating that his research abstract was accepted for a national conference. He has never attended a national academic or professional conference, so he is excited. He asks his faculty mentor for advice. His mentor, Dr. Gannon, tells him that the conference is held in two large hotels located directly across the street from each other in Chicago. The break-out room for his presentation is able to host about 50 conference participants, though he does not expect that there will be that many. There will be a panel of speakers with similar research topics; each presenter has 18 minutes to present their PowerPoint slides.

Mr. Sutton creates 12 PowerPoint slides using the 5 × 5 rule (see **Figure 13-1**). This type of PowerPoint slide allows the audience to easily read the slide as the presenter explains each point.

Mr. Sutton wants to take no more than 2 minutes to explain each slide. He realizes that the title slide takes only a few seconds to read, whereas some slides take a bit more than 2 minutes to explain. Several weeks before the conference, he meets with Dr. Gannon to practice his presentation. He reads from a formal script because he is so nervous. Dr. Gannon realizes that Mr. Sutton is glued to the script and suggests that he reduce his script to a few notecards so he can present the information in a less tense manner. Dr. Gannon believes this tip will also

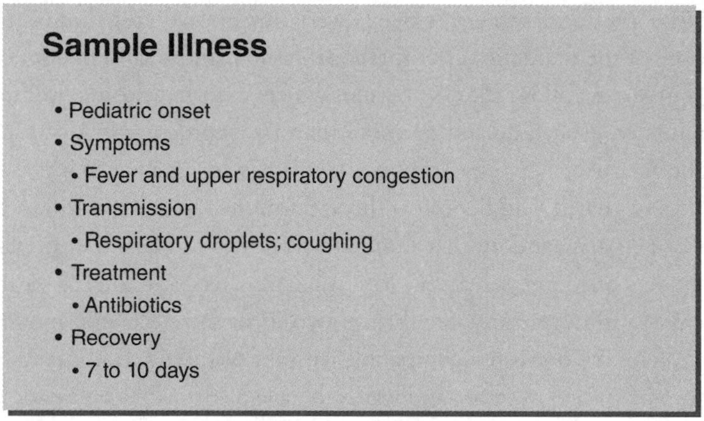

FIGURE 13-1 Sample of 5×5 PowerPoint Slide

help Mr. Sutton relax and make better eye contact with the audience during the presentation.

At the conference, Mr. Sutton dresses in a dark suit and tie. He feels over-dressed, but notices that the other three members of the panel are also dressed in business suits, which is appropriate. His presentation is informative and takes exactly 15 minutes. His precise timing leaves 3 minutes for two audience questions. Mr. Sutton uses the opportunity before and after the presentation to introduce himself to other presenters.

Poster Presentations

As with oral presentations, there are numerous situations in which investigators are asked to present their findings in a poster format. Here are a few examples of poster presentations:

- Poster session presented at a formal conference
- Poster session at a seminar or reception with interested individuals mingling and networking
- Posters displayed in a hallway as a rotating display, such as in a college lobby

Although posters are used for various venues, how a poster is designed influences whether the material is noticed and read or ignored without more than a glance. The next section provides details on how to create a standout poster. For this section, Microsoft PowerPoint is used to show poster development.

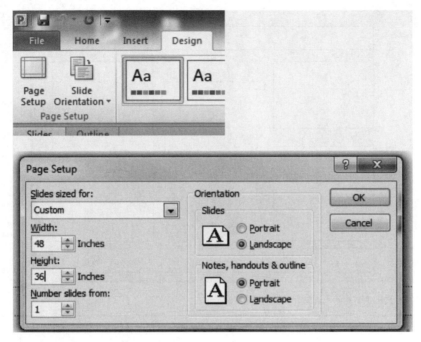

FIGURE 13-2   Poster Size Selection
Used with permission from Microsoft

Step 1: Select a poster size.

Determine the required size of the poster prior starting the development. Note: It is difficult to change the size after the poster is developed. See **Figure 13-2** for an illustration of how to select poster size. First, on the Toolbar, click Design, then Page Setup. Second, select landscape for your slide orientation, then increase the width and height to those of your poster requirements.

Step 2: Select a poster template.

See **Figure 13-3** for details on selecting a poster template. First, on the Toolbar, click Design. Second, select a design. After a design is selected, there are options for colors, fonts, and background styles. Test a few combinations prior to

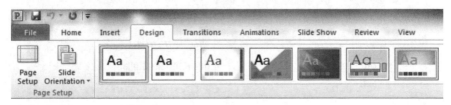

FIGURE 13-3   Selecting a Poster Template
Used with permission from Microsoft

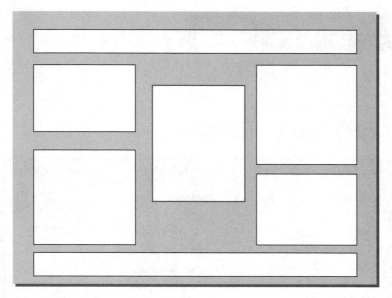

FIGURE 13-4   Information Placement

making the final selection. Keep in mind that the background needs to be simple and not distract from the information on the poster.

Step 3: Place information on the poster.

On a plain piece of paper, draw out approximately where each segment of the poster will be placed (see **Figure 13-4**). Once the placement is drafted, type the information that will be placed in each segment.

Step 4: Select a font style.

The ideal font for a poster is simple and plain. In **Figure 13-5**, note how much space the various fonts use. For a poster, it is important to select fonts from

Column A: Plain, Easy to Read	Column B: Fancy, Harder to Read
1 Information	1 Information
2 Data Analysis	*2 Data Analysis*
3 Background	*3 Background*
4 Recommendations	**4 Recommendations**
5 Conclusion	**5 Conclusion**

FIGURE 13-5   Sample of Font Styles

column A. From column A, select a narrow font, such as font 1 or font 3. A narrow font allows more words per line without compromising the clarity. Column B fonts are not appropriate for posters. The font should never distract from the information presented on the poster.

Step 5: Select a font size.

Font size on a poster is important. Generally, individuals stand about three to four feet from a poster. If the font is too small, individuals will not stop to read the poster. However, if the font is too large, the poster will not have enough space for the necessary information and will look unprofessional. The ideal font size for a poster is as follows:

Title: 60- to 80-point font

Subheadings for each section: 50- to 60-point font

Information under each subheading: 40- to 50-point font

Figures, graphs, and photo captions: 35- to 40-point font

References: 25- to 30-point font

Step 6: Keep it simple.

The most common mistake is trying to fit too much information on the poster. Each segment of the poster should have plenty of blank space so the segments do not run together. It is useful to have the information flow from one section to the next. **Figure 13-6** shows the title in a box with a thicker, bolder frame, whereas the sections are in boxes with lighter frames for contrast. There are hundreds of ways to configure a poster, but simplicity is most important. It is better to have people read the key points with few details than to have the poster ignored with too much information.

Step 7: Create talking points for your poster.

If the poster is presented in person, it is essential for the presenter to have a 2- to 3-minute speech prepared. Individuals walk around the room, reviewing the posters and stopping to chat with presenters who have interesting posters. Presenters should be ready to summarize the key points of the research and to answer questions. There are advantages and disadvantages to having small (8.5 × 11) paper copies of the poster available as a handout. Advantages include the fact that the interested individual receives a copy to review at a later time, and the contact information on the poster allows the person to connect the poster with the presenter. Disadvantages include the possibility that attendees may be carrying food or drinks, so they do not have a place to put the paper copy. In any case, presenters should have business cards available at poster presentations. Attendees are more willing to place business cards in their pockets than take larger pieces of paper. The presenter needs to memorize his or her talking points prior to the poster presentation.

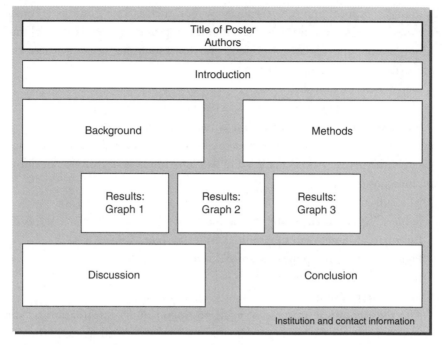

FIGURE 13-6 Simple Poster Design

Tips for Successful Presentations

Let's introduce some tips related to successful presentations. A 2001 Gallup poll found that public speaking was the second biggest (40%) fear among adults, just behind snakes (51%) and in front of heights (36%).[4] This section provides a few tips to help overcome the fear of public speaking and to improve the effect of the presentation.

1. Think about the goal of your presentation.
    Ask yourself these questions:
        Are you being interviewed for an evaluation consulting contract?
        Are you presenting the results of the evaluation?
        Are you persuading the audience to make a decision?
        Are you collecting data as in a focus group?
        Are you demonstrating a product?
2. Determine what you want to say.
    Write the key points of the presentation.
    Use the standard format:
        Tell the audience what you are going to tell them.

Tell them.

Close by telling them what you told them.

Always keep your presentation simple and clear.

3. Write the full script, using the key points as your outline.

Practice each section until you are comfortable and have the key points memorized.

Once each section feels comfortable, practice reading the full script aloud.

If you are stumbling over specific words, change the words. For example, if you stumble with a word such as *phenomenon*, then substitute the word *occurrence*.

Find your comfort zone with the written script.

From the full script, if you intend to use PowerPoint slides or handouts, create them after you are comfortable with the script.

4. Reduce your full script to a few 3 × 5 notecards.

After you have your full script memorized, write the key points and the transition statements that connect the key points on notecards.

Practice with the notecards so you become familiar with looking at the audience and speaking calmly and confidently rather than reading from your script.

Prepare by rehearsing in front of friends. (See step 5.)

5. Rehearse in front of people.

Gather a few friends together and practice a few times.

Time your presentation from start to finish.

Avoid starting over when you are practicing; just go through the full presentation.

Ask your friends for their honest opinions of your presentation, including the quality of the PowerPoint slides.

Look at the audience.

Ask your friends to watch your hand gestures and provide feedback.

6. Practice in different settings.

Practice by standing behind a podium or a conference table. You might be told that your presentation is scheduled for the auditorium; however, the room might be changed to the cafeteria because of a water leak in the auditorium, for example. In this case, you have a conference table instead of a podium.

Practice without a conference table or podium; be prepared for all types of settings.

7. Time management.

   With adequate time management, you will have minimal other duties 48 hours before your presentation so you can relax and practice your notecards one last time.

   All sorts of mishaps may occur, so you should save your full script, notecards, PowerPoint slides, and handouts in at least two electronic formats. Have paper copies of the PowerPoint slides available in case computer equipment has malfunctioned or is not available.

   Have extra copies of handouts in case the emailed file was not received.

8. Focus the audience on you.

   Begin and end your presentation with a "thank you" and a smile; both techniques help you to relax and get settled for your presentation.

   Engage your audience; do not hide behind your slides or handouts.

   If you are passionate about the subject, your presentation will flow with ease.

   Well-prepared presenters are calm and confident; even if you are nervous on the inside, adequate rehearsing allows you to feel comfortable with your information.

9. Think about what you will do after your presentation.

   Be prepared to answer several questions from the audience related to your presentation.

   Answer questions to the best of your ability; do not exaggerate the findings or recommendations.

   If you don't know the answer to a question, tell them you don't, but that you will find out and get back to them.

10. Networking.

   After the presentation, stay in the room for further questions or discussions with individuals.

   Be sure to clean up after your presentation: remove extra handouts or bottled water from the podium or conference table; there may be another speaker following your panel or presentation.

   Have your business cards easily available without digging in your pockets or purse.

   Use this valuable time to network with individuals in the audience to possibly make connections for further research, evaluations, or professional collaboration.

BOX 13-9

Rules of Attire: Top-to-Bottom List

Females

Hair: Freshly washed; pinned up and out of face

Nails: Clean and trimmed with pale polish

Clothing: Dark-colored professional suit

Blouse: Light color; well fitting; no button gaps, low necklines, or bra straps showing

Jewelry: Minimal and small; nothing flashy

Skirt or pants: Well fitting; not too tight or too short; pants length appropriate for shoes

Shoes: Closed toed; no sandals; neutral color; polished; 3-inch or less heels

Makeup: Minimal; avoid bold, bright colors

Males

Hair: Freshly washed and trimmed

Facial hair: Trimmed and neat

Nails: Clean and trimmed

Clothing: Dark-colored professional suit

Shirt: Light color; coordinated tie color; no emblems or sport team ties

Jewelry: Minimal; nothing flashy or bold

Pants: Well fitting; not too tight; appropriate length for shoes

Shoes: Polished; black or brown; matching socks

Your attire during your presentation is also important. See **Box 13-9** for some tips on how to dress.

Summary

This chapter described effective ways to present research and evaluation results in written and oral formats. First, written reports were discussed, including the essential elements of a report, reference styles, and overcoming writer's block. Second, types of oral presentations were reviewed, including creation of informative slide presentations and powerful rehearsal strategies. Lastly, the chapter concluded with techniques to create informative conference poster presentations with key talking points.

Case Study

The Best-Ever Evaluation Team from the University of South State consists of two faculty members, Dr. Marjorie Rhett and Dr. George White. Other team members include Suzanne Cox (qualitative expert), Melissa Wright (health educator with survey design expertise), and Scott Gustafson (statistical analysis expert). Because the team is well known in the community, it frequently receives consulting contracts from local community health facilities. Its most recent contract evaluation was for Shady Trees Center, a local rehabilitation and assisted living residential facility, located in a quiet neighborhood in a small town about 40 miles from the university. On the rehabilitation side of the facility, there are 30 inpatient beds with outpatient physical therapy services available for former patients as well as community members. The assisted living residential side of Shady Trees houses 40 residents. The assisted living residents receive physical therapy as needed on the rehabilitation side for an additional fee for services.

The purpose of the evaluation is to determine the effectiveness of the physical therapy services in rehabilitating elderly patients recovering from knee or hip replacement surgery. The evaluation team was given an adequate budget and six months to conduct the evaluation. All of the patients had their surgeries performed at the University Hospital. Each patient was transferred to Shady Trees 5 days after surgery, so the sample of patients was consistent.

The Best-Ever Team met with the Shady Trees administrative staff to discuss the evaluation design plan.

It was determined that the evaluation would consist of the following:

1. A review of the literature to get an overall perspective of best practices in the physical therapy field for joint replacement surgery among elderly patients
2. A patient medical record review to determine the success of Shady Trees patients over the past two years

continues

CASE STUDY *continued*

3. Interviews conducted with a sample of individuals representing medical billing and finance department staff, nursing and physical therapy staff, patients, and family members

4. Surveys conducted with inpatients during the first week of admission and upon discharge from Shady Trees, patients who participated in outpatient physical therapy services for joint replacement, and former inpatients at least 6 months after discharge

The Shady Trees administration team decided that they wanted the Best-Ever Team to develop a poster with the results, so it could be displayed in the staff lounge (see **Figure 13-7**). The information would be added under each heading after the results were available.

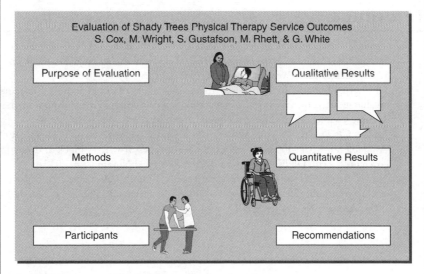

FIGURE 13-7   Shady Trees Evaluation Poster

Case Study Discussion Questions

1. What would be some potential limitations of this evaluation?
2. Where else could the team showcase the results?
3. What would be a possible next phase in this evaluation?

Student Activities

1. Using the information presented in the case study, create a poster to explain the findings of the evaluation.
2. Search the peer-reviewed journals and find a publication with data on a topic of interest to you. Using the demographic data in the publication, practice your skills to make a bar graph and pie chart. Explain why one type of graphic presentation is easier to understand than the other.
3. Using 3 × 5 notecards, outline one section of this chapter and prepare to give a 3-minute presentation without using any other graphic props.
4. Using a copy of your current resume, prepare a 2-minute speech that explains why you are the perfect candidate for a position for which you have applied.

References

1. Virginia Polytechnic Institute and State University. Technical Writing—Progress Reports. Available at: http://wiz.cath.vt.edu/tw/TechnicalWriting/ProgressReports /components4.htm. Accessed November 3, 2012.
2. Northern Illinois University Department of English. Formal Report Elements. Available at: http://www.pearsoned.ca/highered/divisions/virtual_tours/northey /sample_chapter_9.pdf. Accessed November 3, 2012.
3. Anders CJ. The 10 Types of Writer's Block (and How to Overcome Them). IO9. Available at: http://io9.com/5844988/the-10-types-of-writers-block-and-how-to -overcome-them. Published October 6, 2011. Accessed November 3, 2012.
4. Brewer G. Snakes Top List of Americans' Fears. Gallup Poll. Available at: http://www .gallup.com/poll/1891/snakes-top-list-americans-fears.aspx. Published March 19, 2001. Accessed November 3, 2012.

CHAPTER 14

Case Study: University Medical Cancer Care Center

Description

In 2003, the University Medical Cancer Care Center (UMCCC) opened a free-standing cancer care outpatient clinic. This clinic is located in a rural area about 60 miles from the university hospital, which is also located on the main campus of a university in a large metropolitan city in the northern Midwest United States. The clinical staff includes 5 board-certified oncology physicians, 2 board-certified intervention radiology physicians, 3 pharmacists, 3 advanced registered nurse practitioners, and 28 clinical support staff (e.g., registered nurses, social workers, mental health therapists, pastoral care personnel, and registered dietitians). They care for approximately 240 patients per day during the clinic hours from 9:00 a.m. until 4:00 p.m. on Monday, Wednesday, and Thursday. The UMCCC is open Monday through Saturday from 7:00 a.m. to 7:00 p.m. and is staffed by 10 registered nurses (RNs) on rotating shift coverage. They provide 40 to 60 patients with chemotherapy, plasma and blood transfusions, and intravenous antibiotics in the infusion center. About 60 patients receive radiation treatment therapy under the care of board-certified radiology oncologists. In addition, there are a variety of support services offered each day that include pet, art, and music therapy plus patient and family support groups, yoga classes, and mindfulness meditation sessions. There is also a well-stocked lending library of books, DVDs, and music. A café with healthy, fresh food and drink choices is open from 6:00 a.m. until 9:00 p.m. for staff, patients, families, and visitors.

Table 14-1   Employee Summary of University Medical Cancer Care Center (UMCCC)

Employees	Descriptions
Clinical staff (*n* = 13)	5 board-certified oncology physicians 2 board-certified intervention radiology physicians 3 pharmacists 3 advanced registered nurse practitioners
Clinical support staff (*n* = 28)	10 registered nurses 5 social workers 6 mental health therapists 3 pastoral care counselors 4 registered dietitians
Laboratory (*n* = 11)	9 lab technicians 1 licensed medical technologist 1 manager
Nonclinical support staff (*n* = 127)	Full-time and part-time nonclinical employees in departments: Finance Billing Insurance Human resources Continuing education Professional regulations for research and evaluation (e.g., institutional review board, bioethics committee, data management system, and board of directors)
CTPES staff (*n* = 70)	Central supply Technical support Physical plant maintenance Environmental services

The laboratory of the UMCCC houses 9 lab technicians, 1 licensed medical technologist, and 1 manager. On the administrative support side of the UMCCC, there are 127 full-time nonclinical employees in departments such as finance, billing, insurance, human resources, continuing education, and professional regulations for research and evaluation (e.g., institutional review board, bioethics committee, data management system, and board of directors). Lastly, there are 70 individuals employed in central supply, technical support, the physical plant, and environmental services. See **Table 14-1**.

Overview of Evaluation

The UMCCC has been in operation for 7 years. Three years after opening, the UMCCC was inspected by The Joint Commission (TJC). TJC was founded in 1951 with a mission statement as follows:

to continuously improve healthcare for the public, in collaboration with other stakeholders, by evaluating healthcare organizations and inspiring them to excel in providing safe and effective care of the highest quality and value. The Joint Commission evaluates and accredits more than 20,000 healthcare organizations and programs in the United States. An independent, not-for-profit organization, The Joint Commission is the nation's oldest and largest standards-setting and accrediting body in health care.[1]

Four years after UMCCC passed the TJC inspection with high accommodation, the board of directors determined it was time to conduct a thorough evaluation of the center because the next TJC inspection was scheduled to take place in 2 years. To start the preaccreditation process, they hired an evaluation team from the University Institute of Translational Research and Evaluation. The team consisted of Drs. Jessie Abel, Chris Boyle, and Pat Chen. Because they work together so often, they have been named the ABC evaluation team after the first letter of each of their last names. For the UMCCC evaluation, they crafted goals and objectives for the UMCCC board of directors. The ABC evaluation team decided to break down the evaluation into several smaller sections and then develop goals and objectives under each section. The sections include (1) clinical staff and clinical support staff; (2) laboratory; (3) nonclinical staff; (4) central supply, technical support, plant maintenance, and environmental services; (5) finance and accounting; (6) board of directors, executive administration, and management; and (7) patient and visitor satisfaction. The ABC evaluation team started with an example of a basic outline of the evaluation including goals and objectives for three of the seven defined sections (see **Box 14-1**).

BOX 14-1   Example of a Basic Outline of Evaluation Goals and Objectives

Section 1: Clinical Staff and Clinical Support Staff

Goal: The clinical staff and clinical support staff evaluation explores the use of technology, credentials and licensing, employment satisfaction, and retention.

Objectives

1. In the next 12 months, 41 (100%) of the clinical staff and clinical support staff will receive education on the use of electronic medical records (EMRs) and a passing grade on the posttest exam with 100% accuracy.

continues

BOX 14-1

Example of a Basic Outline of Evaluation Goals and Objectives *continued*

2. In the next 12 months, the licensing and credentials of 41(100%) of the clinical staff and clinical support staff will be reviewed for accuracy and compliance.

3. In the next 12 months, 41 (100%) of the clinical staff and clinical support staff will complete employment satisfaction surveys.

4. In the next 12 months, 41 (100%) the clinical staff and clinical support staff personnel records will be reviewed to determine the rate of staff turnover and rate of retention.

Section 2: Laboratory

Goal: The laboratory evaluation investigates the universal biohazard safety precautions and sterile procedures, clean indoor air quality, and disposal of bio hazardous materials.

Objectives:

1. In the next 12 months, the laboratory will maintain 100% of Occupational Safety and Health Administration (OSHA) standards for universal biohazard safety precautions and sterile conditions.

2. In the next 12 months, the laboratory will maintain 100% of OSHA standards for clean indoor air quality.

3. In the next 12 months, the laboratory will maintain 100% of OSHA standards for disposal of biohazardous materials.

4. In the next 12 months, 11 (100%) of the laboratory staff will complete employment satisfaction surveys.

5. In the next 12 months, 11 (100%) of the laboratory staff personnel records will be reviewed to determine personnel retention.

Section 3: Nonclinical Staff

Goal: The nonclinical staff evaluation explores training, employment satisfaction, and retention.

Objectives:

1. In the next 12 months, 127 (100%) of the nonclinical staff will receive education on the use of new software programs linked to EMR and pass the posttest exam with 100% accuracy.

continues

BOX 14-1

Example of a Basic Outline of Evaluation Goals and Objectives *continued*

2. In the next 12 months, 127 (100%) of the nonclinical staff will complete employment satisfaction surveys.
3. In the next 12 months, 127 (100%) of the nonclinical staff personnel records will be reviewed to determine personnel retention.

Budget

After the board of directors approved the final evaluation plan, the ABC evaluation team developed the budget, and it was approved by the board (see **Table 14-2**).

Budget Justification

Personnel

Jessie Abel, PhD, serves as the principal investigator. Salary is requested for 12 months of her salary of $135,000 at a rate of 0.50 FTE and 28% fringe benefits, totaling $86,400.

Chris Boyle, PhD, serves as a co-principal investigator. Salary is requested for 12 months of his salary of $105,000 at a rate of 0.35 FTE and 28% fringe benefits, totaling $47,040.

Pat Chen, PhD, serves as a co-principal investigator. Salary is requested for 12 months of her salary of $117,000 at a rate of 0.40 FTE and 28% fringe benefits totaling $59,904.

Sharad Josey, MS, serves as the computer technician. Salary is requested for 12 months for his salary of $62,000 at a rate of 0.10 FTE and 28% fringe benefits, totaling $7,936.

Graduate Students

Six graduate students serve on this evaluation. Salary is requested for 52 weeks at a rate of $18 per hour at 20 hours per week with fringe benefits of 28%, totaling $122,429.

A tuition stipend of $3,000 for 6 students totals $18,000.

Table 14-2 Evaluation Budget and Budget Justification

Personnel	Salary	Number	Percentage of Time	Weeks	Subtotal	Fringe	Total
Dr. Abel (Principal Investigator [PI])	$135,000		0.5		$ 67,500	$18,900	$ 86,400
Dr. Boyle (Co-PI)	$105,000		0.35		$ 36,750	$10,290	$ 47,040
Dr. Chen (Co-PI)	$117,000		0.4		$ 46,800	$13,104	$ 59,904
Sharad Josey (Computer Technician)	$62,000		0.1		$ 6,200	$ 1,736	$ 7,936
Graduate Students	$18/hour	6 students	20 hours/week	52 weeks	$112,320	$10,109	$122,429
Tuition stipend	$3,000	6 students					$ 18,000
Overtime	$18/hour	6 students	15 hours/week	3 weeks	$ 4,860	$ 437	$ 5,297
Consultants							
Dr. Green	$200		40 hours/week	14 weeks			$112,000
Mr. Sanjay	$175		20 hours/week	6 weeks			$ 21,000
Ms. Jackson	$175		20 hours/week	8 weeks			$ 28,000
Focus Groups							
CTPES focus groups	$25	30 people					$ 750
Satisfaction focus groups	$25	24 people					$ 600
Travel							
Main hospital	$0.49	150 miles	18 trips				$ 1,323
Pilot test site	$0.49	120 miles	9 trips				529
						Subtotal	$511,208
						Indirect costs (12%)	$ 61,345
						TOTAL	$572,553

Overtime payment of $18 per hour for 15 hours per week for 3 weeks plus fringe benefits of $437 totals $5,297.

Consultants

Dr. Green, certified industrial hygienist with specialization in OSHA regulations, is paid $200 per hour for 40 hours per week for 14 weeks, totaling $112,000.

Mr. Sanjay, certified public accountant with specialization in financial audits, is paid $175 per hour for 20 hours per week for 6 weeks, totaling $21,000.

Ms. Jackson, paralegal with specialization in contract law, is paid $175 per hour for 20 hours per week for 8 weeks, totaling $28,000.

Focus Groups

Focus groups conducted with the central supply, technical support, physical plant, and environmental services (CTPES) staff involve a $25 incentive gift card for 30 participants, for a total of $750.

Focus groups conducted for the patient and visitor satisfaction surveys involve a $25 incentive gift card for 24 participants, for a total of $600.

Travel

An estimated 18 round trips to the main hospital at 150 miles at $0.49 per mile total $1,323. An estimated 9 round trips to the pilot test clinic at 120 miles at $0.49 per mile total $529.

Indirect Costs

Indirect costs are calculated at 12% and total $61,345.
   Total: $572,553

Evaluation

After approval, the ABC evaluation team immediately started working on this multifaceted project. Because the entire evaluation had to be completed in 12 months, the team decided to divide the tasks for greater efficiency based on their evaluation expertise. The ABC evaluation team's knowledge includes Dr. Jessie Abel, an expert in survey design; Dr. Chris Boyle, who has extensive experience in secondary data analysis; and Dr. Pat Chen, a human resource and financial management specialist. During the team meeting, they agreed that each team member would hire two graduate students. Lastly, they developed a timeline for the first month of the evaluation so that each person knew what their responsibilities were and when they were expected to accomplish them (see **Table 14-3**).

The last week of the first month, the ABC evaluation team, along with their newly hired graduate students, created a timeline for each section. They found that it was easier to keep track of each section rather than making one comprehensive timeline. For the remainder of the chapter, the evaluation of each section is presented in detail.

Clinical Staff and Clinical Support Staff

Table 14-4 shows the timeline for the goals and objectives for the clinical staff evaluation.

The clinical staff (n = 13) and clinical support staff (n = 28) consist of 41 staff (5 board-certified oncology physicians, 2 board-certified intervention radiology physicians, 3 pharmacists, 3 advanced registered nurse practitioners, and 28 support clinical staff (e.g., registered nurses, social workers, mental health therapists, pastoral care, and registered dietitians). The clinic is open from 7:00 a.m. to 7:00 p.m. Monday through Saturday. Dr. Pamela Sykes, the clinic director, is responsible for clinical and clinical support staff. Prior to becoming clinic director three years ago, she was director of patient services. When this job became too large for one person to accomplish effectively, her position was split into two, and Dr. Melvin Johnson was hired to be director of clinic resources. After being

Table 14-3 Timeline of First Month of the 12-Month Evaluation

Week	Action	Responsible Person
1	Finalize payment schedule of budget for evaluation	Dr. Chen
	Advertise for 6 graduate students	Dr. Abel
	Receive first-quarter budget installment from board	Dr. Chen
	Interview 10 graduate students	Dr. Abel
	Apply for institutional review board approval for data collection at UMCCC	Dr. Boyle
2	Hire 6 graduate students (2 students per team member)	Dr. Abel
	Create the staff, patient, and visitor satisfaction survey; pilot-test with employees at the university	Dr. Abel
3	Schedule meetings with department managers for each section of the evaluation: clinical staff; clinical support staff; laboratory; nonclinical staff; central supply, technical support, physical plant, and environmental services; finance and accounting; executive administration and management; and patient services	Dr. Boyle
	Meet to verify that assigned tasks are complete	Dr. Boyle
	Convert final satisfaction surveys to links for online surveys and paper copies for mailed surveys	Dr. Abel
4	Submission and approval of the UMCCC institutional review board	Dr. Boyle

Table 14-4 Clinical Staff and Clinical Support Staff Evaluation Timeline

Goal: The clinical staff and clinical support staff evaluation explores the level of services, use of technology, credentials and licensing, employment satisfaction, and retention.

Month	Objectives	Action	Outcome	Responsible Person
2	41 (100%) of the clinical staff and clinical support staff receive EMR training.	Schedule all clinical staff and clinical support staff to attend two 90-minute EMR trainings with software technical support team.	41 (100%) of clinical staff and clinical support staff complete EMR training.	Dr. Boyle
3–4	41 (100%) of the clinical staff and clinical support staff pass the posttest exam with 100% accuracy.	Email clinical staff and clinical support staff the EMR posttest seven days after EMR training; clinical staff has 3 days to complete an online posttest exam.	41 (100%) clinical staff and clinical support staff complete and pass the EMR posttest.	Dr. Abel
5–7	The licensing and credentials of 41 (100%) of the clinical staff and clinical support staff are reviewed for accuracy and compliance.	Review personnel files to determine accuracy and compliance of clinical staff license and credential requirements.	41 (100%) of clinical staff and clinical support staff with current license and credential requirements.	Dr. Chen
	41 (100%) of the clinical staff and clinical support staff personnel records are reviewed to determine personnel retention.	Review personnel files to determine clinical staff and clinical support staff retention.	41 (100%) of clinical staff and clinical support staff employed at UMCCC for < 12, 13–24, 25–60, and 61+ months.	Dr. Boyle
8	41 (100%) of the clinical staff and clinical support staff complete employment satisfaction surveys.	Email clinical staff and clinical support staff the employment satisfaction survey; staff has 3 days to complete the online survey.	41 (100%) of clinical staff and clinical support staff complete the employment satisfaction survey; % of clinical staff rating satisfaction as excellent.	Dr. Boyle

notified by the board of directors that the ABC team would be conducting this evaluation, Dr. Sykes was less than supportive. Dr. Sykes had been in support of hiring the XYZ evaluation team because her brother-in-law leads that team. As a result, Dr. Sykes was late for the first meeting with the ABC evaluation team and was not forthcoming with information when asked.

After the first meeting, Dr. Boyle decided to allow the clinical staff to schedule their EMR training instead assigning them to specific sessions. The 3-hour EMR training was offered in two 90-minute blocks to accommodate clinic schedules. There were 12 time slots available over a 2-week period. Dr. Boyle created an online link with the available time slots so that clinical staff could go online and indicate their first and second choices for each of the two 90-minute sessions. The clinical staff managers used the spreadsheet to arrange the staff schedules around the training sessions. Dr. Boyle emailed the clinical staff with their EMR training dates and times; their online schedules reflected the same information.

Dr. Boyle thought that having scheduled the EMR training, he was off to a good start. The computer training room was blocked off for their use, the clinical staff had confirmed their times, and the EMR software tech support was ready for the training. The first training day arrived. An hour early, Dr. Boyle arrived at the computer training room only to discover that the tables, chairs, and laptop computers were stacked at one end of the room. He went to find a few environmental service workers to assist with rearranging the room for training. The workers moved the tables and chairs and he set up the laptops. By the time the clinical staff started arriving, everything was ready. Dr. Boyle was glad he had arrived early enough to handle the unforeseen issues. The first day of training went well after the earlier mishap, but several of the clinical staff failed to attend the training. Dr. Boyle noted the names of the missing staff and sent them emails to schedule another time for their first training session. Before leaving for the day, Dr. Boyle check with Dr. Sykes's administrative assistant to verify that the computer training room would remain set up and ready for training for the next few weeks on designated dates and times. Much to his dismay, Dr. Sykes had intermittently scheduled a few other meetings in the training room. Without showing his frustration, Dr. Boyle noted on his e-tablet when Dr. Sykes had scheduled the room, so he would know when to arrive early to the trainings. It was clear that Dr. Sykes was trying to complicate the EMR training schedule for the ABC evaluation team.

For the next few weeks, Dr. Boyle rearranged the training room, rescheduled training sessions for staff members who missed sessions, and tried to juggle staff requests for changing the time and date of the second training. The training became much more complex than the ABC evaluation team had anticipated. Even though the timeline allowed one month for EMR training of the clinical staff, it actually took more than 5 weeks, putting the whole timeline off.

Over the next few months, Dr. Chen and her two graduate students began to review the licensing, credentials, and retention of the clinical staff. They started the comprehensive review by making a spreadsheet. Each section uses approximately the same spreadsheet, so the data remain consistent across the evaluation (see **Table 14-5**).

Over a few months, the graduate students carefully reviewed the personnel files of every clinical staff individual who had ever been employed at the UMCCC since it opened in 2003. They reported to Dr. Chen a trend of registered nurses leaving after about 12 months of employment at the UMCCC. The reasons given were usually for employment at another healthcare facility or for

Table 14-5   Sample of Clinical Staff and Clinical Support Staff Personnel Credentialing and Retention

Employee ID Number	Date of Hire	Date of Leaving	Reason for Leaving	Type of License/ Credentials	License Current	Date Renewal Required
21795	5/12/03			1	Yes	2015
29035	5/12/03	6/24/09	1	6		
28034	6/30/04			2	Yes	2017
27043	12/10/12	3/17/13	6	3		
27612	1/26/07			5	Yes	2016
28903	3/5/06	6/7/06	8	4		

Codebook: For each section, the codebook expands to enter new items under each category as needed.

Reason for leaving:

    1 = Employment transfer to main campus

    2 = Leaving for personal reasons (e.g., illness, family situation, caregiving)

    3 = Employment in the same field but at another healthcare facility

    4 = Employment outside of health care

    5 = Moving out of state

    6 = Education

    7 = Retirement

    8 = Dismissal from facility

Type of license/credentials:

    1 = Registered nurse

    2 = Social worker

    3 = Mental health therapist

    4 = Clinical psychologist

    5 = Pharmacist

    6 = Physician

Length of service:

    1 = Less than 1 year

    2 = 1–3 years

    3 = 4–7 years

    4 = Over 7 years

further education. After the review process was complete, Dr. Chen analyzed the data and wrote her recommendations for the final report.

In the eighth month of the evaluation, Dr. Boyle emailed the employee satisfaction survey link to the clinical staff. He requested that they complete the anonymous survey within the next 3 days. He was pleased when 39 (95.1%) out of 41 clinical staff and clinical support staff completed the survey in 3 days. Like Dr. Chen, he analyzed the data and wrote his recommendations for the final report. The same employee satisfaction survey was used for all employees, so data remained consistent for the evaluation (see **Table 14-6**).

Table 14-6   Employee Satisfaction Survey

	Strongly Agree*	Agree	Disagree	Strongly Disagree
The UMCCC...				
1. Cares about their employees.	4	3	2	1
2. Tries to retain their employees.	4	3	2	1
3. Offers generous benefits to all employees.	4	3	2	1
4. Only cares about their profit margin.	4	3	2	1
5. Listens to the employees.	4	3	2	1
6. Is focused only on their community image.	4	3	2	1
7. Always wants to improve their patient care.	4	3	2	1
8. Maintains minimal staff to save money.	4	3	2	1
My supervisor...				
9. Cares about me as a person.	4	3	2	1
10. Works with me when I need time off for personal reasons.	4	3	2	1
11. Is always finding ways to improve my skills.	4	3	2	1
12. Does not know how to manage the department.	4	3	2	1
13. Needs training in leadership skills.	4	3	2	1
14. Caters to the board more than the employees.	4	3	2	1
15. Helps the department operate as a team.	4	3	2	1
16. Helps out when the unit is short staffed.	4	3	2	1
17. Finds time to compliment staff when deserved.	4	3	2	1
18. Treats everyone equally.	4	3	2	1
19. Explores ways to improve working conditions.	4	3	2	1
20. Provides adequate training for all employees.	4	3	2	1
21. Is fair in approving vacation schedules.	4	3	2	1

continues

Table 14-6 Employee Satisfaction Survey *continued*

	Strongly Agree*	Agree	Disagree	Strongly Disagree
I intend to stay at UMCCC because...				
22. My salary is competitive.	4	3	2	1
23. I enjoy coming to work each day.	4	3	2	1
24. I appreciate my coworkers.	4	3	2	1
25. The UMCCC offers a generous benefit package.	4	3	2	1
26. I am stuck because of lack of options.	1	2	3	4
27. I need to work and this job is good enough.	1	2	3	4
28. I have relatives who work at the UMCCC.	4	3	2	1
29. I like the mission of the UMCCC to help patients.	4	3	2	1
30. I appreciate the short drive to the UMCCC.	4	3	2	1

Demographics

31. I have been employed at UMCCC for:	Less than 1 year	1–3 years	4–7 years	Over 7 years		
32. My age:	Less than 20 years	21–30 years	31–40 years	41–50 years	51–60 years	61+ years
33. My work schedule is:	Full time (32–40 hours)		Part time (less than 31 hours per week)		Temporary or on-call as needed	
34. My education:	GED or high school	Technical degree	Some college	2-year college degree	4-year college degree	Post-college degree
35. My primary language:			English		Other than English	

36. Any other comments that you would like to share about your employment at the UMCCC:

* Points shown on this example to explain scoring. Points not shown on actual employee survey.

Scoring of Employee Satisfaction Scale: It is important to note that each section has positive and negative statements.

UMCCC: (Questions 1–8)	Positive statements:	1, 2, 3, 5, and 7
Maximum score: 23	Negative statements:	4, 6, and 8
Supervisor: (Questions 9–21)	Positive statements:	9, 10, 11, 15, 16, 17, 18, 19, 20, and 21
Maximum score: 39	Negative statements:	12, 13, and 14
Retention: (Questions 22–30)	Positive statements:	22, 23, 24, 25, 28, 29, and 30
Maximum score: 30	Negative statements:	26, 27

Laboratory

Table 14-7 shows the timeline for the goals and objectives for the laboratory evaluation.

In the second month of the evaluation, Dr. Chen hires a consultant with expertise in OSHA requirements to assist with the review of the UMCCC laboratory. Dr. Green is a certified industrial hygienist in private practice related

Table 14-7 Laboratory Evaluation Timeline

Goal: The laboratory evaluation investigates the accuracy of the equipment, universal biohazard safety precautions and sterile procedures, clean indoor air quality, and disposal of biohazardous materials.

Month	Objectives	Action	Outcome	Responsible Person
3–4	The laboratory maintains 100% of OSHA standards for universal biohazard safety precautions and sterile conditions.	Review the techniques and procedures of laboratory staff to determine compliance with OSHA standards.	100% of laboratory procedures in compliance with OSHA standards.	Dr. Chen and OSHA consultant, Dr. Green
4	The laboratory maintains 100% of OSHA standards for clean indoor air quality.	Test indoor air quality for OSHA compliance.	100% of indoor air quality in compliance with OSHA standards.	Dr. Chen and OSHA consultant, Dr. Green
4	The laboratory maintains 100% of OSHA standards for disposal of biohazardous materials.	Review procedures of disposal of biohazardous materials by 11 (100%) laboratory staff.	100% of disposal of biohazardous materials in compliance with OSHA standards.	Dr. Chen and OSHA consultant, Dr. Green
5	The licensing and credentials of 11 (100%) of the laboratory staff reviewed for accuracy and compliance.	Review 11 (100%) of the personnel files to determine accuracy and compliance of laboratory staff license and credential requirements.	11 (100%) of laboratory staff with current license and credential requirements.	Dr. Chen
	The 11 (100%) laboratory staff personnel records reviewed to determine personnel retention.	Review 11 (100%) personnel files to determine laboratory staff retention.	11 (100%) of laboratory staff employed at the UMCCC for < 12, 12–24, 25–60, and 61+ months.	Dr. Boyle
8	11 (100%) of the laboratory staff complete employment satisfaction surveys.	Email 11 (100%) laboratory staff the employment satisfaction survey; staff have 3 days to complete the online survey.	11 (100%) of laboratory staff complete the employment satisfaction survey; % of laboratory staff rate satisfaction as excellent.	Dr. Boyle

to OSHA standards and compliance. Dr. Green lives in the state capital about 90 miles from the UMCCC and is not associated with the state university system; therefore, he has no conflict of interest. For 2 months, Dr. Green spends each day in the laboratory inspecting procedure manuals, observing the staff, verifying universal biohazard precautions and sterile conditions, testing the indoor air quality, investigating the disposal of biohazardous materials, and testing the quality control standards of various laboratory equipment. He enters volumes of field notes into his laptop. He remains unobtrusive to the laboratory staff except when he needs clarification from them on various procedures or equipment. After 2 months, Dr. Green meets with the laboratory manager and technicians separately to confirm or refute some observations using qualitative interviews. With volumes of data, Dr. Green leaves the UMCCC. After several months, he submits his final report to the ABC evaluation team for inclusion in their final report.

As Dr. Green was inspecting the laboratory, the graduate students completed the clinical staff personnel files and began to review the laboratory staff since the opening of the UMCCC in 2003. They submitted the data to Dr. Chen for analysis. After the laboratory review process was complete, Dr. Chen analyzed the data and added her recommendations to the final report. She found it to be more efficient to add each section to the final report immediately after the analysis, so her findings were fresh in her mind.

In the eighth month of the evaluation, Dr. Boyle emailed the employee satisfaction survey link to the laboratory staff. As with all employees, he requested that they complete the anonymous survey within the next 3 days. He was surprised that 10 (90.9%) out of the 11 laboratory employees completed the survey within 24 hours. Like Dr. Chen, he analyzed the data and wrote his recommendations for the final report.

Nonclinical Staff

Table 14-8 shows the timeline for the goals and objectives for the nonclinical staff evaluation.

After the scheduling issues with training the clinical staff, Dr. Boyle decided to take another approach for the nonclinical staff training. Because the UMCCC clinic is wireless, he was able to convince the president of the board of directors to use the boardroom for the EMR training instead of the one large classroom that was previously used for the clinical staff training. This change meant that he could schedule fewer nonclinical staff at a time for each 90-minute session, but he no longer had to rearrange furniture and juggle a fluctuating schedule. This change also affected the budget because it required more tech support because

Table 14-8 Nonclinical Staff Evaluation Timeline

Goal: The nonclinical staff evaluation explores the level of services, use of technology, training, employment satisfaction, and retention.

Month	Objectives	Action	Outcome	Responsible Person
5	127 (100%) of the nonclinical staff receive EMR training.	Schedule all 127 (100%) nonclinical staff to attend one of the six 3-hour EMR trainings with software technical support team.	127 (100%) of non-clinical staff complete EMR training.	Dr. Boyle
5–6	127 (100%) of the nonclinical staff pass the posttest exam with 100% accuracy.	Email 127 (100%) non-clinical staff the EMR posttest 7 days after EMR training; staff has 3 days to complete an online posttest exam.	127 (100%) of non-clinical staff complete and pass the EMR posttest.	Dr. Abel
6	The 127 (100%) nonclinical staff personnel records will be reviewed to determine personnel retention.	Review 127 (100%) personnel files to deter-mine nonclinical staff retention.	127 (100%) of non-clinical staff employed at the UMCCC for < 12, 12–24, 25–60, and 61+ months.	Dr. Boyle
8	127 (100%) of the nonclinical staff complete employ-ment satisfaction surveys.	Email 127 (100%) of the nonclinical staff the employment satisfac-tion survey; staff has 3 days to complete the online survey.	127 (100%) of non-clinical staff complete the employment sat-isfaction survey; % of staff rate satisfaction as excellent.	Dr. Boyle

there would be more training sessions with fewer staff in each of them. The ABC evaluation team agreed that the room change was worth the extra cost.

Under the direction of Dr. Johnson, the same procedures were followed to schedule the nonclinical staff training sessions. Even though there were 127 non-clinical staff, only 87 employees were in positions that required knowledge of the new EMR software. Because of their more standardized schedule, they were able to leave their duties for 90 minutes more easily than the clinical staff. Dr. Boyle was delighted that 85 (97%) out of the 87 eligible nonclinical staff completed both 90-minute EMR training sessions. As he had previously, he emailed the EMR posttest in 7 days. The data revealed that of the 85 employees who completed the EMR training, 80 (94%) of them completed the posttest. However, of the 80 taking the posttest, only 42 (52.5%) earned a passing score of 70% on the posttest.

It took the graduate students several months to complete the nonclinical staff personnel files. They were able to retrieve the current personnel files with ease, but Dr. Chen had to intervene to obtain the nonclinical personnel files from the opening of the UMCCC in 2003 through 2010. It was reported that during those seven years, Mrs. Hoffman, the director of human resources, was the wife of a past board member. She decided that personnel files should be placed in off-site storage to conserve office space. The storage space was located on the main campus, so it took several weeks to retrieve the dusty boxes. As a result of this delay, the graduate students were behind in their data entry. While the graduate students waited for the personnel files to arrive, they helped the ABC evaluation team with other duties. Once the seven years of nonclinical personnel file boxes arrived, they worked overtime to get the evaluation back on track for the timeline. These overtime hours were paid out of the budget. As before, Dr. Chen analyzed the data and added her recommendations to the final report.

In the 8th month of the evaluation, Dr. Boyle emailed the employee satisfaction survey link to the nonclinical staff. Again, he requested that they complete the anonymous survey within the next 3 days. Unlike with the EMR training, the employee satisfaction survey was emailed to all 127 nonclinical staff. Out of the 127, 80 (63%) nonclinical employees completed the satisfaction survey. Dr. Boyle analyzed the data and wrote his recommendations for the final report.

Central Supply, Technical Support, Physical Plant, and Environmental Services (CTPES)

Table 14-9 shows the timeline for the goals and objectives for the CTPES evaluation.

Dr. Chen invited Dr. Green to return for a portion of the CTPES evaluation. He agreed and returned for another month of data collection. Because the CTPES employees cover a large portion of the plant maintenance operation of the UMCCC, there were numerous OSHA regulations to review. Dr. Green started by conducting focus groups with employees from each unit. For example, in the central supply unit, he asked questions about the required temperature of the autoclave to sterilize equipment. He also inquired as to the new employee training and any periodic training they each received. The technical support employees were asked about training, age of computer equipment, and digital storage space to back up data. Dr. Green spent the most time with employees from physical plant and environmental services, because they used the most chemicals and worked with hazardous equipment such as ladders, floor polishers, and electric hand tools. He questioned them about the literacy level of the OSHA manuals and how the training was conducted prior to the use of new chemicals, cleaning supplies, or paint.

Table 14-9 CTPES Evaluation Timeline

Goal: The CTPES evaluation explores the services, training, employment satisfaction, and retention.

Month	Objectives	Action	Outcome	Responsible Person
5	70 (100%) of CTPES services are reviewed.	Compare CTPES description of services with actual services performed for 70 (100%) of employees.	70 (100%) of actual services performed.	Dr. Chen and OSHA consultant, Dr. Green
6	70 (100%) of CTPES employees are trained to adequately perform job duties.	Review adequacy of CTPES training for 70 (100%) employees.	70 (100%) of CTPES employees trained.	Dr. Chen and OSHA consultant, Dr. Green
7	The 70 (100%) CTPES staff personnel records reviewed to determine personnel retention.	Review 70 (100%) personnel files to determine CTPES staff retention.	70 (100%) of CTPES staff employed at the UMCCC for < 12, 12–24, 25–60, and 61+ months.	Dr. Boyle
8	70 (100%) of CTPES staff complete employment satisfaction surveys.	Email 70 (100%) CTPES staff the employment satisfaction survey; CTPES staff has 3 days to complete the online survey.	70 (100%) of CTPES staff complete the employment satisfaction survey; % of CTPES staff rate satisfaction as excellent.	Dr. Abel

Dr. Green met with the graduate students who were reviewing the personnel files. He wanted to know the license status of professional craft workers. For example, if an individual was employed as an electrician, then he wanted to see if the electrician license was available in the personnel files. The same information was needed for the plumbers and air-conditioning and heating specialists. He suggested that they add several columns to the spreadsheet, including country of origin, first language, and documentation of worker rights status, such as visa or green card status.

In the 8th month of the evaluation, Dr. Boyle emailed the employee satisfaction survey link to the 70 (100%) CTPES staff. Again, he requested that they complete the anonymous survey within the next 3 days. Out of the 70 CTPES employees, 60 (85.7%) completed the satisfaction survey. Dr. Boyle analyzed the data and wrote his recommendations for the final report. This information was included along with the retention rates and other information collected for all employees.

Finance and Accounting

The employees of finance and accounting are nonclinical staff; this section focuses on the profit and loss statements for each department rather than the employees (see **Table 14-10**).

Table 14-10   Evaluation Timeline for Finance and Accounting

Goal: The finance and accounting evaluation explores the profit and loss statements of the UMCCC for the past 12 months.

Month	Objectives	Action	Outcome	Responsible Person
8–10	100% of profit and loss statements for each department of the UMCCC are reviewed.	Obtain copies of profit and loss statements for each department of the UMCCC.	Determine the financial status of the UMCCC.	Dr. Chen and financial consultant, Mr. Sanjay

Dr. Chen hired a financial consultant, Mr. Raj Sanjay, to assist with the review of the profit and loss statements. Dr. Chen requested assistance from the board of directors because several departments were not compliant in furnishing the documents. Although all departments' documents were stored on the UMCCC database, the board of directors thought it would be beneficial for Dr. Chen and Mr. Sanjay to talk to each department individually about their finances (see **Table 14-11**).

Table 14-11   Example of an Annual Profit and Loss Statement for the Laboratory

Expenses			Income		
Salaries			Medicare	$ 324,000	
Manager	$ 123,000		Medicaid	$ 289,000	
Medical technologist	$ 118,000		Private insurance	$1,078,800	
Lab technicians (9)	$ 522,000		Fee for service payment	$ 72,000	
Overtime	$ 33,600		Subtotal		$ 1,763,800
Subtotal		$ 796,600	Sale of used equipment	$ 6,800	$ 6,800
Equipment maintenance contracts	$ 35,000				
New equipment	$ 8,000				
Solutions	$ 22,800				
Glass and paper supplies	$ 408,000				
OSHA inspections	$ 700				
Computer equipment	$ 12,000				
Subtotal		$ 486,500			
Courier service	$ 72,000				
Bad debt	$ 15,600				
Subtotal		$ 87,600			
TOTAL		$1,370,700	TOTAL	$ 1,770,600	
			PROFIT	+$ 399,900	

Board of Directors, Executive Administration, and Management

The employees of executive administration and management are nonclinical staff. This section focuses on the board of directors meeting minutes and contractual agreements for the past 12 months (see **Table 14-12**).

Dr. Boyle hired a legal consultant, Ms. Patti Jackson, to assist with the understanding of the contractual agreements made by the board of directors. After obtaining all the documents, the graduate students matched the meeting minutes with the contractual agreements. This process saved Ms. Jackson time during the legal review. After the review, Ms. Jackson spent one month writing the report for Dr. Boyle. Upon receipt of the legal review, Dr. Boyle saw that it was necessary to interview some of the board members and their staff regarding the contracts. The interviews were not expected, but the ABC evaluation team decided that the qualitative data were essential for greater clarification and interpretation of findings noted in Ms. Jackson's report.

Patient Satisfaction

The patient satisfaction survey was available via use of an information kiosk, online link, or paper survey. The visitor satisfaction survey was available at the information kiosks (see **Table 14-13**).

After Dr. Abel created the patient and visitor satisfaction surveys, she pilot-tested both surveys at a different clinic linked to the main campus hospital. First, she conducted two focus groups: one patient group ($n = 12$) and one visitor group ($n = 12$). After each focus group, she revised the surveys and emailed the link to both groups. To establish validity and reliability, she emailed the link one week later to both groups. Incentives were provided for each step of the process, so she was able to get responses from all 24 participants. Once the surveys were

Table 14-12 Evaluation Timeline for Board of Directors, Executive Administration, and Management

Goal: The executive administration and management evaluation explores the UMCCC board of directors meeting minutes and contractual agreements for the past 12 months.

Month	Objectives	Action	Outcome	Responsible Person
2–6	All the UMCCC board of director meeting minutes and contractual agreements are reviewed for accuracy.	Obtain copies of meeting minutes and contractual agreements.	100% of consistency between meeting minutes and contractual agreements.	Dr. Boyle and a legal consultant, Ms. Patti Jackson

Table 14-13   Evaluation Timeline for Patient and Visitor Satisfaction Survey

Goal: The patient satisfaction evaluation explores all aspects of patient services at UMCCC.

Month	Objectives	Action	Outcome	Responsible Person
6–10	100% of patients, family members, and visitors are invited to complete the UMCCC service satisfaction surveys.	Add the satisfaction survey link to the existing information kiosks located near the main entrance and two waiting areas near the café; place informational displays around the clinic to encourage patients and visitors to complete the satisfaction survey.	100% of patients complete the satisfaction survey using kiosk, link, or paper survey; 100% of patients completing the survey rate UMCCC as excellent.	Dr. Abel
		Mail the link to the satisfaction survey as well as a paper copy with a self-addressed, stamped envelope to each patient after first visit to the UMCCC.	100% of visitors completing the satisfaction survey at the existing information kiosks rate UMCCC as excellent.	Dr. Abel

finalized, Dr. Boyle worked with the creative design team to develop the clinic posters and brochures to encourage patients and visitors to complete the surveys. Also, the technical team developed a link on the information kiosks and an additional link for the emailed survey reminders. The graduate students and the billing department created a partnership in which the satisfaction survey links and paper copy Scantron surveys with a self-addressed stamped envelope were mailed 3 days after a patient completed a series of outpatient cancer treatments. Because the satisfaction surveys were entered into a database, there was limited data entry except for scanning the Scantron surveys. This process saved time, and Dr. Boyle was able to analyze the data quickly and complete this section of the final report.

Draft of the Final Report

The ABC evaluation team worked together to compose the draft of the final report. The report is divided into sections.

Evaluation of Clinical Staff and Clinical Support Staff

The clinical staff and clinical support staff consists of 41 individuals including 13 clinical staff and 28 clinical support staff.

EMR Training for Clinical Staff and Clinical Support Staff Results

- 36 of the 41 (87.8%) clinical staff and clinical support staff completed both EMR training sessions.
- 30 of the 41 (73.1%) clinical staff and clinical support staff completed the online EMR posttest.
- 65% out of 100% was the mean score of the EMR posttest.

Licensing and Credentials of the Clinical and Clinical Support Staff

- 100% of the clinical staff and clinical support staff were current with their licensing and credentials.

Retention of Clinical Staff and Clinical Support Staff

- Of the 41 clinical staff and clinical support staff, 6 (15%) left the UMCCC over the past 12 months.
- Of the 6 individuals, 1 was dismissed as a disciplinary action, 1 returned to employment at the main university hospital, and 4 moved out of state.
- Of the 6 individuals, 1 physician moved out of state, 2 registered nurses returned to school seeking an MSN degree, 1 social worker moved out of state, 1 mental health therapist returned to the main hospital, and 1 one social worker left because of a personal illness.

Employee Satisfaction Survey

Clinical Staff Scores:

UMCCC (maximum score: 23)	Mean score: 18 (78%)
Supervisor (maximum score: 39)	Mean score: 32 (82%)
Retention (maximum score: 30)	Mean score: 28 (93%)

Clinical Support Staff Scores:

UMCCC (maximum score: 23)	Mean score: 16 (70%)
Supervisor (maximum score: 39)	Mean score: 30 (77%)
Retention (maximum score: 30)	Mean score: 24 (80%)

Evaluation of Laboratory

The laboratory staff consists of 11 employees.

Dr. Green's Report

Dr. Green reported several OSHA violations. First, the staff was mixing biohazardous and nonbiohazardous materials in the same red plastic bags. Because the clinic pays by the pound for disposal of the red plastic biohazardous materials, mixing materials causes extra weight and therefore creates extra costs for the clinic. Second, the staff was unable to provide correct responses when asked about safety procedures related to several pieces of equipment. Third, the staff failed to consistently use universal precautions (gloves and goggles) when handling blood products. Fourth, the staff repeatedly reported the lack of training for procedures and OSHA requirements. Fifth, the laboratory failed to have a proper fire extinguisher in place.

Licensing and Credentials of the Clinical and Clinical Support Staff

- 11 (100%) of the laboratory staff were current with their licensing and credentials.

Retention of Clinical and Clinical Support Staff

- Of the 11 (100%) laboratory staff, 7 started employment in the past 12 months.
- Of the current 11 individuals, 1 was dismissed because of disciplinary action.

Employee Satisfaction Survey

Laboratory Staff Scores:

UMCCC (maximum score: 23)   Mean score: 14 (93%)
Supervisor: (maximum score: 39)   Mean score: 12 (96%)
Retention (maximum score: 30)   Mean score: 16 (90%)

Evaluation of Nonclinical Staff

The nonclinical staff consists of 127 individuals, with 87 of those employees required to complete the EMR training.

EMR Training for Nonclinical Staff Results

- 85 of the 87 (97%) nonclinical staff completed both EMR training sessions.
- 80 of the 85 (94%) nonclinical staff completed the online EMR posttest.
- 42 of the 80 (52.5%) earned a passing score of 70% on the posttest.

Employee Satisfaction Survey

Nonclinical Staff Scores:

UMCCC (maximum score: 23)   Mean score: 21 (91.3%)
Supervisor (maximum score: 39)   Mean score: 37 (94.8%)
Retention (maximum score: 30)   Mean score: 28 (93.3%)

Out of the 127, 80 (63%) nonclinical employees completed the satisfaction survey.

Evaluation of CTPES Staff

Dr. Green's Report

Dr. Green conducted focus groups. His report revealed that the employees felt protective of each other because of safety concerns, but the employees expressed a lack of sufficient training related to equipment, use of chemicals, and OSHA regulations. Several employees stated that a few of the employees spoke English as their second language, so these employees feared that the safety guidelines were not understood clearly by the non-English-speaking team members. Even the employees who had worked in the areas of physical plant maintenance knew how to do their jobs well, but could not tell Dr. Green about any of the OSHA requirements. The supervisor of the CTPES staff is Dr. Melvin Johnson.

Licensing and Credentials of the CTPES Staff

- 100% of the CTPES staff was current with licensing and credentials.

Retention of the CTPES Staff

- Of the 70 CTPES staff, 66 had been employed at the UMCCC for more than 5 years.
- Four had left in the last 12 months.
- Of the four that left, all retired from the UMCCC.

Employee Satisfaction Survey

CTPES Staff Scores:

       UMCCC (maximum score: 23)   Mean score: 19 (82.6%)
       Supervisor (maximum score: 39)   Mean score: 37 (94.8%)
       Retention (maximum score: 30)   Mean score: 29 (96.6%)

Out of the 70 CTPES employees, 60 (85.7%) completed the satisfaction survey.

Evaluation of Finance and Accounting

Mr. Raj Sanjay, financial consultant, submitted a report after reviewing the profit and loss statements from each clinic department. His report stated that generally the clinic was fiscally sound. Each department was working within its allocated budget. The only area of concern was the Department of Clinic Staff under the direction of Dr. Pamela Sykes. This department was over budget on overtime for the clinical support staff. This finding was surprising to the ABC evaluation team, because several of the clinical support staff mentioned on the survey that they consistently worked less than 40 hours per week and they would like to have their hours increased. Also, the cost of outpatient clinical services was above average for the geographical location.

Evaluation of the Board of Directors, Executive Administration, and Management

Dr. Boyle and a legal consultant, Ms. Patti Jackson, reviewed the minutes and contractual agreements of each board of directors meeting for the past 12 months. They found three discrepancies between the board meeting minutes and the contractual agreements. First, at the February 16 meeting, the board authorized $157,000 for refurbishing the waiting room of the clinic. The actual cost was $168,000, and there was no record of the reason for the increased cost. However, it is known to the board members that Ms. Hoffman's sister owns a carpet and office furniture store in a nearby town. Second, at the April 26 meeting, the board was notified by the state insurance commissioner that the UMCCC was overcharging for some standard clinic procedures. The board investigated the situation in May and reported to the state insurance commissioner that billing adjustments had been made according to the state requirements. However, Ms. Jackson reported to Dr. Boyle that the reported changes were never implemented and the overcharging continued unchecked. Third, Dr. Sykes had gone to the board in July, requesting an increase to her department's budget to pay increasing overtime charges. The board approved the budget increase per Dr. Sykes's request.

Evaluation of Patient and Visitor Satisfaction

Because it was impossible to accurately calculate the number of patients and visitors, Dr. Abel analyzed all the data received without knowing the exact sample size. Because the patient and visitor survey was anonymous, it was impossible to determine if some individuals completed the satisfaction survey located at the information kiosk more than once. She was able to calculate the return rate of 47% from the mailed paper satisfaction surveys. The combined kiosk and mailed survey patient satisfaction results are reported in **Table 14-14**.

Table 14-14 Results of the Patient Satisfaction Survey (*n* = 683)

	Strongly Agree	Agree	Disagree	Strongly Disagree
I am treated with respect by the clinical staff.	3%	87%	6%	4%
The clinic runs on time for my appointments.	4%	43%	28%	25%
I am given plenty time to ask all of my questions.	22%	34%	31%	13%
I never feel rushed by the clinic staff.	19%	28%	38%	15%
It is easy to get answers by phone after clinic hours.	24%	29%	39%	8%
I have confidence in the care received at the UMCCC.	18%	42%	24%	16%
There are no other choices for care in this geographical region.	92%	8%	0	0
The electronic medical record system works well at the UMCCC clinic.	36%	29%	32%	3%
The valet parking is convenient.	89%	9%	2%	0
The clinic café offers many choices of delicious food.	72%	14%	13%	1%
I appreciate that the clinic is open six days per week.	87%	10%	3%	0
I attend the support groups.	7%	19%	60%	14%
I attend the extra services (e.g., yoga, art therapy, music therapy) on a regular basis.	23%	26%	51%	0
The nurses, social workers, mental health therapists, and support workers are always willing to assist me.	85%	12%	3%	0
The bills that I receive are easy to understand.	0	1%	79%	20%
When I have questions about my bill, I only need to make one telephone call.	0	0	64%	36%
I recommend the UMCCC to friends and family who need clinic services related to cancer.	19%	81%	0	0
I have no complaints about the overall care of the UMCCC.	17%	65%	14%	4%
Other comments that you wish to share:				

The visitor satisfaction survey results are from the information kiosks found in several locations (see **Table 14-15**).

Recommendations for the Final Report

The recommendations for the final report are based on the work of the ABC evaluation team and the following discussion questions:

1. What recommendations are suggested for the Department of Clinical Staff and Clinical Support Staff?
2. What concerns are evident from the Department of Clinical Staff and Clinical Support Staff?

Table 14-15   Visitor Satisfaction Survey Results (*n* = 482)

	Strongly Agree	Agree	Disagree	Strongly Disagree
The clinical staff treats patients with respect.	2%	47%	43%	8%
The clinic runs on time for appointments.	4%	36%	48%	12%
I have confidence in the care received at the UMCCC.	46%	42%	12%	0
There are no other choices for care in this geographical region.	97%	3%	0	0
The valet parking is convenient.	98%	2%	0	0
The waiting room furniture is comfortable.	84%	13%	3%	0
I use the free Wi-Fi when I wait in the clinic.	93%	4%	3%	0
The clinic café offers many choices of delicious food.	88%	9%	2%	1%
It is convenient that the clinic is open 6 days per week.	82%	9%	9%	0
I recommend the UMCCC to friends and family who need clinic services related to cancer.	32%	34%	30%	4%
I have no complaints about the overall services at the UMCCC.	29%	31%	33%	7%

3. How should Dr. Green's two reports be used to improve quality and employee satisfaction?

4. What concerns are evident from Ms. Jackson's report?

5. What are the recommended next steps for the board of directors?

6. Should any further investigations take place? If so, why? If not, why?

7. Using a SWOT (strength, weakness, opportunity, and threat) analysis, review the overall UMCCC services.

8. How should the ABC evaluation team proceed with its recommendations?

9. What does the patient and visitor satisfaction survey indicate?

10. What ethical questions might the ABC evaluation team face in making the recommendations?

Student Activity

Using the data presented and creating the data that were not presented, write one section of the final report.

Reference

1. The Joint Commission. Facts about The Joint Commission. Available at: http://www.jointcommission.org/assets/1/18/Facts_The_Joint_Commission.pdf. Accessed October 12, 2013.

Index

Note: Page numbers followed by *b*, *f* and *t* indicate material in boxes, figures and tables respectively.